UPDATE V

Harrison's

PRINCIPLES OF INTERNAL MEDICINE

UPDATE V

Harrison's
PRINCIPLES
OF INTERNAL
MEDICINE

Editors

ROBERT G. PETERSDORF, M.D., M.A. (Hon.), D.Sc. (Hon.), M.D. (Hon.)
Dean, School of Medicine, Professor of Medicine, Vice-Chancellor, Health Sciences, University of California at San Diego

RAYMOND D. ADAMS, M.D., M.A. (Hon.), D. Sc. (Hon.), M.D. (Hon.)
Bullard Professor of Neuropathology, Emeritus, Harvard Medical School
Consultant Neurologist and Formerly Chief of Neurology Service, Massachusetts General Hospital
Director, Eunice K. Shriver Research Center, Boston
Médicin Adjoint, L'Hôpital Cantonale de Lausanne, Lausanne

EUGENE BRAUNWALD, M.D., M.A. (Hon.)
Hersey Professor of the Theory and Practice of Physic and Herrman Ludwig Blumgart
Professor of Medicine, Harvard Medical School
Chairman, Department of Medicine and Physician-in-Chief
Brigham and Women's Hospital and Beth Israel Hospital, Boston

KURT J. ISSELBACHER, M.D.
Mallinckrodt Professor of Medicine, Harvard Medical School
Physician and Chief, Gastrointestinal Unit, Massachusetts General Hospital, Boston

JOSEPH B. MARTIN, M.D., Ph.D., F.R.C.P. (C), M.A. (Hon.)
Julieanne Dorn Professor of Neurology, Harvard Medical School
Chief, Neurology Service, Massachusetts General Hospital, Boston

JEAN D. WILSON, M.D.
Professor of Internal Medicine, University of Texas Health Science Center at Dallas, Dallas

MCGRAW-HILL BOOK COMPANY

*New York St. Louis San Francisco Auckland Bogotá Guatemala Hamburg
Johannesburg Lisbon London Madrid Mexico Montreal New Delhi
Panama Paris San Juan São Paulo Singapore Sydney Tokyo Toronto*

NOTICE
Medicine is an ever-changing science. As new research and clinical experience broaden our
knowledge, changes in treatment and drug therapy are required. The editors and the publisher of
this work have checked with sources believed to
be reliable in their efforts to provide drug dosage
schedules that are complete and in accord with
the standards accepted at the time of publication.
However, readers are advised to check the product information sheet included in the package of
each drug they plan to administer to be certain
that the information contained in these schedules
is accurate and that changes have not been made
in the recommended dose or in the contraindications for administration. This recommendation is
of particular importance in connection with new
or infrequently used drugs.

UPDATE V:
Harrison's
Principles of Internal Medicine
Copyright © 1984 by McGraw-Hill, Inc. All rights reserved. Printed in the United States of America. Except
as permitted under the United States Copyright Act of
1976, no part of this publication may be reproduced or
distributed in any form or by any means, or stored in a
data base or retrieval system, without the prior written
permission of the publisher.

1 2 3 4 5 6 7 8 9 0 HAL HAL 8 9 8 7 6 5 4

ISBN 0-07-049616-1

This book was set in Times Roman by Ruttle, Shaw &
Wetherill, Inc.; the editors were Robert P. McGraw and
Donna McIvor; the production supervisor was Avé
McCracken; the cover was designed by Edward R.
Schultheis.
Halliday Lithograph Corporation was the printer and
binder.

Library of Congress Cataloging in Publication Data
Main entry under title:

Harrison's Principles of internal medicine. Update V.

  Includes bibliographies and index.
  1. Internal medicine. 2. Internal medicine—Addresses,
essays, lectures. I. Petersdorf, Robert G. II. Harrison,
Tinsley Randolph, date. Principles of internal
medicine. 10th ed. III. Title: Principles of internal
medicine. Update V.
RC45.H323 1933b Suppl.   616   84-4444
ISBN 0-07-049616-1

CONTENTS

The Acquired Immune-Deficiency Syndrome   **1**

Alvin E. Friedman-Kien and Jeffrey B. Greene

The acquired immune-deficiency syndrome (AIDS) is one of the most dreaded diseases in many a year. In this review, one of the discoverers of the association between immune deficiency and Kaposi's sarcoma (Friedman-Kien) and Greene review this syndrome and the management of its complications. The article also includes some exceptionally fine color illustrations of Kaposi's sarcoma.

Recent Advances in Alzheimer's Disease   *Dennis J. Selkoe*   **15**

Alzheimer's disease is the most important neurologic disorder in an aging population. Its cause remains unknown, but recent discoveries have pointed to both specific neurotransmitter abnormalities and to biochemical changes in the neurofilaments contained within the dying nerve cells. These discoveries hold promise for new approaches to research and to treatment of this devastating disorder.

Nine Controversies in the Management of Endocarditis   *David T. Durack*   **35**

Bacterial endocarditis (BE) remains a dangerous disease that is changing rapidly. This article addresses some controversial and sophisticated issues concerning its treatment and prevention. These include duration of treatment, the role of antibiotic tolerance, combination antibiotic therapy, oral versus parenteral prophylactic therapy, the advisability of prophylaxis in mitral valve prolapse, valve replacement for prevention of emboli, and similar questions.

Primary Prevention of Coronary Artery Disease   **47**

Robert I. Levy, Curt D. Furberg, Basil M. Rifkind

Coronary artery disease is the major cause of death and disability in the industrialized world. As a consequence of the demonstrated association between various factors, traits, or habits and increased risk of developing coronary artery disease, there have been many studies attempting to determine whether reduction of risk factors can reduce the incidence of this condition, i.e., whether primary prevention of coronary artery disease is possible. This article reviews the scientific basis for establishing certain traits as risk factors and the results of the major trials directed toward the primary prevention of coronary disease. In some instances, such as in hypertension, the effects of intervention are clear. In other areas, such as in smoking cessation, there is benefit but it is more difficult to quantify. The implications of the results of these epidemiologic studies for primary prevention in healthy individuals as well as in populations are also discussed.

LIST OF CONTRIBUTORS

WAYNE H. AKESON, M.D.
Professor and Head, Division of Orthopedics and Rehabilitation, University of California, San Diego

FERDINANDO S. BUONANNO, M.D.
Assistant Professor of Neurology, Harvard Medical School; Assistant Neurologist, Massachusetts General Hospital, Boston

MARTIN C. CAREY, M.D.
Associate Professor of Medicine, Lawrence J. Henderson Associate Professor of Health Sciences and Technology, and Associate Professor of Physiology and Biophysics, Harvard Medical School; Physician, Brigham and Women's Hospital, Boston

F. RICHARD CONVERY, M.D.
Professor of Surgery in Orthopedics, University of California, San Diego

JEFFREY M. DRAZEN, M.D.
Associate Professor of Medicine, Harvard Medical School; Physician, Brigham and Women's Hospital, Boston

DAVID T. DURACK, M.B., D. Phil.
Professor of Medicine and Microbiology, and Chief, Division of Infectious Diseases, Duke University Medical Center, Durham

LAWRENCE S. FRIEDMAN, M.D.
Research Fellow in Medicine, Harvard Medical School; Clinical and Research Fellow in Medicine, Massachusetts General Hospital, Boston

ALVIN E. FRIEDMAN-KIEN, M.D.
Associate Professor of Dermatology and Microbiology, New York University Medical Center; Director, Dermatology Service, Goldwater Memorial Hospital, New York

CURT D. FURBERG, M.D.
Chief, Clinical Trials Branch, National Heart, Lung and Blood Institute, National Institutes of Health, Bethesda

JEFFREY B. GREENE, M.D.
Clinical Instructor, Department of Medicine, Division of Infectious Diseases, New York University Medical Center, New York

STEPHEN L. HAUSER, M.D.
Instructor in Neurology, Harvard Medical School, Boston

RAYMOND L. HINTZ, M.D.
Associate Professor of Pediatrics and Head, Division of Pediatric Endocrinology, Stanford University School of Medicine, Stanford

RALPH A. KELLY, M.D.
Research Fellow, Harvard Medical School; Associate Physician, Brigham and Women's Hospital, Boston

J. PHILIP KISTLER, M.D.
Assistant Professor of Neurology, Harvard Medical School; Assistant Neurologist, Massachusetts General Hospital, Boston

P. REED LARSEN, M.D.
Professor of Medicine, Harvard Medical School; Investigator, Howard Hughes Medical Institute; Director, Thyroid Diagnostic Center, Brigham and Women's Hospital, Boston

ROBERT I. LEVY, M.D.
Professor of Medicine and Vice President for Health Sciences, Columbia University; Attending Physician, Presbyterian Hospital, New York

JOSEPH B. MARTIN, M.D., Ph.D., F.R.C.P.(C), M.A. (Hon.)
Julieanne Dorn Professor of Neurology, Harvard Medical School; Chief, Neurology Service, Massachusetts General Hospital, Boston

WILLIAM E. MITCH, M.D.
Associate Professor of Medicine, Harvard Medical School; Physician, Brigham and Women's Hospital, Boston

MICHAEL A. O'DONOVAN, M.D., M.B., B.Ch., B.AO., MRCPI
Fogarty International Post-Doctoral Fellow, Harvard Medical School and Brigham and Women's Hospital, Boston; Senior Registrar in Medicine, University College, Regional Hospital, Galway, Ireland

BASIL M. RIFKIND, M.D., F.R.C.P.
Chief, Lipid Metabolism-Atherogenesis Branch; Deputy Associate Director, Atherogenesis, Hypertension and Lipid Metabolism Program, Division of Heart and Vascular Diseases, National Heart, Lung and Blood Institute, National Institutes of Health, Bethesda

STEPHEN H. ROBINSON, M.D.
Professor of Medicine, Harvard Medical School; Chief, Hematology Division and Clinical Director, Department of Medicine, Beth Israel Hospital, Boston

THOMAS H. ROSSING, M.D.
Assistant Professor of Medicine, Harvard Medical School; Associate Physician, Brigham and Women's Hospital, Boston

DENNIS J. SELKOE, M.D.
Associate Professor of Neurology, Harvard Medical School; Associate Neurologist and Neuropathologist, Brigham and Women's Hospital and McLean Hospital, Boston

DAVID A. SHAFRITZ, M.D.
Chief, Molecular Hepatology Unit and Professor of Medicine and Cell Biology, Albert Einstein College of Medicine, New York

MORRIS SHERMAN, M.B., B.Ch., Ph.D., F.C.S. (SA)
Research Associate, Liver Research Centre, Albert Einstein College of Medicine, New York

ARTHUR S. SLUTSKY, MASc., M.D.
Assistant Professor of Medicine, Harvard Medical School, Boston; Associate Physician, West Roxbury VA Medical Center, West Roxbury

JACK R. WANDS, M.D.
Associate Professor of Medicine, Harvard Medical School; Associate Physician, Massachusetts General Hospital, Boston

DAVID M. WARD, M.B., Ch.B., M.R.C.P.
Assistant Professor of Medicine, University of California, San Diego; Director of Dialysis and Apheresis Programs and Chief of Clinical Nephrology, University of California Medical Center, San Diego

HOWARD L. WEINER, M.D.
Associate Professor of Neurology, Harvard Medical School; Director, Multiple Sclerosis Clinical and Research Unit, Brigham and Women's Hospital, Boston

PREFACE

The editors of *Harrison's Principles of Internal Medicine,* encouraged by the positive response of physicians and medical students to the publication of the Updates, have decided to continue the Update series between the 10th and 11th editions of *Harrison's.* The purpose in publishing the Updates remains as it was when the series was first initiated: (1) to review certain clinical topics that could not be covered comprehensively in *Harrison's* and (2) to cover selected new and important medical advances that have become an integral part of medical knowledge since the preparation of the 10th edition.

One Update a year (V–VII) will be published between now and the 11th edition of *Harrison's.* Two of the volumes will have central themes: Update VI will focus on new treatment modalities and Update VII will focus on oncology. For Update V the editors have selected topics in the various clinical disciplines that in their judgment are timely and relevant. Brief explanatory summaries of each article in the table of contents provide insight into the selection process.

ROBERT G. PETERSDORF
RAYMOND D. ADAMS
EUGENE BRAUNWALD
KURT J. ISSELBACHER
JOSEPH B. MARTIN
JEAN D. WILSON

THE ACQUIRED IMMUNE-DEFICIENCY SYNDROME

ALVIN E. FRIEDMAN-KIEN and JEFFREY B. GREENE

The unexpected appearance of opportunistic infections and an aggressive form of Kaposi's sarcoma among apparently healthy homosexual men and intravenous drug users in the latter half of 1980 heralded the recognition of a new clinical entity known as the *acquired immune-deficiency syndrome (AIDS)*. Its sudden occurrence was reminiscent of Legionnaires' disease and the toxic-shock syndrome, but its impact on public health has already exceeded these illnesses. The over 2000 reported cases exhibiting a greater than 50 percent mortality rate represent an as yet undefined fraction of the true number of cases of AIDS.

AIDS, as its name implies, represents a form of secondary immunologic disorder that results in profound depression of cell-mediated immunity. The unique feature of this illness is that the observed abnormalities of immune function are persistent.

The syndrome has become the subject of intensive worldwide clinical and scientific investigation. Its study promises to provide insights into the fundamental mechanisms of immune function, host-parasite relationships, and perhaps the understanding of neoplasia. The clinician is anxiously awaiting the development of diagnostic and therapeutic modalities for use in the ever-increasing numbers of patients afflicted with this life-threatening illness.

DISEASE DESCRIPTION

Experience with AIDS over the past 3 years has led to the recognition that this illness may present to the physician in different ways. At one end of this clinical spectrum is the asymptomatic patient who demonstrates cutaneous anergy, lymphopenia, reversal of the T-helper/T-suppressor cell ratio, and depressed in vitro lymphoproliferative responses to various antigens and mitogens. At the distant end of the spectrum is the patient who presents with fulminant, disseminated Kaposi's sarcoma or with respiratory failure due to *Pneumocystis carinii* infection. Between these extremes are patients suffering from a vague persistent constitutional illness suggestive of a chronic viral disease, or a more characteristic set of symptoms involving the pulmonary, gastrointestinal, or central nervous systems. Other individuals may develop unexplained lymphadenopathy associated with constitutional symptoms. They do not necessarily go on to develop more serious complications of AIDS. It is probably inaccurate to label the less ill patients as "prodromal-AIDS" since many have not progressed from their vague constitutional illness to life-threatening infections or disseminated Kaposi's sarcoma. It is possible that their clinical picture, unaffected by secondary diseases, better depicts the true characteristics of AIDS. Still another group may seek medical attention because of the discovery of a mucocutaneous lesion of Kaposi's sarcoma in the absence of any systemic symptoms.

The diversity of clinical presentations of AIDS is mirrored by the wide range of infectious and noninfectious conditions that are associated with it. Review of the biologic agents that have been reported to cause life-threatening infections in the patients with AIDS gives some insights into the underlying immunologic defect of this disease (Table 1). Many of these infectious agents are ubiquitous and capable of causing mild or subclinical disease in healthy individuals. How-

1

TABLE 1
Biologic agents reported to cause infections in patients with the acquired immune-deficiency syndrome

Parasitic	Fungal	Viral	Bacterial
Pneumocystis carinii	Candida albicans	Cytomegalovirus	Mycobacterium avium-intracellulare
Toxoplasma gondii	Cryptococcus neoformans	Varicella-zoster	M. tuberculosis
Cryptosporidium	Aspergillus spp.	Herpes simplex	Other "atypical" Mycobacterium spp.
Isospora belli	Histoplasma capsulatum	Epstein-Barr	Legionella spp.
Strongyloides stercoralis		Papovavirus* (J-C virus)	Salmonella spp.
			Nocardia spp.

*Agent of progressive multifocal leukoencephalopathy.

ever, because these organisms are known to cause life-threatening infections, especially in the immunocompromised host, they are considered "opportunistic" pathogens. The profound immunosuppression seen in patients with AIDS renders them particularly susceptible to severe infection by these agents (Table 2).

The neoplastic diseases that have been associated with AIDS are shown in Table 3. Prior to the AIDS epidemic, Kaposi's sarcoma, a rare

TABLE 2
Common infectious diseases complicating the acquired immune-deficiency syndrome

Pathogen	Infection
Protozoal	
Pneumocystis carinii	Pneumonia
Toxoplasma gondii	Necrotizing encephalitis
	Disseminated infection
Cryptosporidium	Enteritis
Isospora belli	
Fungal	
Candida albicans	Thrush
	Invasive esophagitis
	Disseminated Moniliasis
Cryptococcus neoformans	Meningitis
	Disseminated (lung, bone marrow, adrenal, renal, central nervous system)
Viral	
Herpes simplex	Extensive, persistent anogenital
	Visceral (pulmonary, gastrointestinal)
Varicella zoster	Severe, localized cutaneous
	Disseminated (cutaneous, visceral)
Human papilloma virus	Condylomata acuminata
J-C Papovavirus	Progressive multifocal leukoencephalopathy
Bacterial	
Mycobacterium avium-intracellulare	Disseminated infection
M. tuberculosis	Localized (pulmonary, cerebrospinal fluid)
	Miliary
Legionella spp.	Pneumonia

TABLE 3
Neoplastic disease associated with acquired immune-deficiency syndrome

Epidemic Kaposi's sarcoma
Undifferentiated lymphoma
Burkitt's-like lymphoma
Immunoblastic lymphoma
Cloacogenic carcinoma
Squamous cell carcinoma of
 the oral cavity

tumor predominantly seen in males, was known to occur in different populations. The classical form of Kaposi's sarcoma is a localized, indolent neoplasm, usually observed in elderly men of Mediterranean or eastern Ashkenazic Jewish European ancestry (Table 4). A more invasive localized variety of this tumor is seen in young black adults in equatorial Africa. In addition, a generalized, lymphadenopathic form is found in black African children. Kaposi's sarcoma has also been observed in the United States in iatrogenically immunosuppressed patients such as renal transplant recipients or patients who had received immunosuppressive therapy for other indications. A newly recognized epidemic form of Kaposi's sarcoma has been identified in association with or as a manifestation of AIDS. While this form is histologically identical to the others, it is a widely disseminated tumor with unique clinical characteristics (see ''Clinical Manifestations'' below). In addition, diffuse undifferentiated lymphomas and Burkitt-type lymphomas have been reported in patients with AIDS. Further study is necessary to establish that these less frequently seen neoplasms are occurring in excess of their expected background incidence.

Certain nonneoplastic conditions appear to be associated with AIDS as well. Autoimmune-like thrombocytopenic purpura, qualitative platelet dysfunction, azoospermia associated with the presence of antispermatozoal antibodies, and an observed ''cotton-wool'' retinopathy are examples.

The foregoing discussion has stressed the diversity of the clinical manifestations of AIDS. Consideration of diagnosis requires a high index of suspicion and familiarity with the epidemiologic risk factors. Clinicians in every field must be prepared for the possibility of having to diagnose this illness.

EPIDEMIOLOGY

Through the reporting of patients by clinicians in New York and California in the early part of 1981, the U.S. Centers for Disease Control

TABLE 4
Clinical variants of Kaposi's sarcoma

Type	Population	Clinical characteristics	Usual course
Classical	Elderly Jewish and Italian individuals; Male/Female = 10–15:1 Iatrogenically immunosuppressed	Localized nodular; lower extremities predominantly involved	Indolent, 10–15 years duration Rarely with late visceral involvement
Localized "florid" aggressive	African Adults; Male/Female = 17:1	Localized; invasive of muscle and bone	Slowly progressive, but fatal over 5–8 years Late visceral involvement
Lymphadeno-pathic	African children age 2–15 years; Male/Female = 3:1	Extensive and generalized lymph node and visceral involvement Rare cutaneous lesions	Rapid, fatal course within 3 years
"Epidemic" disseminated	Acquired immunodeficiency syndrome Iatrogenically immunosuppressed	Mucocutaneous lesions as well as widespread nodal and visceral involvement Males predominantly	Progressive, becomes fulminant, fatal in 2–3 years In patients on immunosuppressive drugs—occasionally tumor regresses after cessation of immunosuppressive therapy

TABLE 5

Neoplasms or infections used as criteria for the diagnosis of acquired immune-deficiency syndrome (AIDS) for surveillance purposes by the Centers for Disease Control

Epidemic Kaposi's sarcoma (in males under 60 years of age)
Lymphoma (central nervous system)
Pneumocystis carinii pneumonia
Mycobacterium avium-intracellulare (disseminated)
Cryptosporidial enteritis
Cryptococcal meningitis
Candida albicans (esophagitis)
Toxoplasmosis (encephalitis, pneumonia)
Strongyloides stercoralis (hyperinfection)
Aspergillosis (central nervous system or disseminated)
Progressive multifocal leukoencephalopathy
Cytomegalovirus (pneumonitis, colitis, encephalitis)
Herpes simplex (anogenital, persisting for greater than 1 month; esophagitis; pneumonitis)

(CDC) became aware of the AIDS epidemic. Since that time this agency has remained the most comprehensive source of epidemiologic information regarding this disease. For the purpose of surveillance, the CDC have formulated an operational definition of AIDS: The finding of any one of a number of infectious diseases or Kaposi's sarcoma, that is "moderately indicative of an underlying cellular immunodeficiency" in a patient where no cause of that immune defect can be found. The diseases that are currently being accepted as being suggestive of the underlying cellular immunodeficiency are shown in Table 5. By September of 1983, over 2600 cases of AIDS fulfilling this definition had been reported. Forty-six states had reported cases, with the largest numbers contributed by New York (43 percent of the total), followed by California and Florida. In addition to cases in the United States, more than 20 countries have reported cases of AIDS. While little epidemiologic data are available from Haiti, this country seems to have a very significant geographic cluster of cases, especially in the vicinity of Port-au-Prince.

In the United States, 93 percent of the reported cases have been in males with a mean age of approximately 37 years (range: 20 to 64 years). Several epidemiologic groups are now recognized as being at risk, including homosexual or bisexual males, intravenous drug users, and Haitians who have recently immigrated to North America. Men of homosexual or bisexual orientation account for 71 percent of the total number

of reported cases of AIDS. Male and female intravenous drug users and recent Haitian immigrants represent 17 and 5 percent of the cases, respectively. All primary racial groups have been represented among the reported patients without any apparent predilection.

Of the 175 cases of AIDS in females, 52 percent occurred in known parenteral drug users and 10 percent in Haitian immigrants. It is interesting to note that among these, only 7 cases of epidemic Kaposi's sarcoma have been reported, all parenteral drug abusers.

A number of other populations are now being suspected of being at risk for AIDS. One such group is patients with hemophilia; 15 cases with severe opportunistic infections have been reported. All of these 15 cases had been transfused with the lyophilized clotting-factor concentrate. A recent study has found low T-helper/T-suppressor lymphocyte ratios in apparently healthy hemophiliacs who had received lyophilized factor VIII concentrate. AIDS has not been diagnosed in hemophiliacs treated only with cryoprecipitate. These observations have been thought to support a theory that there is transmission of an AIDS agent during administration of lyophilized factor VIII but not cryoprecipitate because the former substance is prepared from a much larger commercial donor pool. However, immunosuppression by factor concentrates themselves offers an alternate explanation for this observation.

There have been about 20 cases of AIDS in

patients with no known risk factors who had received blood products up to 3 years before the onset of their disease. In each case blood-product donors with unexplained lymphadenopathy or a nonspecific constitutional illness could be identified. In one instance a blood-product donor was found to have AIDS fulfilling the CDC criteria. Thus, while the possibility of transmission of AIDS via transfusion of blood products is raised by the recognition of this small number of cases, a direct causal relationship has not been established. Over 30 million units of blood were transfused in the United States between 1979 and 1982. It would seem that the risk of developing AIDS in the face of blood transfusion is quite low.

There have been 21 infants or young children reported to the CDC with AIDS-like illnesses. All of these patients have had evidence of depressed cell-mediated immunity. Some of these children were born to mothers with AIDS or to mothers who were at risk for AIDS because of their Haitian origin or history of parenteral drug use. These cases of AIDS-like illnesses in children could be explained by exposure to an AIDS agent prenatally, during parturition, or after birth through intimate household contact (such as breast-feeding). The difficulty in evaluating these children, however, is that it is often impossible to exclude the many congenital causes of immunodeficiency. Therefore, these cases have not been included in the CDC figures.

In addition, eight female sexual partners of AIDS patients who had been parenteral drug users have had immunologic changes similar to those seen in AIDS. One of these women later developed AIDS. Thus female sex partners of AIDS patients may also be at risk.

Of the more than 2600 cases reported to the CDC during the past 3 years, approximately 6 percent cannot be placed into any of the defined epidemiological risk groups. This figure has not changed significantly during the epidemic, suggesting that AIDS remains relatively confined to the recognized risk groups. Some investigators have used this information to suggest that certain susceptibility factors common to the at-risk populations may be a prerequisite for the development of AIDS. The concept of susceptibility factors is consonant with the interesting observation that the mean age for AIDS is 37 years. Relatively few cases of AIDS have been reported in homosexual men aged 18 to 23 years, implying that factors other than the level of sexual activity may be important.

After the recognition that men of homosexual orientation were at risk for AIDS, case-control studies were performed to attempt to identify specific risk factors. The major differences between the AIDS cases and their controls identified sexual activity with numerous partners and the use of various recreational drugs, especially amyl and butyl nitrite, as risk factors. Specific sexual practices, including analingus and passive rectal intercourse, were also more frequently reported among the cases. Recently, however, a greater percentage of homosexual patients are reporting fewer numbers of sexual partners.

Much less attention has been given to the epidemiologic study of other groups at risk, such as Haitians or intravenous drug users. There are some striking differences in the clinical aspects of the illness in these groups compared to homosexual men. An intriguing example is the relative paucity of cases of Kaposi's sarcoma in the nonhomosexual groups. Ninety-five percent of all cases of epidemic Kaposi's sarcoma have been in homosexual or bisexual men. While 48.5 percent of homosexual or bisexual men with AIDS have the epidemic form of Kaposi's sarcoma, only 2 percent of the Haitians and 5.3 percent of the parenteral drug-using AIDS patients demonstrate this complication. No cases of Kaposi's sarcoma in hemophiliacs with AIDS have been reported. The reasons for these differences remain obscure. Other observed differences in the clinical manifestations of AIDS among the various groups at risk concern the infectious complications of the disease. The incidence of tuberculosis, or of toxoplasmosis in Haitians with AIDS, for example, exceeds that of the other defined risk groups. This may reflect a greater likelihood of premorbid exposure to these pathogens.

New cases of AIDS are being reported to the CDC at a rate of three to four cases daily. The number of cases reported thus far has doubled every 6 months. As of September 1983, about 40 percent of the total number of reported cases have died. The mortality rate in patients with opportunistic infections is more than twice that of those with Kaposi's sarcoma alone. The

2-year survival of this illness may be less than 10 percent.

Clusters of cases with direct or indirect sexual contact support the belief that AIDS may be caused by a transmissible agent with similar biologic behavior to hepatitis B virus. Even if the disease is, in fact, transmissible, there is no information regarding the period of communicability, secondary attack rates (the incidence of the disease among contacts), or the precise routes of transmission. However, many nonsexual household contacts and health care personnel caring for cases do not appear to be at increased risk for AIDS. While there remain many unanswered questions regarding the epidemiology of this new syndrome, it does not appear that casual contact with patients represents a significant public health problem.

CLINICAL MANIFESTATIONS

The symptoms and signs in the patient with AIDS may be nonspecific and are often due to the infectious or neoplastic complications rather than to the disease itself. Nonetheless, physicians who have gained extensive experience with this complex illness have come to recognize a number of clinical manifestations that prove useful in the evaluation of putative patients.

Symptoms may be constitutional or may be organ system specific. The AIDS patient has often been aware of ill-health for several months and has usually sought medical attention at an earlier time. The predominant symptoms are marked malaise and pronounced fatigue that interfere with day-to-day activities. The patient often abandons his or her usual physical activity and requires excessive sleep. Patients frequently complain of anorexia and diminished libido. Low-grade fevers and night sweats are common symptoms, as is a moderate weight loss (of approximately 10 to 15 lb over a period of several months). Migratory myalgias and arthralgias that often respond to aspirin are also common.

Medical histories among the homosexual AIDS patients are remarkable for a variety of sexually transmitted diseases, including syphilis, gonorrhea, herpes progenitalis, condylomata acuminata, hepatitis A and B, amebiasis, giardiasis, and lymphogranuloma venereum. Accordingly, many patients have been repeatedly treated under medical supervision with a variety of antimicrobial agents. Moreover, patients may have used self-prescribed antibiotics as infection prophylaxis for sexual activity.

Organ-specific complaints are common and should be sought in the medical history. Persistent lymphadenopathy is frequently recognized by the patient. The lymph node swellings are noted to wax and wane and the nodes are occasionally tender. The adenopathy is often generalized but most often is reported to occur in the posterior cervical, submandibular, or axillary regions.

Skin rashes and generalized pruritus that are new to the patient are also common, as are painful cheilosis, glossitis, and stomatitis. Some patients may report a change in their patterns of preexisting genital herpes infections, with unusually severe, protracted, or more frequently recurring episodes. The occurrence of shingles (herpes zoster) has been observed at an apparently increased rate as well.

Commonly, symptoms associated with opportunistic infections can fall into one or more complexes as indicated in Table 6. Recognition of the significance of these symptom complexes will help the physician direct a diagnostic plan and initiate early therapy.

The pulmonary symptom complex is encountered most often, reflecting the relative frequency of *P. carinii* pneumonia. High fever (102°F or higher), dyspnea on exertion, a nonproductive cough, and vague, nonpleuritic chest discomfort are usually reported. In approximately two-thirds of these patients, respiratory symptoms are of an insidious onset and have been present for 2 to 12 weeks prior to initial evaluation. In contrast, other patients may present with a rapidly progressive pulmonary disease over a period of several days.

Patients with AIDS may present with, or eventually develop, involvement of the central nervous system or an opportunistic infection. Some of these patients will report the occurrence of aphasia, paresis, seizures, or sensory disturbances suggestive of a focal neurologic process. Others develop symptoms consistent with chronic meningitis, such as headache, photophobia, nuchal rigidity, or ocular myalgia. Still others may develop subtle symptoms of memory loss and an inability to concentrate, which may

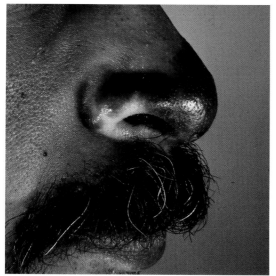

FIGURE 1

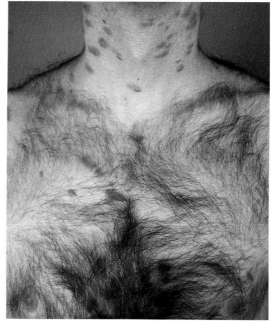

FIGURE 4

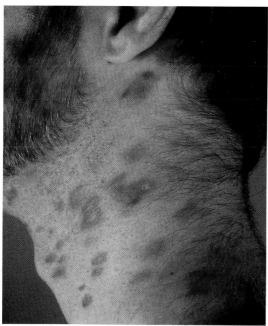

FIGURE 2

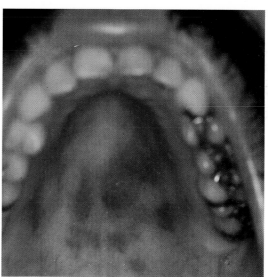

FIGURE 5

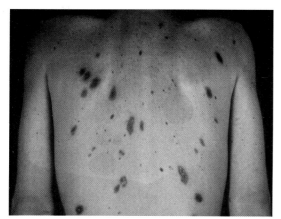

FIGURE 3

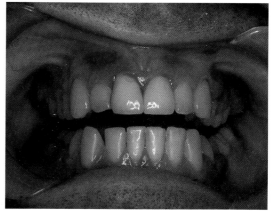

FIGURE 6

FIGURE 1   *Hyperpigmented plaque-stage lesion on nose of a black man.*
FIGURE 2   *Close-up showing pink-red colored lesions. Lesion in occipital region behind the ear is a common site.*
FIGURE 3   *Purple- to blue-colored plaque and nodular lesions on back.*

FIGURE 4   *Widely disseminated patch- and plaque-stage lesions of epidemic Kaposi's sarcoma. Note distribution along lines of skin cleavage and appearance similar to pityriasis rosea.*
FIGURE 5   *Violaceous asymptomatic patch lesions seen on palate of mouth.*
FIGURE 6   *Vascular-appearing asymptomatic tumors on gingiva.*

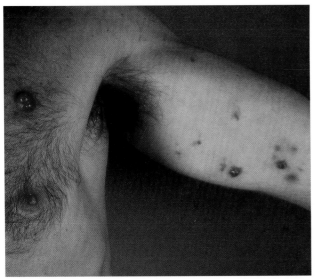

FIGURE 7

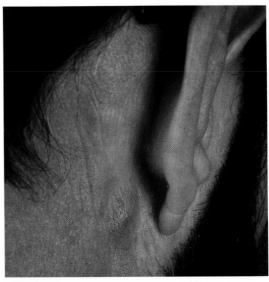

FIGURE 10

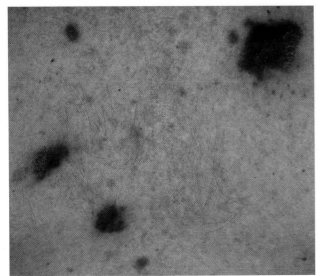

FIGURE 8

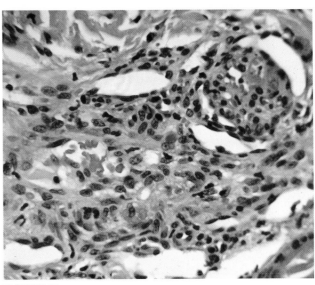

FIGURE 11

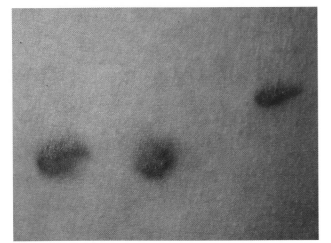

FIGURE 9

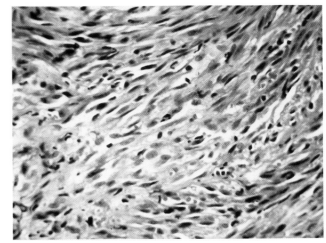

FIGURE 12

FIGURE 7 *Tumor nodules present on chest and inner aspect of forearm 8 months after appearance of disease. Note the faint, early patch- and plaque-stage lesions appearing on arm.*
FIGURE 8 *Purple plaque-stage lesion.*
FIGURE 9 *Ovoid nodular reddish-colored lesions on skin of trunk.*

Photographs by William Slue, Department of Dermatology, New York University Medical Center, Photography Section.

FIGURE 10 *Purple-hued subcutaneous nodular lesion in occipital cervical region.*
FIGURE 11 *Patch and nodular lesions of Kaposi's sarcoma with irregular blood vessels. Note abnormal vascular slits and plasma cells (172×).*
FIGURE 12 *Patch and nodular lesions of Kaposi's sarcoma with irregular blood vessels. Note fasciculi of spindle cells forming around slits. Some extravasated red blood cells are also seen. There are few mitotic figures present (172×).*

TABLE 6
Presentations of opportunistic infections in the acquired immune-deficiency syndrome

Symptom complex	Physical findings	Likely pathogens*
Pulmonary (dyspnea, fever, cough, chest pain)	Tachypnea, cyanosis, occasionally auscultatory findings	*Pneumocystis carinii* *Legionella* spp. Cytomegalovirus Cryptococcosis Pulmonary Kaposi's sarcoma
Central nervous system		
Focal Symptoms	Hemiparesis, aphasia, seizures	*Toxoplasma gondii* (central nervous system lymphoma)
Encephalopathy	Rapid onset of dementia, frontal release signs, occasionally hemorrhagic retinitis	Cytomegalovirus *Toxoplasma gondii* Papovavirus (J-C virus)
Chronic meningitis	Nuchal rigidity, fever, photophobia	*Cryptococcus neoformans* *Mycobacterium* spp.
Gastrointestinal		
Dysentery-like	Cachexia, usually afebrile	*Cryptosporidium* *Isospora* spp.
Colitis-like	Fever, inflamed rectal mucosa, bloody stools	Cytomegalovirus
Fever of unknown origin	Cachexia, remitting temperatures over 102°F, adenopathy, splenomegaly, hepatomegaly	*Mycobacterium avium-intracellulare* *M. tuberculosis* *Toxoplasma gondii*

Most frequently diagnosed pathogens are underscored.

progress to dementia. Occasionally, these patients may complain of visual loss, bowel and bladder disturbances, spastic gait, or sensory and motor problems suggestive of a myelopathy.

Gastrointestinal complaints constitute a third major symptom complex. Many patients will complain of voluminous diarrhea and will exhibit cachexia without fever. In contrast, a second manner in which individuals with a gastrointestinal symptom complex may come to medical attention is with fever and symptoms of colitis, such as tenesmus with stools containing blood and mucus.

Another group of patients will initially complain of a severe febrile illness, associated with persistent, remitting daily temperatures elevated to 102°F or higher. Rigors, drenching sweats, marked weight loss, lymphadenopathy, and hepatosplenomegaly are additional aspects of this clinical picture.

The patients with AIDS who develop Kaposi's sarcoma may come to medical attention after noticing one or more asymptomatic, pink- to purple-colored skin or oral lesions. In some patients Kaposi's sarcoma may occur in lymph nodes or visceral organs without cutaneous manifestations, and although these lesions may appear to be vascular, they rarely bleed when traumatized. Such patients may have associated symptoms attributable to coexistent opportunistic infections. Of interest is the presence of fever in approximately 20 percent of AIDS patients with Kaposi's sarcoma without other detectable disease.

The faint, earliest skin lesions of Kaposi's sarcoma are patchlike and may have to be actively sought in order not to be overlooked. They are flat, may be singular or multifocal, and can appear in clusters or be widely disseminated. These lesions are commonly discrete, ovoid, less than 1 cm in diameter, pink to deep violet in color, and may be hyperpigmented (Fig. 1). When on the neck and trunk, these patch-stage lesions are often oriented along the skin's natural lines of cleavage (Figs. 2 to 4). Such early Kaposi's sarcoma lesions may be mistaken for pityriasis rosea, bruises, vascular nevi, or secondary syphilis. Oral mucosal lesions are sometimes seen on the palate and gingiva (Figs. 5 to 6).

The lesions develop into thickened plaques

(plaque stage) and may continue to develop into tumor nodules ranging from pea-sized to several centimeters in diameter (nodular stage) (Figs. 7 to 10).

A thorough physical evaluation of the patient with suspected AIDS may help to substantiate the diagnosis. Generalized lymphadenopathy may be impressive though there is usually no matting of the nodes and no overlying skin changes. Careful examination of the skin and mucosa is extremely important. The oral cavity may reveal oral thrush, aphthous stomatitis, pyorrhea or herpes simplex labialis. In addition, monilial cheilosis, intertrigo, eczematous patches, hives, or a psoriasiform eruption are seen occasionally. Viral skin infections, such as widespread molluscum contagiosum, severe and extensive varicella-zoster, and anogenital herpes simplex, as well as condylomata acuminata, may also be present.

Ophthalmologic examination may reveal a cotton-wool exudative retinopathy. This finding is of unclear pathogenesis but tends to be associated with the presence of opportunistic infections. A severe hemorrhagic retinitis and papillitis that may be due to cytomegalovirus infection has also been observed.

LABORATORY FINDINGS

There is as yet no specific laboratory test that is diagnostic of AIDS. The diagnosis therefore continues to be made by the clinician at the bedside. The absence of a specific test notwithstanding, the laboratory may provide the physician with information that could be used to either support the diagnosis of AIDS or exclude other illnesses.

The majority of AIDS patients have abnormal hematologic findings. A mild normocytic, normochromic anemia of chronic disease is typical of those patients who have been ill for several months. Severe anemia, with a hemoglobin of less than 10 g/dl can be found in many AIDS patients with Kaposi's sarcoma or opportunistic infections. The white blood cell count is often low (2000 to 4000 cells per cubic millimeter) with an absolute lymphopenia. The platelet count is usually normal but may be markedly depressed due to an autoimmune-like thrombocytopenia. A qualitative defect in platelet function may also be found, and a bleeding time should be obtained in any patient scheduled for a surgical diagnostic procedure. The peripheral blood smear does not usually reveal any atypical lymphocytes or abnormal cells. The erythrocyte sedimentation rate is moderately elevated and can exceed 100 mm per hour in these patients.

Abnormal tests of liver function are nonspecific but may signal the presence of a serious disseminated opportunistic infection with organisms such as *Mycobacterium avium-intracellulare* or *M. tuberculosis.*

Positive serologic tests for syphilis, hepatitis A, hepatitis B, toxoplasmosis, cytomegalovirus, lymphogranuloma venereum, and herpes simplex virus reflect prior exposure to these pathogens in AIDS patients. It is interesting to note that extraordinarily high titers of anti-capsid IgG antibody to Epstein-Barr virus have been measured in AIDS patients.

Determination of histocompatibility types reveals an association between the presence of the HLA-DR5 antigen and Kaposi's sarcoma. Forty-three percent of patients with the epidemic form of Kaposi's sarcoma exhibit this antigen compared to 23 percent of normal controls. Similarly, HLA-DR5 has a frequency of 43 percent among patients with classical Kaposi's sarcoma. A recent study has shown a similar increased association between this haplotype and the syndrome of unexplained lymphadenopathy in homosexual men. No studies bearing on such association have been reported thus far in AIDS patients with opportunistic infections in the absence of Kaposi's sarcoma.

There are a number of abnormalities of immune function that are characteristic, albeit not specific, for AIDS (Table 7). The in vivo evidence for a profound defect in cell-mediated immune function includes cutaneous anergy to multiple recall antigens and poor host responsiveness to multiple opportunistic, intracellular pathogens. Normal delayed-type hypersensitivity response to cutaneous antigens cannot be used to exclude the diagnosis of AIDS because this measure of immune function may be intact early in the disease. For example, approximately 15 percent of AIDS patients with Kaposi's sarcoma are not anergic at the time they are seen by the physician. This observation suggests that patients who are seen with only Kaposi's sarcoma may be less immunocompromised than

TABLE 7

Abnormalities of immune function associated with the acquired immune-deficiency syndrome

Cutaneous anergy to multiple recall antigens
Absolute lymphopenia (decreased circulating T-lymphocyte population)
Decreased natural killer-cell activity
Reversed T-helper/T-suppressor ratio (due to decrease in the circulating T-helper cell population)
Decreased lymphoproliferative responses to mitogens, antigens, and allogenic cells (MLC)
Polyclonal hyperimmunoglobulinemia (IgG, IgA, IgM)
Circulating immune complexes
? Poor serologic response to new antigens (keyhole limpet hemocyanin)

those individuals who have opportunistic infections at the onset of their disease.

A profound lymphopenia (less than 600 cells per cubic millimeter) is frequently observed and is usually attributable to a decrease in circulating T lymphocytes bearing the helper phenotype. These cells are enumerated by recognizing their ability to bind monoclonal Okt 4 (or Leu 3) antibodies. The circulating T-suppressor cell population, bearing Okt 8 (or Leu 2) antigens, may be normal or elevated resulting in a marked reduction in the T-helper/T-suppressor cell ratio. A significant correlation between the number of Okt 4-positive lymphocytes (and the Okt 4/Okt 8 ratio) and in vitro functional assays has been found. There may be a correlation between the degree of reduction of the T-helper/T-suppressor cell ratio and the severity of the clinical illness. Those AIDS patients with opportunistic infections tend to have the lowest Okt 4/Okt 8 ratios, whereas patients with Kaposi's sarcoma without opportunistic infections, or those individuals with the unexplained lymphadenopathy syndrome, often have higher values, though significantly below those of healthy homosexual controls. Nevertheless, the measurement of the Okt 4/Okt 8 ratio in a given patient has not proved useful as a prognostic indicator. It is also important to appreciate that similar numerical abnormalities in this ratio have been seen in a number of other conditions, such as infection with cytomegalovirus, hepatitis B, and the Epstein-Barr virus, as well as in sarcoidosis and pregnancy.

Functional defects in T-cell response can also be measured in the immunology laboratory. Markedly decreased lymphoproliferative response to mitogens, depressed reactivity to allogenic cells, and subnormal natural killer-cell activity are all usually observed in the patient with AIDS.

Laboratory measurements of the humoral arm of the immune system include elevations of circulating immune complexes and high levels of total serum immunoglobulins. Polyclonal hyperimmunoglobulinemia is extremely common, with the IgG isotype most often elevated. These observations may possibly be explained either by decreased catabolism of the circulating immunoglobulins or by nonspecific B-lymphocyte activation. Despite the elevated levels of immunoglobulins in the serum, patients with AIDS may not be able to mount a de novo serologic response to a new antigen, such as keyhole limpet hemocyanin. This may explain the unreliable predictiveness of serum antibody tests for detection of certain clinically important pathogens, such as *Toxoplasma gondii*.

Measurements of serum complement components are usually normal. Recent reports of elevated serum levels of alpha-1-thymosin and beta₂ microglobulins have been observed, as has acid-labile alpha interferon, similar to that found in patients with systemic lupus erythematosus. While these findings may be further indications of altered immune function, more study is required to determine whether these assays will be useful as screening and/or diagnostic tools.

DIAGNOSIS

The clinical diagnosis of AIDS rests on the recognition of an opportunistic infection or Kaposi's sarcoma in a patient with no known cause for immune dysfunction. A comprehensive discussion of the diagnostic approach to the many opportunistic pathogens complicating AIDS is beyond the scope of this discussion. However, a review of some principles as they specifically apply to infections associated with AIDS is in order.

Some of the pathogens encountered in AIDS patients, such as *M. avium-intracellulare* or *Cryptosporidia,* are organisms that were rarely reported to cause life-threatening infections prior to the AIDS epidemic. The patient with AIDS is frequently found to be infected with different pathogens simultaneously. For example, about one-third of diagnostic transbronchial biopsies performed on AIDS patients with pulmonary signs and symptoms reveal more than one pathogen, such as *P. carinii, Legionella* sp., or cytomegalovirus, among others. Therefore, a broadened and more aggressive diagnostic approach is indicated inasmuch as the clinician cannot always rely on the concept of a single unifying diagnosis to explain a patient's clinical course.

It is important to realize that there is an inherently poor host immune response to infectious agents which will alter the anticipated disease manifestations in the patient with AIDS. For example, *Cryptococcus neoformans* may be recovered from acellular spinal fluid having nearly normal chemistries. Similarly, patients with biopsy-proven central nervous system toxoplasmosis may fail to mount the expected serologic response. Probably no better example of the diminished host response is that of the often extensive invasion of bone marrow, liver, or lymph nodes by *M. avium-intracellulare* in the total absence of granuloma formation. It is remarkable that since the clinical signs of infection may be masked by reduced host responsiveness, the isolation of a pathogenic agent may be alarmingly unexpected.

As outlined in the section on clinical manifestations, opportunistic infections often present with a specific symptom complex. The infectious agents most often encountered in each of these patients are specified in Table 6. Awareness of the more characteristic patterns of certain infections as seen in AIDS will assist the clinician in choosing an efficient diagnostic plan.

The diagnosis of Kaposi's sarcoma can be confirmed when a mucocutaneous lesion is identified by biopsy. However, the early patchlike lesions may be so atypical both clinically and histologically that the clinician as well as the pathologist must guard against overlooking the diagnosis. The plaque and nodular mucocutaneous lesions are more typical, consisting of endothelial lined slits. There are an increased number of fasciculi of spindle-shaped cells surrounding irregular thin-walled vascular clefts. Extravasated plasma cells and erythyrocytes are often seen in the intercellular spaces between spindle cells. Nuclear atypia and mitotic figures are uncommon (Figs. 11 and 12). The histopathologic findings of epidemic Kaposi's sarcoma are identical to those seen in all the clinical variants of the tumor seen in other populations. Although when first seen by the physician some patients have no cutaneous involvement of Kaposi's sarcoma, the tumor has been found in the lymph nodes, upper or lower gastrointestinal tracts, and lungs. In time, almost all of the patients will have developed skin and/or oral lesions. Nonetheless, the diagnosis of Kaposi's sarcoma cannot be excluded until extracutaneous sites of tumor involvement are ruled out as well.

TREATMENT

There is no effective treatment for AIDS. Attempts at "restorative immunomodulation" have, to date, met with little established success at reversing the defects in the cell-mediated immune response. Immunomodulators such as cimetidine, isoprinosine, indomethacin, alpha and gamma immune interferon, interleukin 2, thymic hormones (including alpha-1-thymosin and thymopoietin), among others, are currently under study. Bone marrow and thymic transplants have been performed in a small number of patients, but these modalities have not yet been critically evaluated. Until the pathogenesis of the immune defect is better understood, the only available therapeutic regimens will be those aimed at the treatment of the multiple and severe infectious and neoplastic sequelae of AIDS.

The high mortality rate of patients with opportunistic infections exemplifies the clinical observation that successful antimicrobial therapy requires an effective host immune response. Subsequently, the difficulties in treating the opportunistic infections in these patients are many. Because there are few clinical parameters to follow, assessment of response to therapy is difficult. Furthermore, the apparent failure of a therapeutic regimen to elicit a clinical response may be due to the presence of one or more unrecognized pathogens. A successful therapeutic result may require protracted treatment beyond that which would ordinarily be prescribed. For example, in the treatment of *P. carinii* pneumonia, a conventional 10- to 14-day course of trimethoprim-sulfamethoxazole may be inadequate to allow for normalization of clinical symptoms and radiographic findings. A 3- to 4-week course of treatment may sometimes be necessary. An as yet unexplained complication of therapy with trimethoprim-sulfamethoxazole in AIDS patients is the high incidence of adverse drug-related reactions, including allergic skin eruptions (such as erythroderma, erythema multiforme, Stevens-Johnson syndrome), drug-induced fever, and marked leukopenia. One or more of these side effects has been seen in over one-half of the AIDS patients receiving this medication. Although study of the efficacy of trimethoprim-sulfamethoxazole in the prevention of *P. carinii* pneumonia in AIDS has not been undertaken, this high rate of adverse drug reactions may preclude its widespread use for this purpose. Pentamidine isoethionate, exclusively distributed by the CDC, has been a valuable substitute for trimethoprim-sulfamethoxazole.

Another therapeutic problem in dealing with opportunistic infections in AIDS is the high rate of relapse or recurrence of many treated infections. For example, treatment of *P. carinii* pneumonia, systemic cryptococcosis, and central nervous system toxoplasmosis is often attended by a significant rate of clinical recurrence. Clinical trials on the efficacy of long-term suppressive therapeutic regimens for these selected opportunistic infections are required.

For a number of frequently encountered biologic agents, such as cytomegalovirus and cryptosporidiosis, no known effective therapies are available at this time. *M. avium-intracellulare* infection does not respond to treatment with conventional antituberculous drugs. The efficacy of treatment regimens including Ansamycin (an investigational rifamycin derivative) and clofazimine (an antileprosy agent) are currently being evaluated.

The optimal treatment of epidemic Kaposi's sarcoma has not been established. However, several chemotherapeutic regimens have shown effectiveness in treating this tumor. The combination of doxorubicin, bleomycin, and vinblastine will induce partial tumor responses in approximately 80 percent of patients and complete tumor responses in approximately 16 percent. A drug regimen employing the experimental antineoplastic agent VP-16 alone, may achieve results equal to or better than the combination therapy. The concern that chemotherapeutic agents may further depress immune function, thereby increasing the risk of an opportunistic infection, has prompted some investigators to try alternative modalities to treat this neoplasm. One study employing recombinant DNA alpha interferon reported a beneficial effect in a small number of patients. Other therapeutic trials employing alpha- and gamma-interferon preparations, plasmapheresis, interleukin 2, and other thymic hormones are examples of alternative treatment modalities currently under evaluation.

PATHOGENESIS

The pathogenesis of AIDS remains the most fascinating and speculative aspect of this illness.

The most widely held theory is that AIDS is possibly caused or triggered by a yet to be identified biologic agent that can induce a profound state of immune dysregulation. Viral agents have received the greatest attention. Cytomegalovirus was the first organism to be suggested because of its high prevalence among homosexual men and its ability to be transmitted venereally. Seroepidemiologically this virus has also been found to be associated with the classical African and epidemic forms of Kaposi's sarcoma. In addition, cytomegalovirus genome has been demonstrated in tissue cultures of Kaposi's sarcoma by DNA hybridization studies. As mentioned earlier, cytomegalovirus infection alone has been found to cause rather protracted suppression of the cell-mediated immune response.

Other viral agents have been suggested as possible etiologies, including the retroviruses and the Epstein-Barr virus. These organisms are attractive because of their tumorigenic potential and ability to cause diseases with long latency periods. One retrovirus, the human T-cell leukemia virus (HTLV), has recently been linked to patients with AIDS. This virus has been isolated from the circulating lymphocytes of some patients. Furthermore, HTLV genomes were detected by nucleic acid hybridization in a small number of AIDS patients. Finally, preliminary studies have shown that HTLV-specific antibodies were measured in 25 percent of AIDS patients, as well as in homosexual men with unexplained lymphadenopathy, but not in apparently healthy homosexual controls or blood donors. Whether this virus is involved with the pathogenesis of this illness, or whether it is yet another example of an opportunistic pathogen in the face of severe immunosuppression, remains to be established.

Other viral etiologies have been suggested. These include parvoviruses (e.g., Aleutian mink virus, canine parvovirus, minute virus of mice), adenoviruses, or Delta-agent-like viruses. Most recently, attention has been drawn to a fungus (*Thermoascus crustaceus*) recovered in monocyte cultures from a few patients with AIDS. This organism contains a cyclosporin-like compound which would theoretically be capable of inducing many of the immune defects that characterize AIDS. While highly speculative, this observation should serve to remind us to consider nonviral biologic agents as possible etiologies for this disease.

Alternative hypotheses of pathogenesis invoke multifactorial causes including genetic predisposition, environmental factors, or drug exposures. The concept of "immunologic overload" due to serologic responses to multiple sexually transmitted diseases has also been suggested. The recent finding of circulating antisperm antibodies in AIDS patients capable of cross reaction with antigens on the T-lymphocyte surface is being studied as another possible mechanism of immune suppression in the syndrome. The increased association of HLA-DR5 in AIDS patients with Kaposi's sarcoma is one of the first demonstrations of a possible genetic predisposition to a specific neoplasm.

CONCLUSION

The recognition of the AIDS epidemic has allowed this disease to assume its place as one of the most devastating afflictions of modern time. The understanding of the pathogenesis of other recently described illnesses, such as Lyme disease, Legionnaires' disease, and toxic-shock syndrome, has resulted from extensive multidisciplinary research efforts similar to those being applied to the study of AIDS. Nonetheless, it appears that the AIDS puzzle will be a particularly difficult one to solve.

Research endeavors have already brought together investigators from all aspects of medicine. Immunologists are seeking to determine the relationships between the observed numerical and functional immunological abnormalities. Correct assessment of the "causes and effects" may pave the way for effective immunorestorative therapy. Virologists and molecular geneticists are searching for specific etiologies. Animal models must be found to provide a basis for studying disease transmission. Epidemiologists must study other populations at risk for AIDS with the same intensity that they have applied to homosexual patients. The common risk factors need to be identified, and the observed differences in disease manifestations must be explained. In addition, the clinicians must collaborate to establish the most effective therapies of the infectious and neoplastic complications of this disease.

It is particularly timely and essential to develop a sensitive, reliable, and specific laboratory marker of disease in patients with AIDS. Not only will this help in our understanding of the natural course of this illness and of the true breadth of the epidemic, but it will be useful in screening for possible disease in asymptomatic individuals as well.

References

CENTERS FOR DISEASE CONTROL: Kaposi's sarcoma and *Pneumocystis* pneumonia among homosexual men: New York City and California. Morb Mort Week Rep 30:305, 1981

CENTERS FOR DISEASE CONTROL: Update: Acquired immunodeficiency syndrome (AIDS): United States. Morb Mort Week Rep 32:389, 1983

DESTEFANO E et al: Acid-labile human leukocyte interferon in homosexual men with Kaposi's sarcoma and lymphadenopathy. J Infect Dis 146:451, 1982

DREW WL et al: Prevalence of cytomegalovirus infection in homosexual men. J Infect Dis 143:188, 1981

FRIEDMAN-KIEN AE et al: Disseminated Kaposi's sarcoma in homosexual men. Ann Intern Med 96:693, 1982

FRIEDMAN-KIEN AE, LAUBENSTEIN LJ (eds): Proceedings of Symposium on AIDS (Epidemic Kaposi's Sarcoma and Opportunistic Infections), March, 1983. New York University Medical Center, Publ.: Masson, Inc. New York, Jan. 1984

GOLDSMITH JC et al: T-lymphocyte subpopulation abnormalities in apparently healthy patients with hemophilia. Ann Intern Med 98:294, 1983

GOTTLIEB MS et al: *Pneumocystis carinii* pneumonia and mucosal candidiasis in previously healthy homosexual men: Evidence of a new acquired cellular immunodeficiency. N Engl J Med 305:1425, 1981

———— et al: UCLA Conference: The acquired immunodeficiency syndrome. Ann Intern Med 99:208, 1983

GREENE JB et al: *Mycobacterium avium-intracellulare*: A cause of disseminated life-threatening infection in homosexuals and drug abusers. Ann Intern Med 97:539, 1982

HOLLAND GN et al: Ocular disorders associated with a new severe acquired cellular immunodeficiency syndrome. Am J Ophthalmol 93:393, 1982

JAFFE HW et al: National Case-Control Study of Kaposi's sarcoma and *Pneumocystis carinii* pneumonia in homosexual men: 1. Epidemiologic results. Ann Intern Med 99:145, 1983

Joint statement on acquired immune deficiency syndrome (AIDS) related to transfusion. Transfusion 23:87, 1983

KROWN SE et al: Preliminary observations on the effect of recombinant leukocyte A interferon in homosexual men with Kaposi's sarcoma. N Engl J Med 308:1071, 1983

LANDAY A et al: Immunologic studies in asymptomatic hemophilia patients: Relationship to acquired immune deficiency syndrome (AIDS). J Clin Invest 71:1500, 1983

MASUR H et al: An outbreak of community-acquired *Pneumocystis carinii* pneumonia: Initial manifestation of cellular immune dysfunction. N Engl J Med 305:1431, 1981

———— et al: Opportunistic infection in previously healthy women: Initial manifestations of a community-acquired cellular immunodeficiency. Ann Intern Med 97:533, 1982

MILDVAN D et al: Opportunistic infections and immune deficiency in homosexual men. Ann Intern Med 96:700, 1982

MORRIS L et al: Autoimmune thrombocytopenic purpura in homosexual men. Ann Intern Med 96:714, 1982

PITCHENIK AE et al: Opportunistic infections and Kaposi's sarcoma among Haitians: Evidence of a new acquired immunodeficiency state. Ann Intern Med 98:277, 1983

ROGERS MF et al: National Case-Control Study of Kaposi's sarcoma and *Pneumocystis carinii* pneumonia in homosexual men: 2. Laboratory results. Ann Intern Med 99:151, 1983

RUBINSTEIN A et al: Acquired immunodeficiency with reversed T4/T8 ratios in infants born to promiscuous and drug-addicted mothers. JAMA 249:2350, 1983

SEIGAL FP et al: Severe acquired immunodeficiency in male homosexuals, manifested by chronic perianal ulcerative herpes simplex lesions. N Engl J Med 305:1439, 1981

SMALL CB et al: Community-acquired opportunistic infections and defective cellular immunity in heterosexual drug abusers and homosexual men. Am J Med 74:433, 1983

STAHL RE et al: Immunologic abnormalities in homosexual men: Relationship to Kaposi's sarcoma. Am J Med 73:171, 1982

VIEIRA J et al: Acquired immune deficiency in Haitians: Opportunistic infections in previously healthy Haitian immigrants. N Engl J Med 308:125, 1983

RECENT ADVANCES IN ALZHEIMER'S DISEASE

DENNIS J. SELKOE

Rarely in recent medical history has a previously obscure disorder so rapidly engaged the attention of the medical profession and the lay public as has Alzheimer's disease. Alzheimer's disease as a diagnostic entity has evolved from a relatively rare syndrome of presenile dementia, briefly encountered by physicians during their medical training but soon forgotten, into a major, late-life degenerative disease now believed to be the fourth or fifth most common cause of death in the United States. Simultaneously, Alzheimer's disease has become the subject of innumerable newspaper and magazine articles, symposia, and radio and television programs and is rapidly achieving the media status of a "household word."

This dramatic surge of interest in Alzheimer's disease arises from two fundamental developments. First, the steady prolongation of life expectancy during the past several decades, coupled with the lowering of birth rates in many developed countries, has rapidly enlarged the portion of the population surviving beyond the sixth decade and thus subject to late-life neuronal degenerative disease. In the United States, the portion of the population over 65 is currently estimated to be 11 percent (26 million persons) and is expected to climb to approximately 18 percent (50 million) by the year 2020. Second, neuropathologists and other students of the aging nervous system have gradually evolved a major reinterpretation of the pathological basis of common, idiopathic senile dementia. It is now realized that the majority of such cases are not related to cerebral atherosclerosis, as was previously thought, but rather to a progressive degeneration of specific cerebral neurons which, on pathological grounds, appears highly similar if not indistinguishable from the presenile dementia which Alzheimer described in 1907. Thus, the emergence of dementia of the Alzheimer type as a major public health problem in the last decades of this century appears to be related to demographic and medical diagnostic considerations rather than to evidence of fundamental changes in human biology or the environment. The popular description of Alzheimer's disease as an "emerging epidemic" should not be construed to rest on evidence that the currently undefined etiologies of Alzheimer-type neuronal degeneration are actually becoming more prevalent in society.

The purpose of this article is to review recent advances in our understanding of the molecular pathology, diagnostic evaluation, and treatment of presenile and senile dementia of the Alzheimer type, referred to here as *Alzheimer's disease*. The classification of dementias in general (that is, disorders showing gradual loss of memory and other intellectual functions), as well as the clinical features and differential diagnosis of the various degenerative and nondegenerative dementias, is described in the tenth edition of *Harrison's Principles of Internal Medicine*, particularly in Chaps. 21, 22, and 364, and will not be repeated here.

EPIDEMIOLOGIC CONSIDERATIONS AND CURRENT DIAGNOSTIC CLASSIFICATION

Although detailed population surveys are not yet available, current data, largely derived from studies in the United Kingdom, suggest that approximately 5 percent of individuals over 65 have dementia of moderate or severe degree and that an additional 5 to 7 percent have evidence of mild impairment of memory and cognitive functions. The percentage of individuals who are demented rises with age, perhaps reaching 20 percent or more between ages 80 and 90. It is estimated, on the basis of autopsy series, that roughly one-half to two-thirds of these patients with the clinical syndrome of senile dementia will show the changes of Alzheimer's disease on pathological examination of the brain. Based on these data, present estimates of the prevalence of dementia of the Alzheimer type in the United States are projected as approximately 600 cases per 100,000 persons, a figure three times that of Parkinson's disease and about 15 times that of multiple sclerosis. Such data suggest that there are currently more than 1.5 million Americans with Alzheimer's disease. Since the incidence prior to age 65 is relatively low, most patients with Alzheimer's disease fall under the diagnostic term *senile dementia of the Alzheimer type.* The question of whether presenile cases (i.e., onset before age 65) should be considered as a distinct clinicopathological entity remains unsettled. Many investigators believe that a large majority of patients with either presenile or senile Alzheimer's disease are indistinguishable on clinical, neuropathological, or biochemical grounds. Consequently, the two disorders are often considered together under the term Alzheimer's disease; this nomenclature will be used here unless otherwise specified. On the other hand, several authors have pointed to a higher familial incidence, a more rapid progression, and a greater prevalence of certain clinical features in early-onset cases as evidence for considering presenile Alzheimer's disease a separate disorder.

Although Alzheimer's disease is the most common neuropathological basis for late-life dementia, many other neurological and systemic disorders can produce dementia. The great majority of these have clinical and laboratory diagnostic features which allow them to be readily distinguished from Alzheimer-type dementia. After Alzheimer's disease, the most common neuropathological finding in patients dying with senile dementia is the presence of two or more discrete cerebral infarcts. The clinical syndrome associated with this finding, referred to as *multi-infarct dementia*, is distinguished from Alzheimer's disease on the basis of its abrupt onset,

TABLE 1

Diagnostic evaluation of the patient with progressive dementia

Evaluations recommended in all patients
  Neurological history, including family history of dementia
  Medication history
  Neurological examination
  Screening blood tests, including complete blood count, erythrocyte sedimentation rate, blood urea nitrogen, electrolytes, calcium, phosphorus, liver, and thyroid function, vitamin B_{12} and folic acid, serological test for syphilis, and medication blood levels
  Computerized tomography of the brain
Evaluations recommended in selected patients, dependent on neurological history and examination
  Neuropsychological testing
  Psychiatric evaluation
  Electroencephalogram
  Lumbar puncture
  Radionuclide cisternography
  Toxic screen, including central nervous system depressants and stimulants and metallic ions

stepwise progression, and associated focal and generalized signs of cerebrovascular disease. Such cases appear to make up approximately 20 percent of patients with senile dementia, a percentage which may be expected to decrease in view of the declining incidence of stroke. Also, the lesions of Alzheimer's disease can be found together with cerebral infarction in some cases of senile dementia. Among the growing list of treatable and potentially reversible conditions causing intellectual impairment, therapeutic drug intoxication, depression, and metabolic or infectious disorders are the most common. The importance of a careful assessment of the elderly patient's general medical status and medications prior to diagnosing Alzheimer's disease cannot be overemphasized. Table 1 provides a suggested series of evaluations of patients presenting with previously undiagnosed, progressive intellectual impairment after the age of 60.

If one considers only those patients who have a gradually progressive, idiopathic loss of intellectual function with preserved alertness and without major motor signs (i.e., patients who fit research diagnostic criteria for primary degenerative dementia), not all will display the histopathological findings of Alzheimer's disease at autopsy. The accuracy of the clinical diagnosis of Alzheimer's disease reported in pathologically verified series ranges from 70 to 90 percent. Among the remaining cases, other specific neuronal degenerations such as Parkinson's disease and Pick's disease are occasionally found. Indeed, there is growing recognition that the pathological findings of Parkinson's disease may often be accompanied by those of Alzheimer's disease in the same brain. The basis for the coexistence of these two most common neuronal degenerative diseases is not yet known.

In the author's experience, a frequent alternate neuropathological diagnosis in cases of primary degenerative dementia is a constellation of nonspecific findings marked by widespread neuronal loss and gliosis in hippocampus and other limbic structures, cerebral cortex, and certain subcortical nuclei. Such brains appear not to exhibit a characteristic cytopathological signature in degenerating neurons, such as the tangles and plaques of Alzheimer's disease, and are difficult to distinguish from the brains of nondemented aged individuals. These patients seem to have had an illness which falls within the broad and heterogeneous clinical symptomatology of Alzheimer's disease and is thus not readily distinguishable from Alzheimer's disease during life. The inclusion of such cases in clinical or biochemical research investigations of Alzheimer's disease will certainly distort any resulting findings. In coming years, it will be important to attempt to define new forms of primary degenerative dementia on clinical and pathological grounds, as well as to establish subclassifications within the broad spectrum of what is now referred to as Alzheimer's disease. Just as Alzheimer's disease was underdiagnosed 20 years ago, there is little doubt that this disorder is currently overdiagnosed.

NEW METHODS OF DIAGNOSTIC IMAGING IN ALZHEIMER'S DISEASE

The development of innovative techniques for imaging the structure and function of the human brain has provided a series of powerful research tools for studying the pathophysiology of dementia in vivo. These methods, which include high-resolution computerized tomography (CT) scanning, positron emission tomographic (PET) scanning, nuclear magnetic resonance (NMR) scanning, and computerized spectral analysis of the electroencephalogram (EEG), also have proven or potential usefulness in the differential diagnosis of dementing illnesses. They can serve as an adjunct to the neurological history and examination in distinguishing primary degenerative dementias, such as Alzheimer's disease, from many other brain disorders associated with cognitive impairment. Moreover, some of the newer imaging techniques may prove to have the sensitivity to differentiate certain degenerative dementias from each other and perhaps to distinguish the anatomical and physiological changes of normal brain aging from those found in Alzheimer's disease.

CT scanning is invaluable in ruling out various nondegenerative brain diseases presenting with dementia (e.g., multiple infarctions, brain tumor, subdural hematoma, and demyelination). However, several studies have shown that CT scanning is generally not able to distinguish the ventricular enlargement and cortical atrophy that is seen in many elderly individuals with normal mentation from that which occurs in senile dementia of the Alzheimer type. Some investigators have reported initial success in using special parameters in CT scanning (e.g., the mean CT density of subcortical white matter or the ratio between ventricular and brain cross-sectional areas) as a way of separating subjects with normal brain aging from the minority with primary dementia. However, a practical and widely validated formula for the accurate CT diagnosis of senile dementia of the Alzheimer type is not yet available.

PET, which estimates the rate of regional glucose utilization after intravenous administration of $[^{18}F]$2-fluoro-2-deoxy-D-glucose, has been used to measure cortical metabolism in the resting normal state and during various cognitive and motor tasks. The recent application of this methodology to patients with clinically diagnosed Alzheimer's disease has shown that focal areas of diminished cortical glucose metabolism can be seen in cases with prominent lateralized cognitive deficits [e.g., dysphasia (left hemisphere) or visuoconstructive dysfunction (right parietal lobe)]. Patients with memory failure as the major clinical feature showed no cortical metabolic asymmetry. These findings have relevance to the study of localization of specific human brain functions as well as to elucidating the progression of cortical changes in Alzheimer patients.

Other PET studies have demonstrated different patterns of cortical glucose hypometabolism in Alzheimer's disease, Creutzfeldt-Jakob disease, and multi-infarct dementia. The degree of spatial resolution provided by current PET-scanning techniques, particularly in medial and deep structures of the brain, is probably not sufficient to detect and localize early, highly focal metabolic changes that could give clues to the sequence of neuronal degeneration in Alzheimer's disease.

The application of computerized spectral analysis to the waveforms on the EEG can provide highly sensitive and dynamic analyses of brain electrical activity in health and disease. Duffy and colleagues, who have developed a system of computerized brain electrical activity mapping (BEAM), have begun to study normal aged and demented patients with this technique. They find that the frequency distribution of brain electrical activity in patients with senile dementia of the Alzheimer type is shifted toward slower frequencies, while the opposite pattern, an increase in faster frequencies, was observed in subjects of the same age with normal mentation. This observation may enable a more precise and quantifiable distinction between these two groups at the earlier stages of the disease. Similar analyses are also being applied to evoked cortical potentials in Alzheimer patients.

The newest imaging technique to be applied to patients with neurologic diseases is NMR scanning. This exciting technology, which has arisen out of a basic physicochemical method of elucidating the intricate conformation of organic molecules, takes advantage of the fact that hydrogen (or other) nuclei in biological materials generate a miniscule magnetic field due to their inherent property of rotation, or spin. The application of a powerful external magnetic field to the material (in this case, in situ brain tissue) causes a uniform orientation of the millions of tiny magnetic moments given off by the spinning hydrogen nuclei in the tissue. Subsequent application of a much smaller rotating magnetic field at right angles to the major static field will displace the bulk magnetization vector of all the spinning nuclei, giving off a recordable signal. The resulting emitted signals from a complex tissue will depend on the concentration and distribution of hydrogen (and other) nuclei in the

sample, which will differ in tissues of different compositions (e.g., gray matter vs. white matter) and in normal vs. pathological states. Two-dimensional tomographic images of the emitted signals can then be constructed by the computer.

Only a relatively small number of patients with primary degenerative dementia have been examined in the few centers where NMR scanning is currently available. No definitive data about its utility in Alzheimer's disease have been published. Its advantage over CT scanning in distinguishing age-related changes in normal brain tissue from those in neuronal degenerations, such as Alzheimer's disease, and its usefulness as a research tool in Alzheimer's disease remain to be seen. Early results indicate that NMR may be superior to CT scanning in identifying cerebral infarction and thus establishing the diagnosis of multi-infarct dementia.

RECENT ADVANCES IN THE PATHOBIOLOGY OF ALZHEIMER'S DISEASE

Principles of age-related neuronal degeneration

Although the public health implications of a rapidly growing population subject to senile dementia have received much attention, the application of modern molecular and cell biological approaches to the problem of age-related neuronal abiotrophy has only recently begun. The number of laboratories carrying out neurobiological studies of aged human brain tissues or related experimental models remains limited. Due to the complexity of the problem and the difficulty of work on postmortem brain, advances in our knowledge of the events underlying age-related brain dysfunction have come slowly.

The central goal of basic biological research on Alzheimer's disease and other age-linked degenerative diseases is to understand the molecular changes that lead to premature dysfunction and death of certain brain neurons. In contrast to Huntington's disease, in which neuronal loss in the caudate and putamen is unaccompanied by any characteristic ultrastructural change in adjacent neurons that have not yet died, neuronal attrition in Alzheimer brain tissue is associated with marked structural changes in many

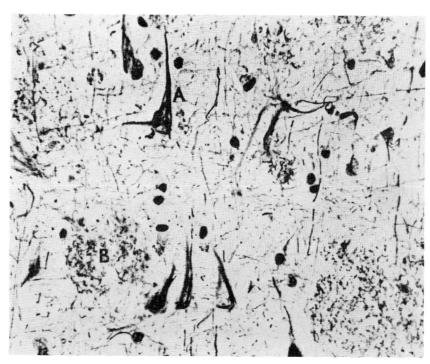

FIGURE 1

Light micrograph of a silver-stained section of cerebral cortex from a case of senile dementia of the Alzheimer type. Numerous nerve cell bodies display bundles of thickened, dark fibrils in their cytoplasm, referred to as neurofibrillary tangles (A). There are also numerous argyrophilic plaques (B) in the neuropil between the nerve cell bodies. (Von Braunmuhl's silver impregnation. 500×) (From Blackwood, Dodds, and Sommerville: Atlas of Neuropathology. Edinburgh, E. & S. Livingstone, 1949, p. 93.)

remaining cells. The two principal neuronal lesions which serve as the basis of the histological diagnosis of Alzheimer's disease are the neurofibrillary tangle and the neuritic (or senile) plaque. Both plaques and tangles are present and often abundant in the hippocampus, amygdala, and cerebral neocortex of virtually all cases of Alzheimer's disease. Some cases show only extensive plaque formation in cerebral neocortex with very few tangles; rarely, the converse is true. In addition to this classical cortical pathology, which Alzheimer originally described, neuropathologists have increasingly recognized the presence of neurofibrillary tangles in various subcortical gray matter structures, including the basal ganglia and nuclei within the brainstem and basal forebrain that contain the cells of origin of cholinergic and noradrenergic fibers widely innervating the cerebral cortex. Besides plaques and tangles, certain other neuropathological changes are characteristic of dementia of the Alzheimer type: the loss of large pyramidal neurons in deeper layers of the cerebral cortex, amyloid deposition within the walls of intracortical blood vessels (congophilic angiopathy), and granulovacuolar degeneration of the cytoplasm of certain pyramidal neurons.

The neurofibrillary tangle (Fig. 1) is a non-membrane-bound mass of abnormal fibrils occupying much of the cytoplasmic area of the neuronal cell body. Electron microscopy indicates that the vast majority of such fibrils consist of a pair of filaments wound into a double helix (Fig. 2). Each of the filaments in a pair bears resemblance to the normal, straight neurofilaments found in all neurons, except for its helical conformation. These fibrils, which are the ultrastructural hallmark of Alzheimer-type neuronal degeneration, are referred to as paired helical filaments (PHF). The senile plaque (Fig. 3) is a complex structure found not inside the neuronal cell body, as is the tangle, but rather within the extensive meshwork of fibers between neurons. The plaque consists of a central core of extracellular amyloid (the chemical nature of which is not yet known) and a surrounding meshwork of abnormal, dilated neuronal processes (i.e., axons and dendrites). By electron microscopy, these axons and dendrites contain abnormal mitochondria and lysosomes, plus some PHF identical to those found in the neurofibrillary tangle. Thus, PHF accumulate both in neuronal cell bodies (i.e., tangles) and in abnormal neuronal fibers (i.e., plaques) in Alzheimer's disease. A major

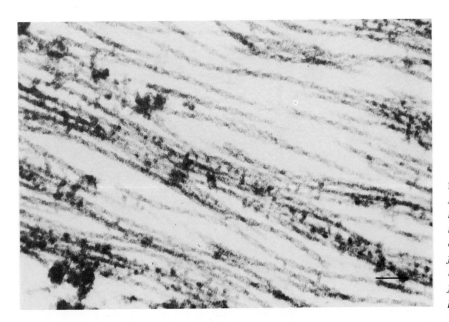

FIGURE 2
Electron micrograph of intra-neuronal paired helical filaments in Alzheimer cerebral cortex. Large masses of these fibers comprise the neurofibrillary tangles and are also found in the neurites of senile plaques. (Bar = 100 nm.)

unresolved issue is the precise anatomical relationship between the tangles and plaques and the relative importance of each in the pathogenesis of intellectual dysfunction.

The striking morphological changes just described in Alzheimer brains are qualitatively indistinguishable from lesions that accumulate in much smaller numbers and in restricted topographical distribution (particularly in hippocampus and amygdala) in the majority of intellectually normal individuals after the sixth decade. Therefore, the neuropathological distinction between normal human brain aging and Alzheimer's disease is essentially quantitative: greater density and wider distribution of the lesions allow the diagnosis of Alzheimer's disease. Painstaking microscopic counting of plaques and tangles in postmortem human cortex has demonstrated a rough but statistically significant relationship between the number of such lesions and the presence and degree of clinical dementia before death. Moreover, the neuronal density in Alzheimer hippocampus is inversely related to the number of tangle-bearing neurons (i.e., the less the number of surviving neurons, the greater the percentage that contain tangles). The density of cortical neuritic plaques also correlates quantitatively with the degree of decrease in acetylcholine synthesis in Alzheimer cortex, the major neurotransmitter alteration discovered to date in this disease. It may be concluded that the plaques and tangles which form the morphological basis for diagnosis are also pathogenetically related to (or at the least a strong marker for) neuronal attrition and subsequent dementia.

It should be emphasized that normal brain aging and Alzheimer's disease are not the only neurological conditions characterized by plaques and tangles. Importantly, a majority of patients with Down's syndrome (trisomy 21) who survive past the age of 40 develop a premature neuronal degeneration morphologically indistinguishable from Alzheimer's disease. Postencephalitic Parkinson's disease and the endemic foci of parkinsonism-dementia complex on the island of Guam and on the Kii peninsula of Japan are characterized by extensive neurofibrillary tangle formation. The syndrome of dementia pugilistica that develops in some individuals, particularly boxers, following multiple head injuries, is also marked by neurofibrillary tangle formation with or without senile plaques. The latter observation raises the issue of a breakdown in the blood-brain barrier as a prerequisite for neurofibrillary degeneration. Certain other degenerative or metabolic brain disorders with diverse etiologies may display occasional neurofibrillary tangles on histological examination of the brain.

Recently, significant progress in characterizing the nature of neuronal degeneration in Alzheimer's disease has occurred. Advances have come in several distinct areas of biochemical and

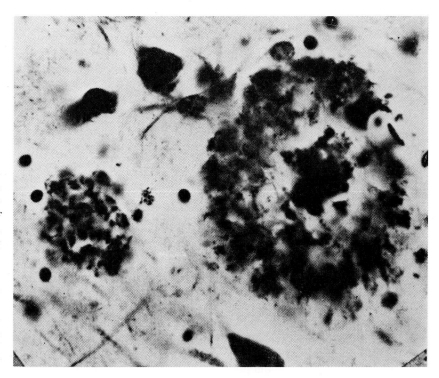

FIGURE 3
Light micrograph of an argyrophilic senile plaque in cerebral cortex in Alzheimer's disease. Central core of amyloid is surrounded by a peripheral ring of abnormal neurites and microglial cells. (Bielschowski's silver impregnation, 800×) (From Blackwood, McMenemy, Meyer, Norman, and Russell: Greenfield's Neuropathology. Baltimore, Williams & Wilkins, 1963, p. 535.)

molecular biological investigation. As often occurs in the formative stages of research on a human disease, it has been difficult to interrelate the diverse experimental observations made to date into a comprehensive or unitary model for the pathogenesis of Alzheimer's disease. In the following section, we will review new information from the investigative area that has received the most attention, namely, the search for changes in neurotransmitter function in Alzheimer tissue. Thereafter, we will consider a series of developments relating to less well-studied aspects of the disease, for example, the cytoskeletal reorganization of the neuron, the role of genetic factors, and the evidence for involvement of toxins or viruses in its pathogenesis.

Alterations of neurotransmitter function

In view of the major contribution that basic studies of neurotransmitters and their synthetic enzymes made to the treatment of Parkinson's disease, it is appropriate that much investigative effort is currently being applied to similar studies in Alzheimer's disease. Interest in this area also derives from rapidly expanding knowledge about

the role of newly discovered putative neurotransmitters (i.e., peptides and amino acids) in the normal brain. Among current investigative approaches to Alzheimer's disease, studies of synaptic biochemistry are most likely to yield new therapies that, although not curative, could control or ameliorate some of the symptoms of the disease in its early and middle stages.

The studies reviewed in this section address the question: What are the neurotransmitter classes of the specific neurons that are dying out prematurely in Alzheimer's disease? It is widely assumed that the neurotransmitter deficiencies observed in idiopathic neuronal degenerations are a result of the neuronal loss and cytologic lesions found in the brain rather than their cause, although the sequence of pathogenesis in this regard is not established. It is possible that the initial loss of one or more specific functional classes of neurons early in the disease (e.g., cholinergic neurons in the basal forebrain) could then lead to widespread secondary neuronal pathology (e.g., tangle formation) and cell death. In such a model, the responsible mechanisms might include transsynaptic degeneration due to the lack of trophic influence of the missing neurotransmitter or other factors secreted by the dying cell on the postsynaptic neuron. However, even if transsynaptic degeneration could be shown to account for much of the neuronal loss in cerebral cortex, the primary cause and mechanism of cell death in the initially dying neurons would still remain unknown.

The first, and to date the most dramatic, neurotransmitter change found in Alzheimer tissue was a marked decline in the activity of the cholinergic synthetic enzyme, choline acetyltransferase (CAT). In 1976, three independent goups in Great Britain reported losses of 50 to 90 percent of cholinergic synthetic capacity in various areas of cerebral cortex. These observations have been widely confirmed, and decreased cortical CAT activity has become a consistent biochemical finding which is considered by many to be a fundamental marker for the disease, like plaques and tangles. The degree of decline of CAT activity in cortical samples has been statistically correlated with the density of tangles and neuritic plaques in the area sampled. It should be noted, however, that 50 percent reductions of CAT activity have also been reported in brain areas (e.g., caudate nucleus) that show neither pathological lesions (i.e., plaques and tangles) nor clinical evidence of involvement in Alzheimer's disease.

Several studies of the postsynaptic side of the cholinergic synapse indicate that muscarinic cholinergic-receptor-binding activity is not depleted in Alzheimer hippocampus and neocortex. Thus, available data suggest that cholinergic neurons are dysfunctional or lost in Alzheimer-type dementia, while cholinoceptive neurons are not markedly affected. These findings provide the rationale for the current intensive effort to develop cholinergic replacement therapies for patients with mild and moderate Alzheimer's disease.

A major advance in understanding the origin of the striking loss of cholinergic function in Alzheimer cortex has come from the work of Price, Whitehouse, and colleagues. Several investigators had shown in recent years that the site of origin of a large majority of the cholinergic terminals in mammalian cerebral neocortex was a relatively small group of magnocellular neurons found in the basal forebrain, ventral to the globus pallidus (Fig. 4). This zone, referred to as the nucleus basalis of Meynert, was specifically examined by Price and associates in the brains of Alzheimer patients. They found a marked decrease in the number of perikaryons in this nucleus in both sporadic and familial Alzheimer's disease compared to age-matched controls. Subsequently, Nakano and Hirano reported a similar attrition of neurons in the adjacent septal nuclei, an area contiguous with the Meynert nucleus that provides the major cholinergic input to the hippocampus. Both groups of investigators observed neurofibrillary tangles in some of the remaining cells in these nuclei.

Price and his colleagues have suggested that the loss of cholinergic cell bodies in the basal forebrain may be anatomically related to the abnormal synaptic terminals in the senile plaques of cerebral cortex. They hypothesize that an as-yet-undertermined process may affect cholinergic terminals in Alzheimer cortex and hippocampus, resulting in senile plaque formation in these areas and a secondary "dying-back" axonal degeneration which eventually kills the cell bodies of origin in the Meynert and medial septal nuclei. However, these investigators have also observed loss of neurons in the Meynert nucleus in Pick's disease, Korsakoff's syndrome, and dementia pugilistica, conditions which are not characterized by widespread senile plaque formation in cortex. Similarly, cell loss in the Meynert nucleus has been reported in patients with the dementia associated with Parkinson's disease. Therefore, basal forebrain cholinergic cell loss, while associated with disorders of memory, appears not to be specific for Alzheimer's disease and can occur in the absence of senile plaque formation in cerebral cortex.

The findings summarized above provide the strongest evidence to date that a transmitter-specific neuronal population is a major target of the pathological processes occurring in Alzheimer's disease. One can readily draw a parallel to the loss of dopaminergic neurons in the substantia nigra in Parkinson's disease. However, it is not yet clear that the loss of cholinergic cells is the initial or essential lesion in the disease, or that it is as selective as the nigral dopaminergic cell loss in Parkinson's disease. Recently evidence has been provided that noradrenergic neurons innervating cerebral cortex, which originate in a small brainstem nucleus called the locus ceruleus, also are markedly decreased in number in at least

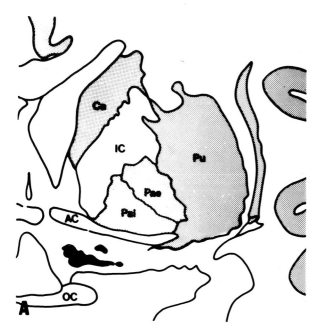

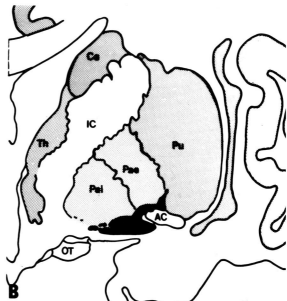

FIGURE 4
Drawing of two sections through the basal frontal lobe of a human cerebral hemisphere showing the position of the nucleus basalis of Meynert (in black) in relation *to other structures. Ca, caudate; Pu, putamen; Pae & Pai, globus pallidus, internal and external segments; IC, internal capsule; AC, anterior commissure; OC, optic chiasm; OT, optic tract.*

some Alzheimer patients. Furthermore, at least one report has described biochemical alterations and structural changes (neurofibrillary tangles) in serotonin-releasing neurons of the brainstem that project to the cerebral cortex. Although there seems little doubt that loss of cholinergic neurons is a major and consistent neurotransmitter abnormality in Alzheimer's disease, there appear to be losses of other monoaminergic neurons in at least some if not all cases. This potentially multisystem degeneration would mitigate against the success of purely cholinergic replacement therapies.

Further complexity regarding the neuropharmacology of the disease occurs when alterations of neuropeptides having putative transmitter function are considered. To date, the most well-documented and reproducible change in neuropeptide levels has been found for somatostatin, cortical concentrations of which are reported to fall by 50 to 75 percent in Alzheimer's disease. Changes for other neuropeptides, for example, substance P, have been reported from some laboratories but have not been widely confirmed. It is known from recent animal studies that somatostatin is not colocalized in cholinergic neurons in cerebral cortex and hippocampus. Therefore, somatostatin-containing neurons may represent another transmitter class which, like cholinergic, noradrenergic, and perhaps serotinergic neurons, is vulnerable to the processes causing premature cell death in Alzheimer's disease.

Cytoskeletal pathology of Alzheimer neurons

The studies reviewed in this section and in the following sections on genetic factors, neurotoxins, and viruses address a different question than the neurotransmitter studies just summarized. The fundamental issue raised here is: what are the molecular mechanisms underlying the premature degeneration of neurons in Alzheimer brain, irrespective of which transmitter class of neurons is primarily affected?

As stated earlier, the progressive accumulation of paired helical filaments in neuronal cell bodies (i.e., tangles) and neurites (i.e., senile plaques) correlates with several parameters of Alzheimer's disease, including degree of dementia, extent of neuronal loss in hippocampus, degree of deficiency of cortical cholinergic function, and the loss of cholinergic neurons in the basal forebrain. In view of these findings, it is important to understand the molecular origin of paired helical filaments and to establish what role their formation plays in accelerated death of neurons during normal aging and in Alzheimer's disease. In setting these goals, we must acknowledge that neurofibrillary degeneration (PHF formation) is presumably a late and somewhat nonspecific event in the course of certain human neuronal degenerations. Nonetheless, understanding the basis for what currently appears to be a remarkable and irreversible restructuring of the neuron's internal skeleton is likely to provide clues to abnormal molecular events that precede PHF formation in neurons destined to die prematurely.

During the past decade, several groups of investigators have used biochemical and immunocytochemical techniques in attempts to derive the composition of paired helical filaments and thereby compare them to the normal filaments and tubules found in neurons. Unfortunately, the results of these studies have been conflicting and inconclusive. Some workers obtained evidence that the PHF might originate from neurofilaments [the normal intermediate-sized (100 Å) protein filaments found in all neurons] while others found a possible relationship to microtubules or microtubule-associated proteins, and still others found no consistent relationship to any normal fibrous protein. It is now known that the principal reason for this confusion derives from the fact that PHF are highly unusual fibrous polymers, unlike any intraneuronal fibrous proteins previously studied. Many, if not all, of the PHF that accumulate in Alzheimer neurons have been discovered to be highly insoluble in the conventional solvents used to break down proteins for biochemical analysis (Fig. 5). As a result, previous biochemical and immunocytochemical studies of PHF faced major, but at the time unrecognized, technical obstacles that could lead to artifactual or uninterpretable results. In the author's laboratory, it has been found that Alzheimer PHF do not readily break down in sodium dodecyl sulfate (SDS) and other reagents used to prepare and separate proteins by gel electrophoresis. Therefore, the PHF re-

main excluded from electrophoretic gels and cannot be analyzed. Furthermore, treatment with a variety of harsh solvents or with strong proteolytic enzymes has so far failed to depolymerize or solubilize these pathological fibers.

These recent and unexpected findings lead to several conclusions. First, PHF are difficult to analyze by conventional biochemical strategies. Second, their insolubility can be used to advantage to partially purify them by the use of harsh solvents. Third, and most important, their apparent high degree of chemical inertness is suggestive of a protein polymer containing strong noncovalent and/or covalent bonds, perhaps analogous, in this regard, to cross-linked structural proteins such as collagen and elastin. Proteins with such properties have usually been found in extracellular fibers such as the keratin found in hair and wool, the fibrin of clotted blood, and the collagen and elastin of connective tissues. The finding that fibers with similar chemical characteristics are present inside human neurons could explain, at least in part, the progressive and irreversible nature of Alzheimer-type neuronal degeneration and the adverse effects that the accumulation of these polymers could have on dynamic processes in the cell, such as axonal transport. Furthermore, we can begin to hypothesize and then search for molecular analogies of this cytoskeletal rigidification in aging human neurons to other age-linked cellular processes in which chemical cross-linking of proteins occurs (e.g., senile cataract formation in the lens and aging of keratinocytes in the epidermis).

Since straightforward biochemical analysis of the origin of PHF will not be possible until they can be completely purified and solubilized, identification of their constituents while still in polymeric form using highly specific antibodies represents an alternate and feasible approach Employing this approach, we prepared highly enriched PHF fractions from Alzheimer brain and used them to immunize rabbits. The resulting antisera displayed strong affinity and specificity for PHF-containing tangles and neurites in Alzheimer brain. Unexpectedly, these anti-PHF antibodies failed to react with normal brain cells or with any normal proteins from human or animal brains tested to date, including the normal neurofilaments and microtubules of brain. This

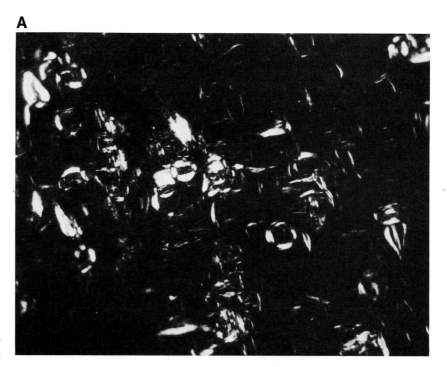

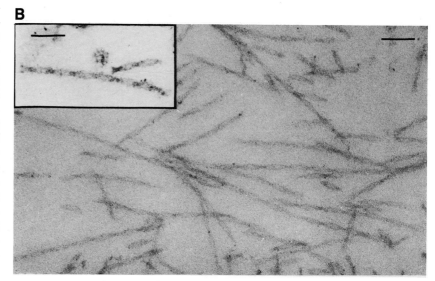

FIGURE 5

Insolubility of neurofibrillary tangles and their paired helical filaments in denaturing solvents. (A) Light micrograph of neurofibrillary tangle-enriched fraction from Alzheimer frontal cortex following prolonged incubation and heating in 2% sodium dodecyl sulfate and 5% β-mercaptoethanol (a reducing agent). Many birefringent tangles of varying size and configuration are seen under polarized light after Congo red staining. (B) Electron micrograph showing intact paired helical filaments following partial purification in the presence of these denaturants. Inset: higher magnification. (Bar = 100 nm.)

high degree of antigenic specificity and failure of cross reaction of PHF with other proteins provides further evidence of their unique molecular nature. The most reasonable explanation for the observations made to date is that the reorganization of the neuronal cytoskeleton in Alzheimer's disease involves a complex series of extensive molecular modifications of normal fibers (most likely neurofilaments) into an insoluble,

end-stage product (the PHF), the progressive accumulation of which might alter irreversibly the metabolism of the neuron and the maintenance of axons and dendrites.

Numerous ongoing studies of the cytoskeletal pathology of Alzheimer neurons suggest that the biochemical pathogenesis may turn out to be extremely complex, involving intermediate or variant fibrous polymers in addition to classical

PHF. Besides contributing to an understanding of neuronal degeneration during aging, such work holds promise for defining metabolic steps in the process of PHF formation which might be blocked pharmacologically, presenting the opportunity for a direct preventive therapy in the early stages of the disease. The primary etiologies (genetic, toxic, infectious) which could serve to trigger such a pathological process in human neurons that have presumably been functioning normally for several decades will be explored in the next sections.

Genetic factors in Alzheimer's disease

An emerging realization among investigators and clinicians interested in Alzheimer's disease is that the importance of genetic factors in the causation of the disease has probably been underestimated. Traditionally, Alzheimer's disease has been considered to be largely a sporadic disorder, in contrast to several other primary neuronal degenerations, such as Huntington's disease and Friedreich's ataxia, which have known patterns of mendelian inheritance. It remains true that the majority of cases of Alzheimer's disease currently seen appear to occur without an identifiable mode of inheritance. However, approximately 10 to 15 percent of patients have a family history indicative of an autosomal dominant trait; this subgroup is correctly referred to as familial Alzheimer's disease. Such cases frequently demonstrate a relatively early age of onset (45 to 65 years) and a more rapid progression and earlier death than do apparently sporadic, "senile" (>65 years) cases. The histopathology of the brain at the light- and electron-microscopic levels in most such autosomal dominant cases is indistinguishable from sporadic presenile and senile dementia of the Alzheimer type, except that the number and density of lesions throughout the cerebral cortex appears to be very high.

Beyond these definitely familial cases, many newly presenting patients with Alzheimer-type dementia have a history of one or more first-degree relatives who had a similar dementing illness in late life. Some authorities believe that the latter patients may represent as many as one-third to one-half of the 85 to 90 percent of Alzheimer cases which are referred to as "sporadic." In these families, a specific pattern of inheritance is not apparent. Moreover, the affected relative(s) of the propositus may have been diagnosed years ago as having "senility," "dementia," or "organic brain syndrome" without pathological confirmation. In other cases, dementia may have been considered as a normal age-related development and not recorded at all. It remains to be seen whether the current movement towards improved clinical and pathological diagnosis and careful record keeping will lead to appreciation of a greater familial incidence of this disorder in the future. Presently, several investigators are attempting to define specific clinical symptoms or signs in an index case (e.g., the early appearance of certain dysphasic disorders) that may correlate with a genetic predisposition for the development of Alzheimer's disease in relatives.

The high incidence of premature, Alzheimer-type neurofibrillary degeneration in middle-aged Down's syndrome patients presents an intriguing clue to a genetic factor. The neuronal lesions in most such cases are morphologically identical to those of sporadic Alzheimer's disease. We have found that PHF from Down's syndrome brains are immunologically reactive with antibodies raised against PHF from sporadic senile Alzheimer's disease; these antibodies also react with PHF from familial (autosomal dominant) Alzheimer's disease. Furthermore, PHF isolated from Down's syndrome cortex display the same unusual chemical properties (e.g., marked insolubility) as those of familial and sporadic Alzheimer's disease. Clinically, there has been some disagreement in the neurological literature as to whether patients with trisomy 21 surviving into their fourth and fifth decades and developing Alzheimer changes in their brains can be shown to have a progressive dementing syndrome in addition to mental retardation. Several workers report that careful psychometric evaluation will reveal the presence of a superimposed dementia.

Although the findings in Down's syndrome raise the possibility of a direct link between Alzheimer-type neuronal degeneration and an abnormal complement of genetic material from chromosome 21, less direct explanations seem more plausible. The fact that neurofibrillary degeneration can occur in a number of disorders and in normal aging suggests that there may be multiple etiologic factors that can lead to a final common neuropathological expression. In the case of Down's syndrome, various kinds of primary metabolic dysfunctions of cells (including neurons) related to the presence of an extra twenty-first chromosome could, over the lifetime of an individual, lead to a secondary or tertiary triggering of premature, age-related neurofibrillary degeneration. A search for cytoskeletal reorganization of intermediate filaments in nonneuronal cells (e.g., keratinocytes, fibroblasts) of young and aged Down's syndrome patients would be of considerable interest.

Molecular genetic analyses of large kindreds with autosomal dominant Alzheimer's disease are currently being planned. Such studies have as their immediate goal the identification of a genetic marker displaying linkage with the Alzheimer trait, providing an indication of the chromosomal locus of the abnormal gene. Successful investigations using this approach have recently been reported in Huntington's disease. They represent an important and methodologically feasible, although difficult strategy for identifying the molecular abnormalities underlying genetically determined Alzheimer's disease and should also have direct relevance to understanding the molecular pathogenesis of sporadic Alzheimer's disease.

Neurotoxins

At present, there is no compelling evidence that an exogenous nutritional or toxic factor plays an important role in the pathogenesis of Alzheimer's disease. However, few epidemiologic studies of Alzheimer's disease in various environmental settings around the world have been completed, and direct neurotoxicological studies of tissues from Alzheimer patients have likewise been limited. The greatest interest in this area of investigation has focused on the finding of excess aluminum levels in the brain tissue of patients with neurofibrillary diseases.

Interest in aluminum in Alzheimer's disease developed via a somewhat serendipitous route. In the 1930s, investigators who were attempting to induce epileptogenic lesions in experimental animals discovered that aluminum salts, in particular aluminum phosphate (Holt's adjuvant),

would produce such foci if injected into the cerebral cortex of cats or rabbits. Some 30 years later, Klatzo, Wisniewski, and colleagues observed that such experimental lesions contained many neuronal cell bodies bearing neurofibrillary tangles which, by light microscopy, resembled those seen in Alzheimer's disease. However, electron microscopy demonstrated that the tangles consisted of masses of straight 100-Å filaments rather than paired helical filaments. Subsequent biochemical and immunocytochemical studies confirmed that the aluminum-induced filaments were similar to normal neurofilaments. Aluminum-induced neurofibrillary degeneration, although of interest in its own right, does not provide a close neuropathological model of Alzheimer's disease; indeed, such a model does not presently exist.

In the early 1970s, Crapper-McLachlan and colleagues decided to assay aluminum levels in Alzheimer cerebral cortex and age-matched normal cortex. They found three- to fourfold elevations in Alzheimer patients and in cases of Down's syndrome with Alzheimer-type degeneration. These workers also observed an association between the density of neurofibrillary tangles in a cortical sample and the level of tissue aluminum. Recently, Perl and coworkers have employed a combined morphological-microanalytical technique which uses scanning electron microscopy and x-ray spectrometry to detect intracellular levels of metallic ions. They found elevations of intraneuronal aluminum in neurons containing neurofibrillary tangles (both in Alzheimer's disease and in aged controls) but not in immediately adjacent neurons without the cytoskeletal pathology (Fig. 6). These studies have been extended to patients from the endemic focus of Alzheimer-type pathology on Guam (so-called Guamanian parkinsonism-dementia complex). Tangle-bearing neurons in these cases also displayed peaks for excess aluminum; in addition, the same neurons had elevated calcium concentrations. The question of whether patients with sporadic Alzheimer's disease in the United States also have increased calcium in their tangle-bearing neurons is currently under investigation.

The most conservative interpretation of the available data is that already damaged neuronal cell bodies in Alzheimer's disease take up and

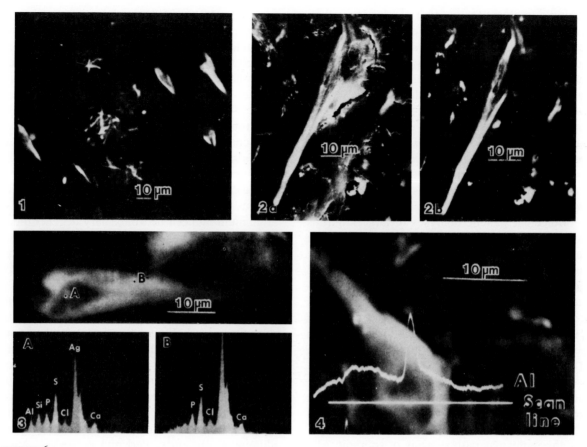

FIGURE 6

(1) Scanning electron micrograph-secondary electron surface imaging of modified Bielschowski silver-stained section of Alzheimer hippocampus, showing several neurofibrillary tangles (NFT) and a senile plaque. (2) Scanning electron micrograph-secondary electron surface image (a) and backscattered electron image (b) of neuron containing a NFT. (3) Scanning electron micrograph-backscattered electron image of a silver-stained neuron containing a NFT. Points A and B indicate the areas subjected to elemental analysis. Partial x-ray energy spectra are shown below corresponding to these two points. Note the prominent peaks for aluminum and silicon present in point A but not detected in point B. The counting time was 100 s. (4) Scanning electron micrograph-backscattered electron image of a silver-stained neuron with a NFT. A line scan is passed through the nuclear region. The superimposed tracing demonstrates the distribution of energy detected along the line scan at the x-ray wavelength characteristic for aluminum. Note the focal intranuclear concentration of aluminum. (From Perl and Brady: Science 208:297–299, 1980.)

sequester certain cations, including aluminum and calcium. Excess levels of these ions, particularly calcium with its numerous critical effects on neuronal metabolism, would then contribute to progressive cell injury and death. Markesbery and colleagues have found no elevation of brain aluminum levels in their cases of Alzheimer's disease in Kentucky. It may be that the presence or absence of excess aluminum in Alzheimer's disease relates to the degree of exposure to aluminum in the patient's environment, particularly in the local tap water. There is no evidence at present that neuronal degeneration in Alzheimer's disease is primarily initiated by neurotoxic concentrations of aluminum. Aluminum is the third most common element in the earth's crust and is ubiquitous in the environment, so that unusual sources of exposure to the element need not be postulated. Presumably, any patient who accumulates aluminum in brain cells, including patients with Alzheimer's disease and patients with the syndrome of chronic renal failure and progressive dialysis encephalopathy, must have a preexisting cellular defect that allows the accumulation of excess amounts of this ion. Thereafter, the aluminum may well cause additional neuronal injury, since it is clear that aluminum is toxic to mammalian neurons. To complicate matters further, the cerebral cortexes of patients dying with dialysis encephalopathy, which contain aluminum concentrations even higher than those found in Alzheimer cortex, do not show neurofibrillary tangles.

In summary, the fact that at least some patients with Alzheimer's disease accumulate excess levels of aluminum in tangle-bearing neurons seems clear. However, the role of aluminum, calcium, and other neurotoxic chemicals in the pathogenesis of the disease is entirely unknown.

Virologic studies

The possibility of viral etiologies for various neuronal abiotrophies of late life has become increasingly attractive in the years since the discovery by Gajdusek and coworkers that Creutzfeldt-Jakob disease and kuru are caused by a transmissible agent. Neither the identity of this agent nor the natural mode of transmission has been established. Of potential importance is the observation that Creutzfeldt-Jakob disease developed in a patient who received a corneal transplant 18 months previously from a donor who had died of the disease. This finding and extensive experience with the laboratory transmission of Creutzfeldt-Jakob disease and kuru in experimental animals suggest that parenteral inoculation and prolonged exposure to the causative agent are necessary to induce symptomatic disease. It is also of interest that approximately 15 percent of all cases of Creutzfeldt-Jakob disease have a positive family history consistent with an autosomal dominant mode of transmission. The onset of the disease in such familial cases is significantly earlier than in sporadic cases. The mechanisms of spread of the agent within affected families is unknown, but it has been hypothesized that there is a genetically determined susceptibility to infection, which is then acquired in infancy or early childhood. In addition to Creutzfeldt-Jakob disease and kuru,

another rare human dementing illness has recently been shown to be caused by an unconventional transmissible agent; this disorder is referred to as the Gerstmann-Straussler syndrome.

In the case of Alzheimer's disease, there is at present no convincing evidence implicating a viral etiology. Viruslike particles have not been found in brain affected with Alzheimer's disease, although such negative results appear to be characteristic for slow infections of humans caused by unconventional viruses (e.g., Creutzfeldt-Jakob disease). The clinical syndrome and neuropathology of Alzheimer's disease are generally distinguishable from the known viral encephalopathies of humans. However, neurofibrillary tangles that are ultrastructurally identical to those in Alzheimer's disease have been found in rare, long-surviving cases of subacute sclerosing panencephalitis (a postmeasles encephalopathy) and are a prominent feature of the syndrome of postencephalitic parkinsonism which arose after the pandemic of influenza in 1919–1927.

In two cases of familial Alzheimer's disease, brain injected into New World monkeys produced, after a 2-year latent period, a clinical and pathologic syndrome typical of the primate spongiform encephalopathy that occurs after inoculation of Creutzfeldt-Jakob tissue. However, no histologic features of Alzheimer's disease were produced. Brain tissue from many other familial and sporadic cases of Alzheimer's disease has been inoculated into a variety of primates, and to date no animal has developed any neurological disease, despite latent intervals of up to 12 years in some instances. Although these and numerous other studies provide no support for a causative virus in Alzheimer's disease, negative transmission studies are not sufficient to exclude the possibility of an unconventional viruslike particle in a brain degenerative disease.

A laboratory model of potential relevance to the question of a viral basis for certain histopathological changes of the Alzheimer type is the scrapie-infected mouse. Certain susceptible strains of inbred female mice have been shown by Wisniewski and colleagues to develop neuritic plaques in gray matter almost 2 years after brain inoculation with certain strains of the agent causing scrapie, a naturally occurring slow-virus infection of sheep. Electron microscopy of these induced lesions has shown them to be highly similar to classical senile plaques of humans, although their abnormal neurites do not contain the paired helical filaments seen in Alzheimer's disease. This model has been used in experimental studies of the pathogenesis of amyloid deposition in the brain.

Finally, mention should be made of current attempts to detect autoimmune phenomena in Alzheimer's disease. Although circulating immune globulins that react selectively with brain cells in vitro have been observed in the sera of aged humans and lower mammals, their cytotoxicity, mechanism of access to the brain, and role in neuronal degeneration have not been established. The search for specific antibodies that could either initiate or participate secondarily in Alzheimer-type brain degeneration is an important area for further study.

MANAGEMENT AND PROSPECTIVE THERAPY

The application of new techniques in neurobiology and biochemical pathology has provided some intriguing clues to the pathogenesis of Alzheimer's disease. Yet, an understanding of the etiology and molecular basis of this disorder is not at hand. That this should be so is not surprising, since clinical and laboratory investigations of the late-life dementias are in their infancy compared to the cumulative research efforts that have been directed at still-unresolved neurological diseases such as multiple sclerosis.

Fortunately, the lack of an etiologic understanding does not preclude advances in the therapy of the disorder. New knowledge about changes in cholinergic neurons and their synaptic projections provides the theoretical basis for current intensive efforts to design an effective cholinergic replacement therapy. Numerous trials have shown that administration of large doses of the choline precursor, lecithin (phosphatidylcholine), does not significantly improve intellectual function or behavior in Alzheimer patients. Recently, however, two groups have reported preliminary results of the combined administration of lecithin and physostigmine, an acetylcholinesterase inhibitor that crosses the blood-brain barrier and presumably decreases the hydrolysis of acetylcholine in the synaptic cleft. In double-blind crossover trials, both Davis and coworkers

and Thal and colleagues have observed reproducible and statistically significant improvement in certain memory functions in a majority of the Alzheimer patients they treated. In the study of Thal et al., the improvement in one psychometric test was strongly correlated with the degree of inhibition of cholinesterase activity in cerebrospinal fluid, suggesting a direct relationship of enhanced memory function to an effect of physostigmine on brain cholinergic neurons. Several other groups have also reported preliminary evidence of transient improvement in selected aspects of memory after administration of physostigmine and lecithin to small numbers of Alzheimer patients.

Several points are worthy of comment. In these recent trials the optimal dose of physostigmine was carefully selected for each patient in a preliminary open study prior to the blinded trial, since doses above or below this optimal level may impair memory, even in normal subjects. In some of the studies reporting beneficial results, the physostigmine was given intravenously; although oral administration appeared to be effective in other trials, it is not yet clear which route is optimal in most Alzheimer patients. Further complicating the usefulness of physostigmine in routine therapy is the fact that its short half-life requires very frequent administration (every 2 h). Although the importance of lecithin in the clinical response to physostigmine therapy is unknown, theoretical reasons for administering both agents concurrently have been proposed.

The initial success of studies using cholinesterase inhibition plus choline precursors is encouraging and supports the notion of a prominent role for altered cholinergic function in the memory disorder of Alzheimer's disease. However, these results do not yet translate into a practical therapeutic regimen which can provide effective treatment for a large number of Alzheimer patients. The effects noted in the physostigmine trials were temporary; continued treatment of some of the subjects for several months did not prevent a further decline in their overall intellectual function. Replacement therapy would not be expected to alter the progressive attrition of cholinergic neurons in Alzheimer's disease, just as levodopa therapy does not prevent late-stage Parkinson's disease. Indeed, as cell loss continues, physostigmine and lecithin will become less effective, since they require the presence of functional presynaptic terminals which can synthesize and release acetylcholine. Furthermore, Bowen and Davison have shown that the activity of the high-affinity choline-uptake system is markedly reduced in biopsied cortex from some Alzheimer cases. Therefore, precursor and anticholinesterase treatment may only be useful in early stages of the disease. Administration of cholinergic agonists (e.g., arecoline), which directly stimulate the cholinoceptive neuron, would theoretically provide a more effective long-term therapy. The search for new muscarinic cholinergic agonists that can cross the blood-brain barrier is under way.

Attrition of neurons releasing neurotransmitters other than acetylcholine may preclude the development of a clinically useful cholinergic treatment in Alzheimer's disease. On the basis of evidence gathered to date, Alzheimer's disease appears to be characterized by a more complex pattern of neuropharmacological deficits than is idiopathic Parkinson's disease. It may be exceedingly difficult to design practical multitransmitter therapeutic regimens that avoid significant adverse interactions and side effects.

Nonspecific pharmacologic treatment

For many years, vasodilating agents such as papaverine hydrochloride and ergot alkaloid derivatives were widely used in elderly patients with dementia. The proposed rationale for administering these drugs was that a diffuse, atherosclerotic narrowing of cerebral arteries was responsible for most cases of senile dementia. The realization that the majority of patients display primary neuronal degeneration and that even those with a vascular etiology have a series of discrete, focal infarcts in brain has eliminated the theoretical basis for chronic vasodilator therapy. More importantly, several controlled trials of such agents in idiopathic senile dementia have failed to demonstrate their benefit. There is currently no theoretical or practical justification for advocating their use in Alzheimer's disease.

A useful axiom in the management of elderly patients, particularly the cognitively impaired, is to exercise great care in prescribing any drugs that stimulate or depress central nervous system

function and, in all cases, to begin with the lowest possible doses and advance slowly. Many patients with Alzheimer's disease display agitated, compulsive, or aggressive behavior during certain stages of their disease. Low doses of anxiety-reducing medication may be necessary to afford relief to the patient and those caring for him or her. Haloperidol or thioridazine in low doses may be useful in such situations. Monitoring for adverse behavioral effects and frequent reevaluation of the need for continued treatment are important.

The issues of distinguishing primary depression from degenerative dementia and of treating the mild to moderate depression which sometimes accompanies Alzheimer's disease are complex. Consultation with a geriatric psychiatrist and appropriate use of psychometric assessment are often necessary in such cases. Although cautious treatment with antidepressant medication can be useful in these settings, tricyclic antidepressants, through their anticholinergic action, may worsen intellectual function in Alzheimer patients. Newer antidepressants chemically unrelated to tricyclic and tetracyclic agents, such as trazodone hydrochloride, have less anticholinergic activity and may eventually prove to be more useful for treatment of depression in patients with Alzheimer's disease.

Caring for the patient with Alzheimer's disease

In a progressive degenerative disease which lacks any definitive or even palliative treatment, the optimal day-to-day management of the patient becomes a subject of utmost importance. Physicians, nurses, and especially the relatives of the patient experience intense frustration in trying to deal with the myriad psychosocial problems encountered during the course of Alzheimer's disease. This anxiety is often heightened by the lack of readily available written information or professional consultation regarding the management of the elderly demented patient. Fortunately, the situation is now changing. A major factor bringing about an improved understanding of how to care for the Alzheimer patient has been the effort of affected families to organize into self-help or support groups, often with the assistance of concerned professionals. These groups encourage the beleaguered family member to share directly her or his anger, experiences, and suggestions for care with others similarly afflicted. It is often appropriate to refer the family of a newly diagnosed patient with Alzheimer's disease to a local support group. This task has become much easier since the coalescence in 1979 of various local Alzheimer support groups into a national organization, the Alzheimer's Disease and Related Disorders Association (ADRDA), with headquarters at 360 North Michigan Avenue, Chicago. Chapters of ADRDA are now found in many states and can provide the names and locations of local support groups.

A full discussion of current ideas regarding the day-to-day care of the patient with Alzheimer's disease is clearly beyond the scope of this chapter. The reader is referred to monographs dealing with this aspect of the disease; one currently popular example is The 36 Hour Day by Mace and Rabins. However, a few basic guidelines are worthy of mention. Any changes in the patient's daily routine should occur gradually and preferably one at a time. Patients with cognitive impairment often show an abrupt worsening of behavior with changes in their immediate environment (e.g., the arrival of a new member of the household or a move from one residence to another). It is well to maintain as much routine as possible in the patient's daily activities and to introduce necessary changes gradually and with psychological support. A sudden worsening of the patient's mental status in the absence of any obvious environmental stress signifies the onset of a new medical complication (e.g., infection, metabolic abnormality, or drug toxicity).

In moderate and advanced stages of the disease, the disintegration of the patient's personality requires that he or she receive almost constant supervision. Activities that could be harmful to the patient and those nearby (e.g., cooking, working with hand tools) must be restricted or closely supervised. If left alone even briefly, the patient may inadvertently wander outside of the house and become lost for hours or even days. The burden of setting limits for the Alzheimer patient and yet trying to maintain a semblance of normal activity becomes monumental. Early referral of the family to community agencies that can provide home health aides or homemaking assistance is critical; the patient's relatives must be allowed some time away from the home on a regular basis. In many cities and towns, day-care centers have been established to provide a structured outlet for the patient's energies and to encourage continued socialization, while allowing a respite for care givers. The decision as to whether and when nursing home placement is appropriate is perhaps the most difficult issue facing Alzheimer families. Consultation with social workers and other professionals who are experienced in managing the disease should begin as early as possible. This enables the family to receive ongoing support as they come to grips with this painful decision and also allows the often lengthy process of finding an appropriate facility to proceed on a nonemergency basis. It is also frequently advisable to suggest that the family seek early consultation with an attorney regarding the legal aspects of establishing custody of the patient and managing her or his financial affairs.

CONCLUSION

Major demographic changes that have occurred in recent decades, both in the United States and abroad, have led to a dramatic acceleration of interest in the biomedical and social problems of human aging. Among the most affected by these emerging problems are physicians and other health professionals concerned with the care of patients with age-related neuronal degenerative diseases. A major obstacle to progress in discerning the basis of dementia of the Alzheimer type has been the previous failure to separate this entity from the cerebrovascular disorders that often accompany senescence. Clinical research and advances in diagnostic imaging have helped to resolve this difficulty and have also sharpened the distinction between brain aging as a normal biological process and the selective and malignant neuronal degenerations that affect a minority of the elderly population. The principal challenge in the study of Alzheimer's disease now rests in the proliferation of seemingly unrelated clues regarding its pathobiology. This fact precludes the development of a unitary hypothesis for the etiology of Alzheimer's disease at present and requires the simultaneous direction of resources at various lines of evidence. It is hoped that the increasing attention that age-related human neuronal degeneration is receiving from both clinical and basic science perspectives will soon provide a clearer understanding of this common and devastating disease.

References

ALZHEIMER: Über eine eigen artige Erkrankung der Hirnrinde. Allg Zeit Psychiatrie und Psychisch-Grichtlich Medicin 64:146, 1907

BESDINE RW et al: Senility reconsidered: Treatment possibilities for mental impairment in the elderly. (NIA Task Force) JAMA 244:259, 1980

BESSEN JAQ et al: Differentiating senile dementia of Alzheimer's type and multi-infarct dementia by proton NMR imaging. Lancet 1983:789, 1983

BLASS JP, WEKSLER ME: Toward an effective treatment of Alzheimer's disease. Ann Intern Med 98:251, 1983

BLESSED G et al: The association between quantitative measures of dementia and of senile change in the cerebral gray matter of elderly patients. Br J Psychiatry 114:797, 1968

BOWEN DM: Biochemical assessment of neurotransmitter and metabolic dysfunction and cerebral atrophy in Alzheimer's disease, in *Biological Aspects of Alzheimer's Disease*. R. Katzman, (ed). Cold Spring Harbor Laboratory, Banbury Report 15, pp 219–231, 1983

CRAPPER DR et al: Brain aluminum distribution in Alzheimer's disease and experimental neurofibrillary degeneration. Science 180:511, 1973

DAVIES P et al: Reduced somatostatin-like immunoreactivity in cerebral cortex from cases of Alzheimer disease and Alzheimer senile dementia. Nature 288:279, 1980

DAVIS KL, MONS RC: Enhancement of memory processes in Alzheimer's disease with multiple-dose intravenous physostigmine. Am J Psychiatry 139:1421, 1982

DUFFY FH et al: Brain electrical activity in patients with presenile and senile dementia of the Alzheimer's type. Ann Neurol (in press)

GAJDUSEK DC: Unconventional viruses and the origin and disappearances of Kuru. Science 197:943, 1977

GOUDSMIT J et al: Evidence for and against the transmissibility of Alzheimer disease. Neurology 30:945, 1980

IHARA Y et al: Antibodies to paired helical filaments in Alzheimer's disease do not recognize normal brain proteins. Nature 304:727, 1983

KATZMAN R (ed): *Biological Aspects of Alzheimer's Disease*. Cold Spring Harbor, NY, Cold Spring Harbor Laboratory, 1983, Banbury Report 15

—— et al: *Aging*, vol 7: *Alzheimer's Disease: Senile Dementia and Related Disorders*. New York, Raven Press, 1978

KRAL VA: Senescent forgetfulness: Benign and malignant. Can Med Assoc J 86:257, 1962

MANN DM et al: The noradrenergic system in Alzheimer and multi-infarct dementias. J Neurol Neurosurg Psychiatry 45:113, 1982

MARKESBERY WR et al: Instrumental neutron activation analysis of brain aluminum in Alzheimer disease and aging. Ann Neurol 10:511, 1981

MASTERS CL et al: The familial occurrence of Creutzfeldt-Jakob disease and Alzheimer's disease. Brain 104:535, 1981

—— et al: Creutzfeldt-Jakob disease virus isolation from the Gerstmann-Straussler syndrome, with an analysis of the various forms of amyloid plaque deposition in the virus-induced spongiform encephalopathies. Brain 104:559–587, 1981

NAKANO I, HIRANO A: Loss of large neurons of the medical septal nucleus in an autopsy case of Alzheimer's disease. J Neuropath Exp Neurol 41:341, 1982

PERL DP, BRODY AR: Alzheimer's disease: X-ray spectrometric evidence of aluminum accumulation in neurofibrillary tangle-bearing neurons. Science 208:297, 1980

—— et al: Intraneuronal aluminum accumulation in amyotrophic lateral sclerosis and parkinsonism-dementia of Guam. Science 217:1053, 1982

PERRY EL et al: Correlation of cholinergic abnormalities with senile plaques and mental test scores in senile dementia. Br Med J 2:1457, 1978

SELKOE DJ et al: Alzheimer's disease: Insolubility of partially purified paired helical filaments in sodium dodecyl sulfate and urea. Science 215:1243, 1982

SELTZER B, SHERWIN I: A comparison of clinical features in early- and late-onset primary degenerative dementia. Arch Neurol 40:143, 1983

SULKAVA R et al: Accuracy of clinical diagnosis in primary degenerative dementia: Correlation with neuropharmacological findings. J Neurol Neurosurg Psychiatry 46:9, 1983

TERRY RD, DAVIES P: Dementia of the Alzheimer type. Ann J Rev Neurosci 3:77, 1980

THAL LJ et al: Oral physostigmine and lecithin improve memory in Alzheimer's disease. Ann Neurol 13:491, 1983

WHITEHOUSE PJ et al: Alzheimer's disease and senile dementia: Loss of neurons in the basal forebrain. Science 215:1237, 1982

WISNIEWSKI HM et al: Infectious etiology of neuritic (senile) plaques in mice. Science 190:1108, 1975

NINE CONTROVERSIES IN THE MANAGEMENT OF ENDOCARDITIS

DAVID T. DURACK

In the four decades since the advent of antibiotics, the management of endocarditis has been a field notable for steady accumulation of new information, shifting opinion, and active controversy. This essay will address nine specific topics, all of which are subject to current debate:

1 Is 2 weeks long enough to cure uncomplicated viridans streptococcal endocarditis?

2 Is antibiotic tolerance among viridans streptococci a significant factor in therapy and prophylaxis?

3 Should an aminoglycoside be added to a penicillin for treatment of *Staphylococcus aureus* endocarditis?

4 For prevention of endocarditis, should antibiotics be given parenterally or orally?

5 Is prophylaxis for bacterial endocarditis indicated in patients with mitral valve prolapse?

6 Can anticoagulants be administered during active endocardial infection?

7 Can cardiac catheterization be performed safely during active endocarditis?

8 Should valve replacement be undertaken during active endocardial infection?

9 Should an infected valve be replaced to prevent emboli?

1. IS 2 WEEKS LONG ENOUGH TO CURE UNCOMPLICATED VIRIDANS STREPTOCOCCAL ENDOCARDITIS?

Background

This is probably one of the longest-running debates in the management of endocarditis and,

indeed, in the whole field of antimicrobial chemotherapy. The question extends back to the very beginning of the penicillin era. A few early failures of low-dose, short-term penicillin therapy for endocarditis during World War II were reported by Florey's team in Oxford and by Keefer's committee, which studied the response to penicillin of 500 patients with various infections. The first paper providing good evidence that endocarditis could be cured with penicillin was published early in 1944. During the next 6 years, many patients were cured with low doses of penicillin (100,000 to 300,000 units per day) given for various periods ranging from 10 days to several months. The cure rate for series of patients treated during this period (before valve replacement or renal dialysis became available) ranged from about 66 to 75 percent. This experience established that streptococcal endocarditis often could be cured by low-dose penicillin given for only 10 to 14 days, but the relapse rate after such regimens was significant (about 5 to 20 percent). To overcome this problem, various medical centers took differing approaches: many raised the dose of penicillin (to as much as 2 million units per day); some relied upon increasing the duration of therapy to 4 to 6 weeks; others added streptomycin to take advantage of its synergistic action with penicillin against viridans streptococci; still others used a combined approach, administering penicillin plus streptomycin for the first 2 weeks, followed by treatment with penicillin alone for a further 2 weeks. During the same period, it became evident that 6 weeks' treatment with high-dose penicillin (20 million units per day) plus streptomycin was required for treatment of *Streptococcus faecalis* (enterococcal) endocarditis. These various events eventually gave rise to the common practice of treating subacute endocarditis with 20 million units of penicillin a day for 6 weeks. Actually, it is a misconception to extrapolate the treatment needed to cure enterococcal endocarditis to uncomplicated viridans streptococcal endocarditis. Unfortunately, even today confusion on this point has not been entirely eradicated; in many community hospitals, uncomplicated viridans streptococcal endocarditis is still treated for 6 weeks.

Most current discussion centers on the relative merits of three leading regimens for uncomplicated viridans endocarditis:

1 Penicillin alone for 4 weeks (P_4)

2 Penicillin plus streptomycin for 2 weeks (P_2S_2)

3 Penicillin for 4 weeks, plus streptomycin for the first 2 weeks (P_4S_2)

A committee of the American Heart Association has recently reviewed this question and concluded that all three of these regimens are entirely acceptable from the point of view of cure rates and patient safety. The choice among them depends upon individual circumstances and opinion.

Arguments for

While penicillin alone for 2 weeks is not sufficiently reliable, there is good evidence that P_2S_2 therapy is adequate to cure uncomplicated viridans streptococcal endocarditis, while assuring extremely low relapse rates. This regimen has been used for about 30 years at the Mayo Clinic; good records are available on more than 170 selected patients treated with this regimen. In this large, well-documented series there has been only one relapse, and that one is questionable. Patients excluded from this group included those with major complications such as shock, intracranial infection, or mycotic aneurysm; those infected with nutritionally variant streptococci; and patients with prosthetic valves. Within this carefully selected group, the results of P_2S_2 therapy have been so good that it would be impossible to show statistically that any other regimen was better. Several other medical centers have

achieved equally good results, although with smaller numbers of patients.

The greatest advantage of 2-week regimens today is the enormous savings in the cost of hospitalization compared with 4-week regimens. Patients with uncomplicated streptococcal endocarditis often become afebrile and feel well within a few days after penicillin therapy is instituted; naturally, these people find unnecessary hospitalization financially and emotionally onerous. Additional advantages of shorter therapy include reduced risk of nosocomial infections and other undesirable side effects of hospitalization. Another advantage of the combined, streptomycin-containing regimen is that relatively penicillin-resistant strains can usually be treated without alteration of the basic treatment program.

Arguments against

Viridans streptococcal endocarditis can be cured reliably without using two drugs; the cure rate after P_4 therapy is excellent. In other words, it is impossible to show any statistically significant difference in outcome between this regimen and the P_2S_2 regimen. The P_4 regimen avoids the risk of vestibular side effects from streptomycin, while the risk of a penicillin reaction in the final 2 weeks of a 4-week regimen is low. Proponents of the P_4 regimen argue that it is simple and safe, and that the extra time and expense of 2 weeks more in hospital are a small consideration in the face of such a serious disease as bacterial endocarditis.

Author's opinion

The author believes that there is ample evidence to convince even prudent and conservative physicians that 2 weeks of treatment with penicillin plus streptomycin is adequate for treatment of streptococcal endocarditis, *always provided* that the following conditions are met:

1 The organism is properly identified as one of the common viridans streptococci, not a related species or a nutritional variant. Moreover, although rare, group A β-streptococcal endocarditis is an acute and more dangerous disease which should not be treated with the 2-week regimen.

2 The organism is fully sensitive to penicillin [minimal inhibitory concentration (MIC) ≤ 0.2 mg/ml] and not tolerant [ratio of MIC to minimal bactericidal concentration (MBC) ≤ 1:16].

3 The patient has no major complications such as serious heart failure (which requires valve replacement), intracerebral infection, mycotic aneurysm, valve ring abscess, or recurrent embolization.

Old age (> 65 years) and renal impairment are relative contraindications to the use of strepto-mycin. Therefore, in elderly patients with cre-atinine clearance less than 50 ml/minute, the physician may choose to use penicillin alone. However, streptomycin has little toxicity at the standard dosage of 0.5 g intramuscularly twice daily, and in practice the P_2S_2 regimen can often be used in older patients without danger or dif-ficulty.

If these criteria are applied, approximately two-thirds of patients with streptococcal endo-carditis should qualify for treatment with the P_2S_2 regimen. If the P_2S_2 regimen were used more widely, the saving of time and money for patients currently receiving 4- or 6-week regi-mens would be considerable.

Because relapse, though very rare, can occur after any appropriate treatment regimen for en-docarditis, all patients should be followed care-fully after treatment is completed. Finally, there is no place for 6 weeks of treatment for uncom-plicated, penicillin-sensitive viridans streptococ-cal endocarditis occurring on a native valve in the modern era.

2. IS ANTIBIOTIC TOLERANCE AMONG VIRIDANS STREPTOCOCCI A SIGNIFICANT FACTOR IN THERAPY AND PROPHYLAXIS?

Background

The term *tolerant* is used to describe certain organisms that are inhibited by penicillin but are not killed by concentrations of the drug that are usually achieved in the bloodstream. To put it in simple terms, penicillin behaves like a bac-teriostatic drug for tolerant strains. Tolerance is quantitated by the MIC/MBC ratio, which varies greatly between strains. This phenomenon was first observed among staphylococci and has now been described with various streptococci, includ-ing enterococci and viridans strains. Approxi-mately 20 percent of strains of viridans strepto-cocci from the mouth or from patients with endocarditis are tolerant to the killing action of penicillin.

Arguments for

In experimental endocarditis, penicillin is much less effective for both prophylaxis and treatment if the infecting strain of viridans streptococcus is highly tolerant to penicillin. Both treatment failures and relapses after penicillin therapy do occur in human cases; these may be due to tol-erant strains. There is some clinical evidence, based upon series of case reports, that tolerant strains of staphylococci are more difficult to treat than nontolerant strains. A number of cases of staphylococcal endocarditis are included among these reports. The same could be true for strep-tococcal endocarditis, but cases to demonstrate this have not been reported during the relatively short period since tolerance was recognized among viridans streptococci.

Arguments against

The clinical significance of tolerance among staphylococci remains somewhat controversial, even after more than 5 years' observation. The clinical significance of streptococcal tolerance in endocarditis remains unsubstantiated. Al-though tolerant strains of streptococci are fairly common (about 20 percent, see above), treat-ment failures and relapses after penicillin treat-ment are rather rare (less than 5 percent of cases). This observation argues against the fact that tolerance is a critical factor in the outcome of penicillin treatment.

Author's opinion

The clinical significance of tolerance is unknown at the time of writing. More investigation will be required before this question can be answered, including further documentation of the incidence of tolerant strains in (1) the normal flora, (2) cases of endocarditis, and (3) cases of prophylaxis failure, treatment failure, or relapse.

It is intriguing to speculate that tolerance could be one of the main reasons why relatively long-term treatment is needed for endocarditis. We know that most cases of pneumococcal pneumonia are cured with penicillin within a few days. Perhaps the same is true for endocarditis that is caused by organisms that are exquisitely sensitive to penicillin; certainly the early experience with penicillin indicated that some patients with subacute bacterial endocarditis (SBE) were cured within 10 days, a fact that is obscured by the current practice of treating for several weeks. Perhaps only the subgroup of tolerant strains requires treatment for 2 to 4 weeks to achieve cure.

Because only a small percentage of an inoculum from the mouth or other sources may be tolerant to penicillin, tolerance is more likely to be clinically significant in *treatment* than in *prophylaxis*. The aim of attempted prophylaxis is to prevent bacteremia and to prevent colonization of the surface of a cardiac valve by a very small inoculum of organisms. In contrast, treatment must succeed against the large inoculum of streptococci concentrated in the vegetation. If a tolerant strain is involved, a few highly tolerant cocci are likely to be present at the start of treatment but none may be present in the setting in which prophylaxis is employed.

Potential problems in therapy due to tolerance could probably be avoided by use of combined penicillin plus streptomycin, which acts synergistically against tolerant as well as nontolerant strains of viridans streptococci.

3. SHOULD AN AMINOGLYCOSIDE BE ADDED TO A PENICILLIN FOR TREATMENT OF *STAPH. AUREUS* ENDOCARDITIS?

Background

Staphylococcal endocarditis is a serious infection with a high incidence of complications. Its clinical manifestations and outcome are highly variable. For example, in elderly patients with preexisting diseases such as diabetes or obstructive airway disease, the mortality rate is high (in excess of 50 percent). On the other hand, for young intravenous drug addicts the prognosis is much better, with a death rate of less than 5 percent.

Staphylococci are classical primary pathogens having the capacity to seed other tissues from the bloodstream and to cause serious infections such as staphylococcal pneumonia, osteomyelitis, and cerebritis. For this reason, staphylococcal endocarditis must be regarded as being disseminated staphylococcal infection. The immediate aim of treatment is to sterilize the bloodstream, reverse dissemination, and reduce the patient's risk of death in the acute stage of disease. Once this has been achieved, the next objective is to cure the endocardial infection before irreversible valvular damage develops.

Arguments for

The patient with staphylococcal endocarditis usually has a severe systemic illness, with high-grade, continuous bacteremia originating from a large population of staphylococci concentrated in the vegetation. Under these circumstances, it is logical to seek a bactericidal regimen whose effect is both as *rapid* and as *complete* as possible. Most staphylococci are sensitive to both semisynthetic penicillins and to gentamicin. Combined exposure of staphylococci to these agents results in synergism in vitro, producing an enhanced rate of bacterial killing. Gentamicin plus a semisynthetic penicillin cures rabbits with experimental staphylococcal endocarditis more rapidly than the penicillin alone, although the improvement due to addition of the aminoglycoside is modest. Synergism can be achieved without using high doses of gentamicin, and renal toxicity due to gentamicin is usually reversible and can be managed with ease in most patients.

Arguments against

The combined regimen is somewhat more toxic than a semisynthetic penicillin alone. The final outcome of treatment is not significantly different for either regimen. The combined regimen is more costly than a single-drug regimen, due not only to the price of the aminoglycoside itself but also to administration charges and the cost of laboratory tests done to check for toxic side effects.

Author's opinion

Combination therapy is not required for most cases of staphylococcal endocarditis, especially in young drug addicts. Nafcillin, or a similar semisynthetic, penicillinase-resistant penicillin alone should suffice. In severely ill patients with overwhelming staphylococcal bacteremia and/or multiple metastatic infections, the author uses gentamicin for the first 3 days in order to realize the potential benefit of synergism in clearing the bloodstream of staphylococci in the shortest possible time. Unless there is persistent bacteremia, fortunately a rare event, the author is able to discontinue the gentamicin after 3 days and to complete treatment with a semisynthetic penicillin alone.

4. FOR PREVENTION OF ENDOCARDITIS, SHOULD ANTIBIOTICS BE GIVEN PARENTERALLY OR ORALLY?

Background

The practice of administering prophylaxis to humans with congenital or acquired heart disease is based on the unproven presumption that it will prevent endocarditis. In the past, most antibiotics given to prevent endocarditis have been administered orally. This is still true today, despite the fact that the American Heart Association and the American Dental Association, in their 1977 recommendations, favored parenteral prophylaxis whenever this is practical.

Arguments for parenteral administration

Bacterial endocarditis is a serious disease, with significant mortality and morbidity. Obviously, every reasonable effort should be made to prevent it. Anecdotal reports of apparent failure of endocarditis prophylaxis are not unusual; about 20 such cases had appeared in the literature by 1980. More recently, a series of 52 cases of apparent failures of endocarditis prophylaxis was collected by a national registry sponsored by the American Heart Association. Most of the early and recently reported patients with presumed prophylaxis failures developed endocarditis despite administration of oral penicillin.

In the laboratory, studies on prophylaxis of streptococcal endocarditis in rabbits consistently indicate that a high and prolonged level of penicillin in the blood is desirable for effective prophylaxis.

Arguments against parenteral administration

Although apparent prophylaxis failures have been recorded, the actual rate of failure cannot be quantitated because the denominator is unknown. However, because this denominator must be large, the risk of prophylaxis failure must be very low, even if antibiotics are given orally.

Oral medications are much easier to administer than parenteral drugs. Injections are unpopular with patients, and, as a general rule, dentists cannot or will not administer parenteral prophylaxis in their offices. In practice, this means that patients must visit a physician before going to the dentist, or must be treated in a hospital setting, either as inpatients or as outpatients. Parenteral drugs are more likely to cause serious reactions, including anaphylaxis, than oral treatment.

Author's opinion

In our present state of knowledge, the choice between oral and parenteral administration for prophylaxis of endocarditis remains moot. It is unlikely that we shall obtain the answer to this question by means of controlled clinical trials; because an enormous number of patients would be required to show statistical differences, the expense and difficulty of such trials would be excessive. Therefore, an empirical approach is required, based upon secondary sources of information such as the degree of risk for endocarditis posed by a patient's underlying cardiac lesion, the likelihood of bacteremia, and the circumstances under which the patient is being treated.

The author's practice is to use parenteral prophylaxis for high-risk situations (for example, patients with prosthetic valves and patients who have had multiple previous episodes of endocarditis), or when a physician or patient specifically requests maximum possible protection. For virtually every patient who is in the hospital (mak-

TABLE 1
Author's current recommendations for prophylaxis of endocarditis*

STANDARD REGIMEN	
For dental procedures and oral or upper respiratory tract surgery	Penicillin V 2.0 g orally 1 h before, then 1.0 g 6 h later†

SPECIAL REGIMENS	
Parenteral regimen for high-risk patients; also for GI or GU tract procedures	Ampicillin 2.0 g IM or IV *plus* gentamicin 1.5 mg/kg IM or IV, 0.5 h before†
Parenteral regimen for penicillin-allergic patients	Vancomycin 1.0 g IV slowly over 1 h, starting 1 h before; *add* gentamicin 1.5 mg/kg IM or IV if GI or GU tract involved†
Oral regimen for penicillin-allergic patients (oral and respiratory tract only)	Erythromycin 1.0 g orally 1 h before, then 0.5 g 6 h later†
Oral regimen for minor GI or GU tract procedures	Amoxicillin 3.0 g orally 1 h before, then 1.5 g 6 h later†

* *Note that (1) these regimens are empirical suggestions; no regimen has been* proved *effective for prevention of endocarditis, and prevention failures may occur with any regimen, (2) these regimens are not intended to cover all clinical situations; the practitioner should use his or her own judgment on safety and cost-benefit issues in each individual case, (3) one or two additional doses may be given if the period of risk for bacteremia is prolonged.*

† *Pediatric dosages: ampicillin 50 mg/kg; erythromycin 20 mg/kg for first dose, then 10 mg/kg; gentamicin 200 mg/kg; penicillin V and amoxicillin, for children who weigh more than 60 lb, use same as for adults; for children less than 60 lb, use one-half the adult dose; vancomycin 20 mg/kg.*

ing parenteral injections easy to administer and monitor for side effects), the author would choose parenteral prophylaxis in order to achieve the greatest possible margin of preventive efficacy. On the other hand, for most low-risk, outpatient settings such as dental cleaning and scaling in a patient with mitral valve disease, the author would use oral prophylaxis. See Table 1 for a summary of the author's recommendations.

5. IS PROPHYLAXIS FOR BACTERIAL ENDOCARDITIS INDICATED IN PATIENTS WITH MITRAL VALVE PROLAPSE?

Background

Mitral valve prolapse is a common underlying cardiac lesion in patients with SBE. Various estimates put the prevalence of mitral valve prolapse at 10 to 30 percent among patients with SBE. It has been calculated that the presence of mitral valve prolapse increases a person's chance of developing endocarditis by five to eight times. However, mitral valve prolapse is so common in the general population that the risk that any one individual will develop bacterial endocarditis on this lesion is very low.

Arguments for

Endocarditis is a serious disease that should be prevented whenever possible. Antibiotics are relatively cheap and relatively safe. Physicians and dentists believe that prophylaxis works, even though this has never been demonstrated in proper clinical trials. In fact, the standard of medical practice in the United States for patients with underlying cardiac lesions requires recognition of the risk of endocarditis and administration of antibiotics to prevent it. This practice is perpetuated in part by habit and in part by fear of claims of malpractice if antibiotic is not given to such patients.

Arguments against

Because the risk of developing endocarditis in a patient with mitral valve prolapse who undergoes a dental procedure is so low, the risk of death from anaphylaxis may well be greater than the risk of death from endocarditis. And, based upon similar arguments, the cost of prophylaxis ·may well outweigh the cost of the disease; in other words, institution of prophylaxis would not be cost-effective. The application of decision analysis to these questions by Clemens and Ransohoff led them to conclude that *parenteral* prophylaxis itself was probably more dangerous for patients with mitral valve prolapse than the chance of developing endocarditis. They also concluded that prophylaxis, while possibly justified in older patients, would not be cost-effective. It is also possible that excessive use of prophylaxis might deter patients from seeking necessary dental care and detract from their dental health.

Author's opinion

While accepting the argument that prophylaxis for mitral valve prolapse may not be cost-effective, the cost of a single course of oral prophylaxis is extremely low. Therefore, the author would not wish to deprive the patient of the possible benefit of endocarditis prophylaxis with oral penicillin. For both patients and physicians, the increased peace of mind and the possible reduction in the risk of endocarditis can be purchased at a very low price, in terms of both dollars and side effects. Therefore, the author uses an oral antibiotic regimen in selected patients with mitral valve prolapse, especially if mitral regurgitation is present. The chance that a serious or fatal anaphylactic reaction will occur, though small, is an order of magnitude greater for parenteral than for oral prophylaxis. In view of this fact, as well as the findings of the analysis performed by Clemens and Ransohoff, the author personally would not choose to use parenteral prophylaxis for uncomplicated mitral valve prolapse.

6. CAN ANTICOAGULANTS BE ADMINISTERED DURING ACTIVE ENDOCARDIAL INFECTION?

Background

The vegetations of bacterial endocarditis are primarily thrombotic lesions in which bacterial colonies grow in a matrix of fibrin and platelets. Therefore, many authors have discussed the the-

oretical value of treatment with anticoagulants or thrombolytic agents.

There are two reasons why anticoagulant therapy might be considered in patients with bacterial endocarditis: (1) as a therapeutic measure and (2) for treatment of another related or unrelated condition, such as pulmonary embolus, for which anticoagulants are usually given. As to the first reason, even before the advent of penicillin, treatment of endocarditis with heparin had been attempted without success. However, all seven of the first series of patients to be treated successfully with penicillin received heparin *as well*. It was another 5 years or so before physicians realized that heparin was hindering, not helping, the outcome of penicillin treatment for endocarditis. This realization was based upon the appearance of a number of case reports documenting serious or fatal intracerebral hemorrhage in patients receiving heparin during treatment of endocarditis.

Experimental studies in rabbits indicate that warfarin (Coumadin), heparin, and streptokinase all can alter the natural history of the infection. For example, streptokinase can actually lyse experimental vegetations. However, it has not been demonstrated that these drugs offer any therapeutic advantages over antibiotics alone, while they certainly pose potential risks. Therefore, at present there is no role for anticoagulation or thrombolysis in the *primary treatment* of endocarditis. This leaves the use of anticoagulants for treatment of other conditions during active endocarditis to be considered.

Arguments for

Anticoagulants are usually given for life-threatening diseases such as pulmonary embolism. Therefore, it could be argued that any risks posed by anticoagulation during active endocarditis must be accepted. In general, these risks have not been quantitated, but in the case of heparin there seems to be a real risk of serious intracerebral hemorrhage or of bleeding elsewhere. For this reason, for a period of about 25 years after 1950, many physicians taught that anticoagulants were absolutely contraindicated during treatment of active endocarditis. However, in the 1970s well-documented experience at the Mayo Clinic indicated that patients with prosthetic valves who received Coumadin during antibiotic treatment did as well as, or better than, those in whom anticoagulation was discontinued or was not used at all. This experience with a high-risk group of patients with prosthetic valve endocarditis showed that anticoagulants were safe and helped to avert formation of thrombi on the prosthetic valves. Whether thrombus formation can be prevented or mitigated on native valve endocarditis is not clear. What can be said is that laboratory control of anticoagulation has improved over the years, reducing the risk that overdose will occur and lead to bleeding.

Arguments against

The arguments against administration of anticoagulants have been summarized above. A patient with active endocarditis who is given anticoagulants may die of cerebral hemorrhage or may suffer an incapacitating stroke. Serious bleeding could also occur elsewhere in the body. In view of the absence of a modern controlled trial, the effect of heparin on the outcome of infection can not be assessed.

Author's opinion

Although controlled trials are lacking, the available evidence indicates that it would be prudent to regard active endocarditis as being at least a relative contraindication to heparin therapy. The only exceptions might be for the emergency treatment of a massive pulmonary embolism or extensive lower extremity thrombophlebitis if the diagnosis were reasonably certain and there was a high risk that the patient would die from the thrombotic or embolic complication. Coumadin may be given during active endocarditis *provided* that (1) a definite indication for anticoagulation exists and (2) the dose is carefully controlled at a therapeutic level by appropriate, repeated laboratory tests.

7. CAN CARDIAC CATHETERIZATION BE PERFORMED SAFELY DURING ACTIVE ENDOCARDITIS?

Background

There are many obvious reasons why diagnostic cardiac catheterization is useful in management of endocarditis: to define preexisting and new valvular lesions; to quantitate pressures and hemodynamic function; to detect complications of endocarditis such as mycotic aneurysms or rupture of a sinus of Valsalva; and to detect possible coexisting coronary artery disease. Diagnostic catheterization is a frequent and proper prelude to valve replacement.

Arguments for

Valve replacement constitutes a critically important measure in management of many cases of endocarditis. To achieve the best possible results, it is important that the surgeon should be in possession of as much information as possible before surgery and should not encounter any unexpected conditions during surgery.

Arguments against

The primary argument against diagnostic catheterization during active endocarditis is based on the fear that the catheter will dislodge a vegetation, causing a serious embolus to a vital organ. The data available on this question, while not extensive, indicate that this rarely occurs.

Author's opinion

Catheterization of the right side of the heart can nearly always be undertaken, because any emboli that might be generated will go to the lungs (except when there is a right-to-left shunt). Vegetations are usually too small to cause serious trouble when they migrate to the pulmonary arteries. On the left side, the author believes that if cardiac catheterization is indicated, the benefits outweigh the theoretical risks. Arterial emboli occur unpredictably at any time during treatment of active endocarditis. Even if an embolus occurred soon after cardiac catheterization, it is uncertain whether this would not have happened anyway. Therefore, if the team managing the patient believes that useful information could be gained by passing a catheter across the aortic valve, this should be done. If adequate information is available without passing a catheter across the aortic valve, then even the theoretical risks of precipitating an embolus should be avoided.

8. SHOULD VALVE REPLACEMENT BE UNDERTAKEN DURING ACTIVE ENDOCARDIAL INFECTION?

Background

This question has been discussed many times during the past 20 years. A fairly clear answer has emerged during the past decade, but the question still arises frequently in management of individual patients. The development of acute congestive heart failure is the most common and generally accepted indication for valve replacement during endocarditis occurring on native valves, and the discussion will address primarily this issue. However, it should be recognized that other indications for surgery exist in native valve endocarditis. These include valve ring abscesses and unremitting infection. While not discussed here in detail, firm indications for surgery have been formulated for prosthetic valve endocarditis, including congestive heart failure, paravalvular leaks, and infection with organisms other than streptococci.

Arguments for

The greatest single advance in treatment of endocarditis since the discovery of penicillin unquestionably has been the development of valve replacement surgery. This operation permits the "rescue" of the patient whose valvular infection can be eradicated by antibiotics but whose valve is so badly scarred that continuing heart failure is inevitable. If valve replacement is delayed too long, the patient's heart failure may worsen to a point where surgery cannot be performed. If this happens, the patient may have been deprived of the best chance for survival. This alone constitutes a strong argument for valve replacement despite presence of active infection.

Arguments against

It is usually undesirable to perform an elective operation on a patient with a systemic bacterial infection. The patient's strength and healing ability may be lowered by the catabolic state caused by active infection. There may be renal failure or other complications that increase the morbidity and mortality of any major operation such as valve replacement. Cardiac function may be impaired in several ways: by the presence of myo-

cardial lesions caused by endocarditis, such as valve ring abscesses or focal infiltrations of inflammatory cells known as Bracht-Wächter bodies; by the nonspecific effects of fever and protein catabolism; or by arrhythmias generated by spread of infection from the valve into regions of the myocardium adjacent to the conduction system. Any of these factors might exacerbate the hemodynamic stress placed upon the myocardium by a malfunctioning valve.

There is some risk that a prosthetic valve implanted in the presence of active infection will immediately itself become infected with the same organism. If this were to happen, the patient's physicians would have substituted early prosthetic valve endocarditis for native valve endocarditis. This theoretical risk is probably at its highest when a myocardial abscess is present.

Author's opinion

The timing of valve replacement remains a delicate and difficult decision. Ideally, it should be made in a tertiary-care setting which can offer the best consultative and support services. The degree of heart failure and its cause should outweigh all other considerations. Individual factors must be evaluated in each case; for example, acute valvular incompetence, especially involving the aortic valve, is a stronger indication for early surgery than chronic regurgitation or regurgitation involving the mitral valve.

It is a surprising fact that prosthetic valves implanted during active infection *rarely* become infected with the same organism. The frequency with which this occurs is well under 5 percent. Even if an abscess is present, the rate of immediate infection of the newly implanted valve is low. While the presence of an abscess obviously increases the technical difficulty of valve implantation and makes the overall prognosis worse, its presence does not constitute an argument for delay in valve replacement because abscesses in the heart as in other sites are unlikely to resolve on antibiotic therapy alone.

The author is unaware of any useful data concerning the significance of the nonspecific myocardial dysfunction that might be present during active infective endocarditis, but there is ample practical experience to show that improvement in hemodynamics following valve replacement will more than likely occur following surgery. Of course, this is dependent to some extent on the chronicity of the heart failure and the functioning state of the ventricle(s).

Because the greatest reduction in the number of organisms on an infected valve occurs within the first few days of treatment, leaving only a small number of slowly replicating survivors to be eradicated during the last weeks of therapy, there may be some advantage to delaying operation until at least 2 or 3 days of antibiotic treatment has been given. This is a theoretical argument, however, and even a short delay is subject to the danger that heart failure may worsen. The reasonable desire to treat patients with antibiotics for at least 2 to 3 days prior to surgery should not be used as a reason to postpone operation in patients with serious heart failure.

It is important, of course, not to become so aggressive that unnecessary valve replacements are performed. Prosthetic valves have a limited life and entail a predictable morbidity and mortality, which is especially important in young patients. In patients with mild or moderate heart failure, it is often prudent to begin nonoperative treatment for heart failure while continuing antibiotic therapy. Those who do not respond to conservative measures should undergo valve replacement. For those who do respond well, the decision whether to replace the valve can be postponed. For some patients, surgery will prove unnecessary; the remainder will enjoy the theoretical advantages of undergoing surgery after the infection has been cured.

In summary, the answer is clear: when valve replacement is needed, the morbidity and mortality associated with delay are usually greater than the risk of surgery. This is especially true when a patient experiences sudden onset of aortic regurgitation during the active stage of endocarditis. Valve replacement should be regarded as an emergency rather than an elective operation in such patients.

9. SHOULD AN INFECTED VALVE BE REPLACED TO PREVENT EMBOLI?

Background

In the author's experience, this is one of the most troublesome questions in management of endocarditis, equalled in difficulty only by the prob-

lems of managing intracerebral mycotic aneurysms. Arterial emboli can occur before, during, or after treatment for native valve or prosthetic valve endocarditis. The risk is relatively high in untreated patients, diminishes during treatment, and is low after cure. It is said that the risk of embolization falls to near normal when 2 years have passed since cure.

Arguments for

Many physicians find it psychologically easier to act than to wait. The concept of removing the source of emboli that have caused a stroke by excising the infected valve and inserting a prosthetic valve is attractive. The physician knows that emboli can be fatal (e.g., myocardial infarction) or permanently incapacitating (e.g., stroke). The risk of operation is fairly low, and the cure of infective endocarditis itself may be effected or aided by valve replacement. Some advocates of valve replacement for embolic disease are more likely to propose the procedure when organisms that are prone to form large vegetations and large emboli such as fungi, *Haemophilus aphrophilus*, and *H. parainfluenzae* are causing the infection.

Arguments against

The chance of arterial embolization in an individual patient is highly unpredictable, even after one or two emboli have already occurred. The patient may experience none, one, or many more emboli. It follows that the risk of significant ill effects from emboli is also highly unpredictable. On the other hand, the mortality and morbidity of valve replacement, although low, is appreciable and predictable. Even if surgery goes well, the prosthetic valve has a limited life span: it is likely to require replacement within 10 years. This is a significant consideration for young patients, who may require several such valve replacements during their lifetime, each with its attendant risks. Some patients with infective endocarditis suffer only minor valve damage and enjoy a normal life after cure, while patients with prosthetic valves cannot be considered normal at any time after the operation.

Author's opinion

Valve replacement for the *sole purpose* of preventing emboli should seldom be undertaken. If this is done repeatedly in a medical center, physicians there should ask themselves whether they may be replacing some valves unnecessarily. The author's approach is to avoid valve replacement for this indication unless there has been *more than one* major embolus with significant sequelae. The management team should be especially reluctant to implant prosthetic valves into young people without heart failure for prevention of emboli. Clearly, emboli should rank as a much lesser argument for valve replacement than heart failure.

References

BISNO AL: *Treatment of Infective Endocarditis.* New York, Grune § Stratton, 1981

—— et al: AHA Committee Report: Treatment of infective endocarditis due to viridans streptococci. Circulation 63:730A, 1981

BRENNAN RO, DURACK DT: Therapeutic significance of penicillin tolerance in experimental streptococcal endocarditis. Antimicrob Agents Chemother 23:273, 1983

CLEMENS JD et al: A controlled evaluation of the risk of bacterial endocarditis in persons with mitral valve prolapse. N Engl J Med 307, 1982

——RANSOHOFF DF: Pre-dental antibiotic prophylaxis for mitral valve prolapse: Cost and effect, abstracted (no 768). Read at the *Twenty-second Interscience Conference on Antimicrobial Agents and Chemotherapy.* Washington, DC, American Society for Microbiology, 1982

COHEN PS et al: Infective endocarditis caused by gram-negative bacteria: A review of the literature, 1945–1977. Prog Cardiovasc Dis 22:205-242, 1980

CORRIGAL L et al: Mitral valve prolapse and infective endocarditis. Am J Med 63:215, 1977

DURACK DT: Prophylaxis of infective endocarditis, in *Principles and Practice of Infectious Diseases,* GL Mandell et al (eds). New York, Wiley, 1979

——: Infective and noninfective endocarditis, in *The Heart,* JW Hurst (ed). New York, McGraw-Hill, 1982

—— et al: Apparent failures of endocarditis prophylaxis: Analysis of 52 cases submitted to a national registry. JAMA 250:2318, 1983

FREEDMAN LR: *Infective Endocarditis and Other Intravascular Infections.* New York, Plenum, 1982

HESS J et al: Significance of penicillin tolerance in vivo: Prevention of experimental *Streptococcus sanguis* endocarditis. J Antimicrob Chemother 11:555, 1983

PRUITT AA ET AL: Neurologic complications in bacterial endocarditis. Medicine 57:329, 1978

RAHIMTOOLA SH (ed): *Infective Endocarditis.* New York, Grune § Stratton, 1978

SANDE MA, SCHELD WM: Combination antibiotic therapy of bacterial endocarditis. Ann Intern Med 92:390, 1980

SCHELD WM, SANDE MA: Infective endocarditis, in *Principles and Practice of Infectious Diseases,* GL Mandell et al (eds). New York, Wiley, 1979

WEINSTEIN L: Infective endocarditis, in *Heart Disease,* E Braunwald (ed). Philadelphia, Saunders, 1980, p 1166

WELTON DE et al: Value and safety of cardiac catheterization during active infective endocarditis. Am J Cardiol 44:1306, 1979

WILSON WR et al: Anticoagulant therapy and central nervous system complications in patients with prosthetic valve endocarditis. Circulation 57:1004, 1978

PRIMARY PREVENTION OF CORONARY ARTERY DISEASE

ROBERT I. LEVY, CURT D. FURBERG, and BASIL M. RIFKIND

THE MAGNITUDE OF THE PROBLEM

Coronary heart disease (CHD) remains the major cause of death and disability in the United States and in other industrialized countries despite recent welcome declines in its mortality. CHD accounts for more deaths each year than any other disease, including all forms of cancer combined. CHD ranks first in terms of social security disability, second only to all forms of arthritis for limitation of activity, and second only to all forms of cancer combined for total hospital-bed days. In health care costs and lost wages and productivity, CHD costs this country over $60 billion a year. Over 1 million new heart attacks occur each year, and despite a recent decline, over 0.5 million people still die as a result. Many of these deaths occur in otherwise healthy, productive, middle-aged men.

PREVENTION OF CHD

A great deal of effort and money has been expended to try to prolong life in subjects who already have manifestations of CHD, so-called *secondary prevention*. The introduction of coronary care units is a major example of this. Although many advances have been recorded, there are limits to the impact that such an approach can have on the overall CHD death rate since so many CHD deaths are sudden. The frequent onset of death within minutes or hours of the first symptom means that there is often little or no opportunity to bring medical care to bear on a high proportion of subjects. Furthermore, subjects who have survived a myocardial infarction have a much greater subsequent mortality

rate than prevailed before the event. After a heart attack, the location and extent of heart muscle damage becomes the major determinant of long-term survival.

Such considerations have increasingly focused attention on the so-called *primary prevention* of CHD, namely, the prevention of the onset of the initial clinical manifestations of CHD. Efforts have been made to identify individuals who are free of symptoms or signs of CHD but who possess factors, traits, or habits which place them at increased risk, in order to apply interventions that would reduce this risk. Another preventive and more ideal approach, *primordial prevention*, attempts to prevent the development of these various risk factors themselves.

MAJOR RISK FACTORS FOR CHD

The incidence of CHD increases in both sexes with age, and is much higher in men than in women, especially below age 70. While such age and sex relationships are of importance in directing attention to possible underlying mechanisms, they offer little direct opportunity to derive a prevention strategy. However, several major and many other potentially correctable risk factors for CHD have been identified. Knowledge of these risk factors permits the identification of individuals who have a much greater than average risk of developing CHD in the subsequent years. The three major classical risk factors for CHD, identified mainly by prospective epidemiological studies, are the levels of total serum cholesterol, blood pressure, and cigarette smoking (Fig. 1). The greater the level of any one of these, independent of the level of others,

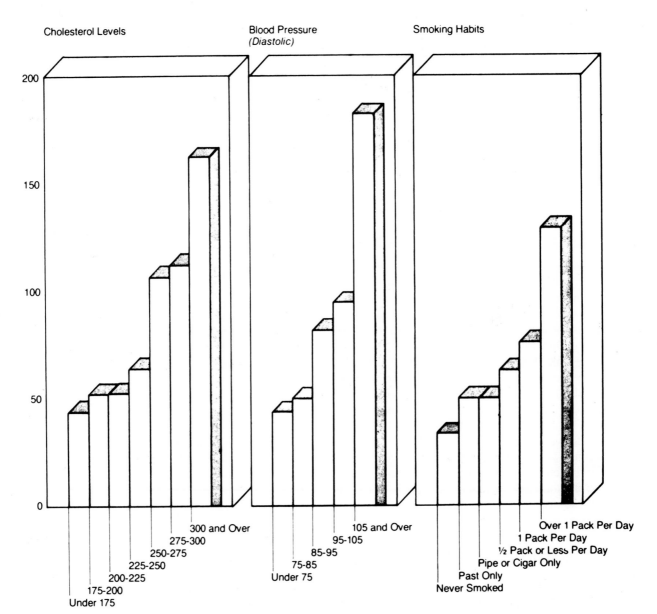

Cholesterol Levels

Blood Pressure
(Diastolic)

Smoking Habits

300 and Over
275-300
250-275
225-250
200-225
175-200
Under 175

105 and Over
95-105
85-95
75-85
Under 75

Over 1 Pack Per Day
1 Pack Per Day
½ Pack or Less Per Day
Pipe or Cigar Only
Past Only
Never Smoked

FIGURE 1
Rates of first heart attack per 1000 males for the three major risk factors for coronary heart disease.

the greater the risk of developing CHD. For example, an individual with a total serum cholesterol over 300 mg/dl has three to four times the risk of developing a heart attack than an individual with a cholesterol of under 175 mg/dl. These risk factors act in aggregate. A heavy cigarette smoker who is hypertensive and has a very high serum cholesterol has 30 to 40 times the risk of a nonsmoker with low cholesterol and blood pressure levels. The level of high-density lipoprotein (HDL) has also emerged as a major CHD risk factor (Fig. 2). In contrast to the classical factors, the correlation is negative (i.e., the lower the level of HDL, the greater the risk of CHD).

Other CHD risk factors

Diabetes Diabetes more than doubles CHD risk. Its greatest impact is on occlusive peripheral arterial disease, but CHD is still its most

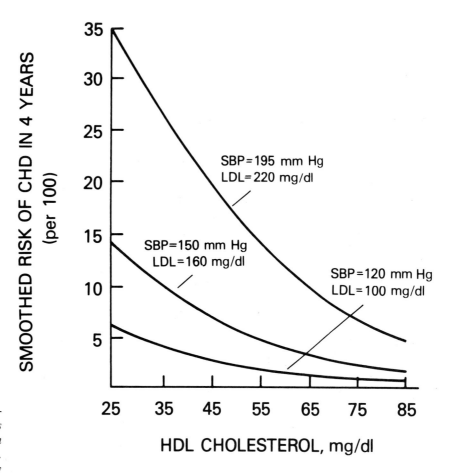

FIGURE 2
Risk of coronary heart diseases according to levels of high-density lipoprotein (HDL) levels in men aged 55. (From the Framingham Study 24-year follow-up.)

common sequela. Diabetes also causes myocardial damage predisposing to cardiac failure. Its cardiovascular effects are more severe in women than in men and tend to diminish with advancing age.

As in the nondiabetic patient, levels of cigarette smoking, hypertension, and hypercholesterolemia influence the subsequent risk of developing CHD. While diabetic tendency may be genetically determined, factors such as obesity and physical inactivity play a role in whether or not it will become manifest. Some evidence suggests that the risk of cardiovascular sequelae can be reduced by rigid control of hypoglycemia, but this remains to be verified by controlled clinical trials. The evidence at hand, however, clearly justifies attention to the other risk factors associated with diabetes.

Lesser risk factors

Predisposition to CHD also results from excessive intake of calories with unrestrained weight gain, a sedentary life-style, and other factors such as alcohol intake, stress, and gout.

Obesity Obesity is a powerful determinant of the major atherogenic traits. Weight gain or obesity are associated with increases in blood pressure, blood glucose, and blood cholesterol, and a worsening of the low-density lipoprotein (LDL)/HDL ratio. Weight loss is accompanied by improvements in all these atherogenic traits. Overweight people have twice as much congestive cardiac failure as lean people, but only a little more CHD. In women, the general cardiovascular effect of obesity is more severe, particularly for cardiac failure and cerebral infarction;

its effect is mediated largely through other risk factors that obesity promotes, and diminishes with age. In men, obesity increases the risk for all cardiovascular disease except occlusive peripheral arterial disease.

Sedentary life-style Physical inactivity is directly related to CHD and overall mortality. In the Framingham Study, the evidence of a protective effect of exercise was confined to men and was significant only for CHD. The potential benefit is modest in comparison with modification of other risk factors but persists when the other risk factors are controlled.

Physical activity has a definite role in a comprehensive risk-reduction program. It helps to control such other risk factors as obesity, low HDL, impaired glucose tolerance, and possibly hypertension. It also appears to improve myocardial functioning.

Alcohol Excessive alcohol may damage the myocardium and predispose to hypertension and stroke. However, moderate drinking appears to increase HDL.

Stress Persons with the so-called type A personality have exaggerated feelings of time-urgency, drive, and competitiveness. They also have an increased risk for CHD. In men this association seems confined to white collar workers; in women it has been noted for both homemakers and those in outside employment. In both sexes, where this association has been found, it has been independent of other risk factors.

It is unknown whether type A or CHD-prone behavior can be effectively altered and whether this would reduce risk. In such persons, other risk factors known to be modifiable would seem to warrant more attention.

Gout and hyperuricemia These factors are associated with modest increase in CHD risk thought largely to be due to their association with hypertension, obesity, and hypercholesterolemia. In gouty patients, these associated risk factors should be corrected, since there is no evidence that correcting the hyperuricemia per se reduces the risk of CHD.

Oral contraceptives Use of oral contraceptives is associated with increased risk of myocardial infarction particularly with prolonged use, use after age 35, and use in conjunction with cigarette smoking or coexisting hypertension, hypercholesterolemia, or diabetes.

Unmodifiable risk factors

Age and sex The incidence of CHD increases markedly after age 45 in men and age 55 in women. Women with hypercholesterolemia, hypertension, or who smoke are somewhat protected from CHD relative to their male counterparts. This protection is only relative because, compared to normal women, risk is greatly increased. However, at any age, in either sex, some persons are clearly more vulnerable than others.

Postmenopause Both the incidence and severity of CHD increase with menopause. Twice as many menopausal women have CHD as women of the same age who are still menstruating. This holds true for either natural or surgical menopause.

Hereditary susceptibility Innate susceptibility to CHD may be indicated by a strong family history of premature CHD, diabetes, gout, or hypertension. A myocardial infarction in a younger brother is significantly related to comparable experience in older brothers, suggesting a shared tendency to hypertension, hypercholesterolemia, and smoking. History of premature CHD (before age 60) in a parent or older sibling generally doubles a patient's CHD risk. Such persons deserve careful surveillance for early and vigorous correction of any modifiable CHD risk factors.

Significance of risk factors

The use of risk factors is a powerful tool in predicting prognosis. It has been shown that those subjects aged 40 to 65 who fall into the top 20 percent of the population distribution of the major risk factors represent 40 percent of the population who will subsequently develop a first myocardial infarction. It has been estimated that 55 to 70 percent of all cases of CHD are attributable to the three major risk factors. However, 30 to 45 percent of subjects, whose risk-factor levels are not unusually high, will also develop a heart attack. These considerations suggest that a strategy to prevent CHD should direct attention not only to high-risk subjects but also to subjects whose risk-factor levels are not so evident.

Pathogenic significance of risk factors

Although the measurement of risk factors is important in identifying both individuals and populations at risk for CHD, a cause-effect relationship between the various risk factors and CHD cannot automatically be assumed. Whether given risk factors are of etiological significance depends on other types of evidence. Furthermore, because the level of a given factor correlates well with the subsequent risk of CHD, it does not follow that correction of this factor by whatever means will lower the individual's risk even if the risk factor is of pathogenic significance. The critical method for determining whether a cause-effect relationship exists is demonstration that risk-factor modification will reduce CHD mortality and morbidity in a controlled clinical trial. A properly planned and executed clinical trial is the most powerful experimental technique for assessing the effectiveness of an intervention. A *clinical trial* is defined as "prospective study comparing the effect and value of intervention(s) against control in human subjects." A clinical trial must contain a control (reference) group against which the intervention group is compared. The ideal trial is one that randomly assigns subjects to the treatment groups and is double-blind.

Clinical trials in the primary prevention of CHD are associated with many difficulties, especially since CHD risk factors are closely bound up with behavioral and life-style attributes which are not easy to reverse. Additional primary prevention trials require a large number of subjects and long periods of observation, involve problems of compliance, and often do not lend themselves to a double-blind design.

CHOLESTEROL, LDL, AND HDL AS RISK FACTORS

Numerous case-control, prevalence (cross-sectional), and, most importantly, prospective epidemiological studies in the United States and elsewhere have consistently demonstrated that the level of serum cholesterol is directly related to the subsequent risk of CHD. Multivariate analysis has shown that this relationship is independent of any relationship between serum cholesterol levels and the levels of other risk factors. About 60 to 70 percent of the total serum cholesterol is carried in the LDL fraction in normal subjects so that LDL and total serum cholesterol levels are strongly correlated. In fact the direct relationship of total serum cholesterol to CHD risk is largely a reflection of the very strong direct relationship between CHD and LDL cholesterol. Within the range of cholesterol levels encountered in studies of industrialized populations, CHD risk is continuous (i.e., there is no level below which risk disappears).

From 20 to 25 percent of the serum cholesterol is normally carried in the HDL fraction. Many case-control and several prospective studies in recent years have found HDL to be a powerful and inverse predictor of CHD risk (i.e., the higher the HDL levels, the less the risk). HDL levels correlate poorly with those of LDL but are closely related to levels of several other risk factors such as cigarette smoking, obesity, and sedentary behavior. However, when statistical adjustment is made for these various relationships, HDL levels still retain their predictive power. Accordingly, both HDL and LDL are independent predictors of CHD risk, so that knowledge of both of them results in better prediction of risk than knowledge of either one of them alone. Various indexes have been recommended which combine information on levels of both of these fractions. The LDL/HDL ratio (or its more conveniently obtained surrogate, the total serum cholesterol/HDL ratio) appears to be as good an index as any.

The findings of epidemiological studies relating total serum and LDL cholesterol to CHD are consistent with findings from many other experimental approaches. For example, studies of humans and of various animals have shown cholesterol to be a major component of the atherosclerotic plaque. Cholesterol feeding, supplemented with other measures to induce hypercholesterolemia, results in the production of atherosclerotic lesions in a variety of species such as rabbits, cockerels, and non-human primates and has provided considerable insights into the pathogenesis of the atherosclerotic lesion. Regression of induced atherosclerotic lesions has been observed in non-human primates by reversal of hypercholesterolemia using diet or drugs. That raised plasma cholesterol levels are involved in the production of early CHD is also strongly suggested by observations on the natural history of genetic hyperlipidemias, such as familial hypercholesterolemia. In this disorder, high levels of LDL are associated with severe premature CHD to the extent that, in the rare homozygous form, death usually occurs within the first or second decade of life.

In families with the more common heterozygous forms of familial hypercholesterolemia, affected males have been shown to have a 52 percent chance of developing nonfatal or fatal CHD by age 60.

Although much remains to be learned, detailed studies of lipoprotein metabolism in normal and hyperlipidemic subjects reenforce the view that high levels of LDL are atherogenic, leading to the deposition of cholesterol in the arteries, and that HDL may play a "protective" role in facilitating the removal of cholesterol from the arterial wall or preventing its deposition in the first place.

Clinical convention often designates subjects with cholesterol (or LDL) levels above the 95th percentile as abnormal and hypercholesterolemic, necessitating advice and treatment, and subjects below the 95th percentile as having "normal" cholesterol levels not requiring further attention. This approach should be discarded on the grounds of both the continuous relationship of cholesterol levels and CHD and the recognition that levels of cholesterol in industrialized populations such as the United States are generally higher than those found in societies in which CHD is much less common. For example, the average cholesterol level in U.S. middle-aged males is about 210 to 220 mg/dl; in Japanese males, only about 180 mg/dl. Coronary disease is much rarer in Japan than in the United States.

Although subjects with high levels of cholesterol have a greatly increased risk of CHD, they are relatively few in number and account for only a small proportion of all myocardial infarctions. To have an impact on the overall prevalence of disease, a primary preventive approach must consider subjects throughout the cholesterol distribution and not merely those concentrated at its upper end. Such considerations emphasize the need for the clinician not only to recognize, identify, and treat the high-risk subject, but also to seek a downward shift in the population's cholesterol distribution. Such considerations apply equally to other risk factors such as hypertension and cigarette smoking.

Diet and plasma cholesterol levels

Dietary factors play an important role in determining the levels of plasma and LDL cholesterol in U.S. populations. The quantity and type of dietary fat are important in this respect as is the intake of dietary cholesterol. Dietary saturated fat and cholesterol increase serum cholesterol levels. Replacement of saturated fat by polyunsaturated fat leads to a reduction in serum cholesterol. Removal of a given amount of saturated fat from the diet has twice the cholesterol-lowering effect as the introduction of a corresponding amount of polyunsaturated fat. Such influences of dietary fat have been confirmed in many clinical and epidemiological studies, and have become part of the standard treatment for control of hyperlipidemia. Rigorous application of a low cholesterol, low saturated fat diet in the metabolic ward results in serum cholesterol lowering of from 15 to 25 percent. Numerous trials in which cholesterol lowering has been attempted by dietary means in populations containing hundreds or thousands of subjects have frequently obtained an average reduction of 10 to 15 percent, maintained for several years, pointing to the feasibility of such measures.

In addition to the influence of the amount and type of dietary fat, obesity appears to influence serum cholesterol levels. Several studies have now shown that moderate weight reduction often results in significant reductions in serum and LDL cholesterol levels. An additional benefit may be an increase in HDL.

In the United States over 40 percent of total

calories is consumed in the form of fat, of which over one-third is saturated and less than one-sixth is polyunsaturated. This high saturated fat intake, which is paralleled by a high cholesterol intake, is typical of industrialized societies consuming a "western type" diet. It is not inevitable. For example, about 70 years ago fat constituted approximately 32 percent of the total U.S. caloric intake, a level similar to that currently consumed by westernized Israeli populations. The Japanese eat a diet in which the total fat intake provides less than 10 percent of total calories. This almost certainly relates to the low cholesterol levels and relative freedom from CHD that the Japanese enjoy.

A slight improvement in the U.S. diet appears to be occurring. The Lipid Research Clinics, in a study of diet and lipids in various North American populations, measured dietary intakes employing the 24-h dietary recall method in a series of population studies from 1972 to 1976. They observed a dietary cholesterol intake of 350 to 450 mg per day and a P/S (polyunsaturated fat/saturated fat) ratio of 0.4 to 0.5. In the 1960s the U.S. diet provided 600 to 700 mg per day of cholesterol and a P/S ratio of 0.1 to 0.2. These findings are consistent with studies by the U.S. Department of Agriculture based on estimates of food entering the marketplace. These modest trends could account for a fall in the total plasma cholesterol of about 5 to 10 mg/dl, a finding consonant with evidence that there has been a slight reduction in plasma cholesterol levels in the United States over the past decade or so.

Determinants of HDL

The identification of the level of HDL as a powerful, independent predictor of CHD risk has led to a search for the various factors which relate to, and may determine the levels of, HDL. Females have higher levels of HDL than males after puberty, possibly due to their higher estrogen levels. HDL increases only slightly with age. Factors which are associated with lower levels of HDL include obesity and cigarette smoking. Higher levels are associated with moderate alcohol consumption and physical exercise.

It seems reasonable to assume that changing the levels of those factors capable of alteration such as weight, cigarette smoking, or level of physical activity would result in an increased level of HDL. Such measures have a considerable theoretical potential for altering HDL. For example, it has been calculated that a physically inactive, obese, cigarette-smoking, middle-aged male might raise his HDL from 38 mg/dl to 58 mg/dl by becoming physically active, reducing weight, and stopping smoking (Fig. 3). Changes of this magnitude might in theory markedly reduce CHD risk.

However, changes in these various behaviors have not yet been clearly shown to result consistently in the predicted rise in HDL, and secondly, there is little or no information on whether raising HDL actually prevents CHD. Nevertheless, since obesity and cigarette smoking have many other adverse consequences, and since their correction, together with moderate, regulated increases in physical activity, is generally safe, it seems wise to promote correction of these risk factors. Thought has been given to developing drugs that raise HDL in an attempt to prevent CHD. Much more development and evaluation work is required before such drugs can be considered for use in humans.

As mentioned earlier, moderate alcohol intake has also been shown to directly relate to the levels of HDL in several studies. However, it has not been advocated for use in view of its many toxic consequences when taken in excess.

Correction of hyperlipidemia by diet and drugs

The relationship between dietary fats and blood lipids has led to widespread advocacy and use of dietary treatment as a means of reducing raised cholesterol levels due to high levels of LDL. In many subjects, substantial reduction of cholesterol levels can be achieved by restriction of both total and saturated fat, replacement of some of the saturated fat by polyunsaturated fat, dietary cholesterol restriction, and, when necessary, weight reduction. Even severely hypercholesterolemic subjects, who are relatively resistant to dietary manipulation, often achieve a useful reduction by such means. However, such subjects may also require the addition of drugs. A variety of drugs has been advocated for the treatment of hyperlipidemia; few consistently produce marked reductions in total cholesterol

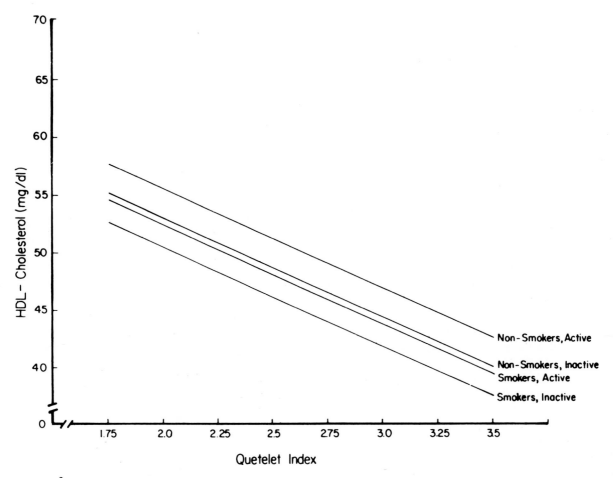

FIGURE 3

Relationship between physical activity and smoking and high-density lipoprotein (HDL) levels in middle-aged males.

and LDL levels without toxicity. Only the biliary sequestering agents, cholestyramine and colestipol, are unabsorbed and act solely in the intestinal tract. Their use is often complicated by compliance problems due to their bulk and taste and their frequent tendency to constipate. Other systemic drugs such as clofibrate may occasionally produce marked falls in LDL. More often they produce only moderate reductions. Fortunately most forms of hypertriglyceridemia require weight-reduction diets and only occasionally does drug use have to be considered. Since treatment of hyperlipidemia is lifelong, it is important, even if benefit is ultimately shown to be conferred through drug therapy, to exclude drugs that produce long-term toxicity; such toxicity

may obviate the drug's benefits. Systemic drugs like clofibrate, nicotinic acid, and dextrothyroxine, have each been found to be associated with a variety of toxic effects in long-term studies. More recently introduced drugs such as gemfibrozil and probucol have yet to be fully evaluated.

Trials of efficacy of CHD prevention through lipid lowering

The strong direct relationship between cholesterol and LDL levels in CHD, and the ability to reduce these levels by dietary means and/or drugs, has encouraged studies to evaluate whether CHD may be prevented by such treatment. Many of these studies have been on subjects with symptomatic heart disease (secondary prevention). Their results have been encouraging in some respects but inconclusive. The rationale for such studies is much weaker than for primary prevention since it has been shown that cholesterol levels are weaker predictors of survival in subjects who have already experienced a myocardial infarction. The subsequent history of such subjects appears to be primarily determined by the status and function of the myocardium following the myocardial infarction.

Clinical trials designed to assess the efficacy of cholesterol lowering in preventing CHD must meet rigorous design standards. Two prerequisites of such trials are the use of randomization (to ensure comparability of treatment and control groups) and of a double-blind design (to avoid confounding of the data through affects of many other factors which potentially influence CHD incidence). Few such studies have been conducted; most primary prevention trials of cholesterol lowering have used dietary treatment and have produced encouraging results. Dietary studies are inherently attractive since they represent an attempt to correct a major risk factor which is thought to have been produced in the first place through undesirable dietary practice. They also have the advantage of assessing a therapy which, if adopted, is likely to be nontoxic, in contrast to the problems that are often associated with long-term drug use.

However, it is virtually impossible to design a satisfactory study to evaluate cholesterol lowering by dietary means to prevent CHD. Impediments to a successful trial of diet, other than those concerned with maintaining a double-blind design, were recognized in the decision of the National Heart, Lung and Blood Institute (NHLBI) Task Force on Arteriosclerosis. After consideration of the Diet/Heart Feasibility Studies and other evidence, this task force was not in favor of a major national dietary prevention study in a free-living population as a means of testing whether cholesterol lowering prevents CHD. Such a study was thought not to be feasible and to be likely to fail in its objectives of providing conclusive results. Special concerns were the large size of the required population (which was estimated to range from 24,000 to 115,000 subjects, with its attendant managerial problems), the huge predicted expenditures ($0.5 to 1 billion in 1970 dollars), confounding of the study by likely modifications in other risk factors, and doubts about the degree of lipid low-

ering that could be achieved in a free-living population. Several major primary prevention trials of lipid lowering through diet have been reported and have, in the main, produced encouraging results. However, they have not been regarded as conclusive.

A number of primary prevention trials employing the simultaneous correction of several risk factors have been conducted recently. These studies also do not employ a double-blind design and are limited in their ability to identify which, if any, change in risk factor was responsible for the observed benefits. The results of the recently reported Oslo Study simultaneously reduced cigarette smoking and serum cholesterol levels. An encouraging 47 percent reduction in the incidence of fatal and nonfatal myocardial infarction and sudden death was obtained. Analysis showed that the reduction in incidence was correlated to a greater extent with the reduction in total cholesterol than with that in smoking. The Multiple Risk Factor Intervention Trial has also recently reported its findings. Its ability to speak to the efficacy of cholesterol lowering is severely limited by the small (2 percent) differential in plasma cholesterol produced between the two treatment groups, partly due to the fact that the control group experienced a greater than predicted fall in cholesterol. This trial is discussed in more detail below.

Primary prevention trials of lipid-lowering drugs

There have been surprisingly few primary prevention trials of lipid-lowering drugs and only one, the World Health Organization Clofibrate Study, meets many of the design requirements for such studies. This double-blind, randomized, multicenter, primary prevention trial involved 10,000 men in the upper one-third of the serum cholesterol distribution, half of whom received clofibrate and the other half a placebo. A mean reduction of approximately 9 percent of the initial serum cholesterol levels was achieved in the treatment group. The incidence of ischemic heart disease was lowered by 20 percent in the clofibrate group, but this fall was confined to nonfatal myocardial infarction which was reduced by 25 percent. The incidence of fatal heart attacks was unchanged. A disquieting feature was a significant increase in deaths due to causes other than CHD, mainly to an increase in cancer deaths, and deaths due to other medical causes. Explanation for the adverse findings in the clofibrate study are not apparent. Consideration has been given to their being due to a long-term toxic effect of clofibrate itself.

In summary, clinical trials of the benefits of cholesterol lowering for the primary prevention of CHD have provided evidence of benefit but have not been conclusive. Given the difficulty of conducting such studies and the impressive amount of other evidence relating dietary fat, serum cholesterol, and CHD, many authorities and organizations have suggested that there is a strong case for recommending cholesterol lowering to the general public. Others, while generally impressed with the evidence for such interrelationships, prefer to await the results of well-designed and conducted clinical trials before advocating changes that could affect virtually the whole population with wide socioeconomic ramifications. The Lipid Research Clinics Coronary Primary Prevention Trial is a double-blind, randomized clinical trial of drug-induced cholesterol lowering in 3810 middle-aged men with type II hyperlipoproteinemia. Its results are expected in January 1984 after 7 to 10 years of observation and are hoped to clarify some of the issues regarding the desirability of cholesterol lowering. The gradual development of better noninvasive methods for the assessment of the progress of atherosclerotic lesions offers considerable promise that future clinical trials of lipid lowering may be easier to design and implement.

Cholesterol levels and cancer incidence

Recently, focus has been directed to the lower end of the plasma cholesterol distribution. A few population-based studies have suggested that there may be an inverse relationship between low plasma cholesterol levels and noncardiovascular mortality in general and cancer of the colon in particular. Studies in places as disparate as Evans County, Ga., and the south Pacific found an increased mortality from cancers in groups with the lowest levels of cholesterol, less than 195 mg/dl. These relationships were reviewed at an NHLBI workshop, which con-

cluded that there seemed to be a somewhat inconsistent and weak relationship between low cholesterol levels and colon cancer in men but not in women. Recently an international collaborative group reported findings consistent with the hypothesis that lower cholesterol levels in cancer decedents are due to the effect of undetected disease on cholesterol level rather than an effect of low cholesterol level on development of cancer. The evidence relating low cholesterol levels to a possible increased cancer incidence within certain populations also has to be reconciled with previous observations that certain cancers, including colon cancer, are more prevalent in countries where fat intake and blood cholesterol levels are high.

The NHLBI workshop issued a unanimous opinion that the data which were reviewed did not preclude, countermand, or contradict the current public health message that recommends that those with elevated cholesterol levels seek to lower them through diets lower in saturated fat and cholesterol.

HYPERTENSION AS A RISK FACTOR

Hypertension is one of the most prevalent chronic conditions known to increase the risk of CHD. It has been demonstrated consistently that both systolic blood pressure (SBP) and diastolic blood pressure (DBP) are strong independent predictors of CHD risk. In addition, elevated blood pressure, like the other major risk factors, is associated with greatly increased risk of cerebrovascular and peripheral vascular diseases. This relationship between risk and blood pressure level is a continuous one. In some populations studied in the United States, subjects in the upper 20 percent of the blood pressure distribution have a fourfold greater relative risk of CHD than those in the lower 20 percent.

The SBP increases with age, from a mean level of 120 mmHg at the age of 30 to approximately 140 mmHg at the age of 70 years. The DBP increases from approximately 75 mmHg at the age of 30 to slightly over 80 mmHg at the age of 50. There is a little further change of DBP with age. For people 25 to 74 years of age, hypertension is sometimes classified, based on the level of DBP, as *mild* (90 to 104 mmHg), *moderate* (105 to 114 mmHg), and *severe* (115 mmHg).

This stratification is arbitrary because the blood pressure is a continuum with increased risk at higher levels.

Approximately 30 percent of the U.S. adult population meets the criteria of having hypertension if the definition of mean SBP and DBP of greater than 140/90 on two occasions is applied. This prevalence estimate drops to 14.5 percent if the critical levels are set at 160/95 mmHg. The prevalence rate of moderate to severe hypertension (i.e., DBP of at least 105 mmHg) is 2.8 percent.

Several factors are known to be related to elevated blood pressure, although the underlying cause of hypertension is unknown in more than 90 percent of hypertensives, so-called essential hypertension. Epidemiological studies have shown that obesity, sodium intake, and alcohol consumption are positively related to blood pressure. Each of these relationships suggests a potential for dietary intervention in the management of hypertension. Other factors associated with high blood pressure are family history, race, diabetes, and low educational and socioeconomic status. In the remaining hypertensives, so-called secondary hypertension, an underlying cause can be demonstrated (e.g., renal parenchymal disease, renovascular disease, primary aldosteronism, and pheochromocytoma). This form should be suspected in patients whose hypertension is refractory to drug therapy and in patients with accelerated or malignant hypertension.

Elevated blood pressure is often asymptomatic, and perceived symptoms are not reliably associated with blood pressure level. Therefore detection of hypertension requires mass screening, often in the context of comprehensive community control programs.

Antihypertensive therapy

The modern era, in the treatment of hypertension, began with the introduction of thiazide diuretics and methyldopa in the 1950s. Today, the physician can choose from a spectrum of antihypertensive drugs, the most commonly used of which are still the various types of diuretics. In the treatment of hypertension, beta-adrenergic blocking drugs have become the drug of choice in many European countries. Other drugs with

peripheral sympatholytic action are *Rauwolfia*-derived alkaloids and alpha-adrenergic blocking agents. Methyldopa and clonidine represent a third category, drugs with central sympatholytic action. Hydralazine belongs to the so-called arteriolar dilators. More recently introduced antihypertensive drugs are the angiotensin-converting enzyme inhibitors and the calcium channel blockers.

Treatment is usually instituted with a thiazide-type diuretic. If the response is inadequate, a beta-adrenergic blocking agent may be added. A third drug, hydralazine, is often chosen in resistant cases. In many centers, a selective beta-adrenergic blocking agent such as atenolol is used as the initial drug with thiazides, and then other drugs are added if needed. With this "stepped care" treatment, DBP can effectively be reduced below 90 mmHg in almost all patients with essential hypertension.

A decade ago it was estimated that every other subject with hypertension in the United States was unaware of the condition; that of those who were aware, half were treated; and that of those treated, half were adequately controlled. As a result of massive screening and educational programs, those figures have improved substantially. Today less than 20 percent of hypertensives do not know they have elevated blood pressure, and as many as one-third may be under effective control.

Because antihypertensive therapy is lifelong, and millions of people are receiving treatment in the United States alone, special consideration must be given to the occurrence of side effects. Besides the well-recognized adverse effects, both the diuretics and the beta-adrenergic blocking drugs have metabolic effects. Diuretics increase the levels of serum lipids (total cholesterol and triglycerides), uric acid, and blood sugar, whereas beta-adrenergic blockers affect lipids (HDL cholesterol and triglycerides). Although these metabolic changes are small to moderate, they could counteract the beneficial antihypertensive effect of these drugs.

Because of the large number of subjects with mild hypertension, the many young hypertensives, the cost of therapy, and the uncertain consequences of lifelong drug therapy, special attention has been directed at nonpharmacological interventions. Weight reduction in obese individuals and sodium restriction (0.5 g of salt daily) appear to lower blood pressure in a moderate proportion of subjects. Dietary management, which also might include reduction in alcohol consumption, appears to be a reasonable initial therapeutic alternative in selected persons and could be considered an adjunctive in all hypertensives. Biofeedback, psychotherapy, and relaxation are behavioral methods which may reduce blood pressure in some subjects. These methods should still be considered experimental. The apparent freedom of adverse effects makes nonpharmacological intervention an attractive alternative. Large-scale clinical trials are needed to determine its role in the management of hypertension.

Randomized clinical trials

The first evidence of benefit from antihypertensive therapy came from a series of Veterans Administration (VA) trials. The first trial involved patients with severe hypertension (DBP > 115 mmHg). The drop in DBP of approximately 30 mmHg caused a statistically significant reduction in so-called terminating events. In a second trial, it was demonstrated that patients with mild and moderate hypertension (DBP 90 to 114 mmHg) experienced a reduction in cardiovascular mortality of 56 percent over an average follow-up period of almost 4 years. The blood pressure decrease in this trial was 17.4 mmHg in the intervention group. The benefit was observed predominantly among the subjects with moderate hypertension (DBP 105 to 114 mmHg). These trials were conducted in middle-aged men with sustained blood pressure elevations and high prevalence of cardiovascular and renal damage. The active intervention consisted of a combination of hydrochlorothiazide, reserpine, and hydralazine given in dosages to achieve blood pressure control. The VA trials convincingly documented the value of treating moderate to severe hypertension, and antihypertensive therapy became part of standard care.

The benefit of treatment of predominantly mild hypertension was examined in the Hypertension Detection and Follow-up Program (HDFP). This trial was a community-based, controlled clinical trial that involved 10,940 subjects. Half of the subjects were randomly assigned to

a 5-year systematic-treatment program, stepped care (SC); the other half, to their regular community source of medical therapy, referred care (RC). Control of blood pressure was consistently better for the SC than the RC participants. The group difference in mean DBP was 5 mmHg. The majority of the hypertensives were controlled by step 1 medication (diuretics, predominantly chlorthalidone) or step 2 medication (diuretics and an antiadrenergic drug).

The 5-year mortality for the SC group was 17 percent lower compared to the RC group. An almost 45 percent reduction in cerebrovascular deaths was noted in the SC group. There were fewer deaths (26 percent) attributed to acute myocardial infarction but no difference in deaths from other CHD. Analyses of subgroups (sex, race, age groups) of the HDFP population have shown findings generally in accordance with the overall results. In the cohort of participants with mild hypertension (DBP 90 to 104 mmHg) the 5-year mortality for the SC group was 20.3 percent lower than for the RC group (Fig. 4). This benefit was consistent for the three blood pressure strata 90 to 94, 95 to 99, and 100 to 104 mmHg, and was independent of the presence of end-organ damage. These findings support the recommendation that antihypertensive treatment is beneficial in patients with mild hypertension, even before evidence of end-organ damage occurs.

Recent findings in the Multiple Risk Factor Intervention Trial (MRFIT) have clouded the situation. In this trial involving 12,866 high-risk men, half of the men were randomly assigned to a special intervention (SI) program which included counseling for cigarette smoking, stepped-care treatment for hypertension, and dietary advice for lowering blood cholesterol levels. The other half of the participants, the control group, were referred to their usual sources of health care in the community (UC). Those assigned to the SI program had only a 7.1 percent lower CHD mortality during the average follow-up of 7 years than those assigned to the UC program. Three possible explanations for the insignificant effect on mortality have been considered by the MRFIT investigators. Most likely, one or more components of the intervention program had a favorable affect on survival in some subgroups that was offset by an unfavorable affect in others. Measures to reduce cigarette

CUMULATIVE MORTALITY (%)
Mild Hypertension (DBP 90 to 104 mmHg)

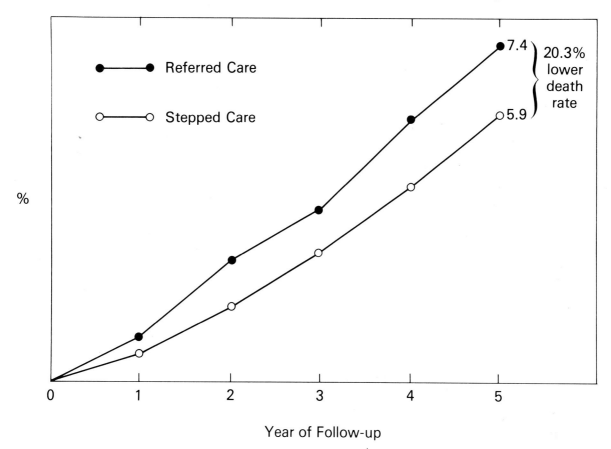

Year of Follow-up

FIGURE 4
Cumulative mortality rate associated with mild hypertension (diastolic blood pressure of 90 to 104 mmHg) over 5 years in the Hypertension Detection and Follow-up Program.

smoking and blood cholesterol levels may have lowered the mortality from CHD within subgroups of the SI men. This apparent benefit seems to be countered by a possibly unfavorable response to antihypertensive therapy in *some* but not all antihypertensive SI participants. Posthoc analyses have revealed three different patterns of response. In hypertensives with initial DBP of 95 mmHg or higher and no resting electrocardiogram (ECG) abnormality, treatment seemed to have a favorable effect. In the SI men with DBP of 90 to 94 mmHg and normal resting ECGs at base line, there was no apparent benefit. Finally, in hypertensives with resting ECG abnormalities, the mortality from CHD was substantially higher in the SI group compared to the control group. The mechanism of this possible negative effect is not known. A large proportion of the SI

men received thiazide diuretics which can induce hypokalemia, rhythm disturbances, and even hyperlipidemia. Therefore, some of the recommendations regarding antihypertensive treatment may require reassessment.

In summary, it has been convincingly demonstrated that drug treatment for moderate to severe hypertension lowers CHD risk. Future research is needed to determine whether subjects with modestly elevated blood pressure and ECG abnormalities benefit from drug therapy and to determine more firmly the role of nonpharmacological intervention.

SMOKING AS A RISK FACTOR

The first official warning that "cigarette smoking is dangerous to your health" was issued by the U.S. surgeon general in 1964. Smoking affects health in many ways and probably contributes more than any other factor to the nation's health care cost. Cigarette smokers have higher death rates from cardiovascular and cerebrovascular diseases, leading to an estimated 188,000 excess deaths from these diseases in the United States each year. Organ systems other than the cardiovascular system are also affected. Of the estimated 60,000 persons who die of lung cancer annually in the United States, 90 percent smoke cigarettes. Smokers have a 3 to 20 times higher risk of developing chronic bronchitis and pulmonary emphysema than nonsmokers, depending on age and amount smoked. People who smoke also have a higher number of other cancers, peripheral vascular diseases, and peptic ulcers.

Cigarette smoking is one of the strongest independent risk factors for CHD. Among males, the CHD death rate is on average 70 percent higher for smokers than for nonsmokers. Men aged 45 to 54 who are heavy smokers have a threefold increase in CHD mortality rate compared to nonsmokers. For female smokers in the same age group, the rate is twice that of nonsmoking women. The relationship between cigarette smoking and CHD mortality is proportional to smoking dose and duration of exposure, greater in men than women and in younger compared to older ages. Pipe and cigar smoking generally are less strongly associated with risk of CHD than cigarette smoking. Epidemiological evidence suggests that the negative effects of smoking are associated primarily with the acute precipitating event (myocardial infarction and sudden death) rather than the underlying atherosclerosis. In countries with low fat intake and low serum cholesterol levels such as Japan, the relationship between cigarette smoking and CHD mortality is less convincing.

The total cigarette consumption in the United States (expressed as prevalence of smoking among adults, especially males, and per-capita consumption) has shown a decline in the last two decades. The pattern of smoking has also changed. There has been a marked decline in consumption among adult males who are at the highest risk of developing CHD, while consumption has increased among females and young people. Nevertheless 30 billion packages of cigarettes were sold and 54 million adults continued to smoke or took up the habit in the United States in 1982. Recent survey data indicate that the proportion of persons who regularly smoke 25 or more cigarettes per day has increased during the last decade.

The inhaled cigarette smoke contains many substances that are known to be hazardous, such as tar, nicotine, and carbon monoxide. The tarry compounds are cancer-producing and lead to the development of the crippling lung diseases. The mechanisms by which smoking influences CHD are not yet clear. Nicotine increases sympathetic discharge, which is reflected in higher heart rate and increased contractility, which leads to higher oxygen demand. This is obviously more of a problem for a heart already threatened by narrowed coronary arteries. Moreover, nicotine is related experimentally to cardiac arrhythmias, endothelial damage, and thrombus formation. Carbon monoxide's affinity to hemoglobin impairs oxygen transport; this becomes most apparent during exercise. In addition, carbon monoxide may induce vascular damage and act through relative hypoxia.

Cessation of smoking

The antismoking campaign initiated by the surgeon general in 1964 initially had a major impact. However, as the intensity of the campaign eased, so did its effectiveness. Continued public education is essential to the health of the nation. The objective of education is to inform the public of the health hazards of smoking and to motivate the smokers to quit. Even more important than stopping smoking may be the efforts directed at preventing young persons from ever taking up the habit. Recent evidence would indicate that all smoking-induced damage may not be reversible.

Most smokers shed their habit without formal treatment. For those seeking treatment, three broad types of smoking cessation methods are currently employed. The first is based on the use of aversive-conditioning techniques aimed at creating a desire not to smoke in certain situations.

Electric shock is a common form. The second relies on self-control which is based on self-administered treatment, including environmental planning and behavioral programming. The third uses pharmacological treatment (nicotine) during the initial withdrawal period to reduce withdrawal symptoms. The immediate success rate for smokers who decide to quit is over 90 percent. Relapses are common, particularly during the first 3 months, and surveys have shown that only approximately one-third of quitters are successful in avoiding cigarettes for 1 year.

Among participants in clinical trials, the success rate has been higher. As described above, the men in the SI half of the MRFIT received counseling for cigarette smoking. Ten-week group sessions at the beginning of the trial turned out to be particularly successful. Dosage reduction, including switching to cigarettes low in nicotine and tar, was recommended only as an intermediate step to cessation. Five-day quit clinics, hypnosis, and aversive techniques were used in the treatment of the hard-core group of smokers during the final years of the trial. Of the 64 percent of SI men who reported themselves as current smokers at screening, approximately one-half reported that they were no longer smoking at 6 years. The 29 percent reduction in the UC group (which was unanticipated in the design) implies an increased health awareness in the past decade.

Quitting and subsequent CHD risk

Observational studies The evidence from most prospective epidemiological studies suggests that smoking cessation is associated with a severalfold decreased risk of CHD mortality. However, such studies have several methodological limitations. The quitters are usually self-selected, and comparing them to those who continue to smoke may introduce bias. A recent study has shown that quitters differ from nonquitters with respect to many characteristics. Quitters, on average, smoke fewer cigarettes, have a shorter duration of exposure, and inhale less. In addition, they have less chest pain, a lower prevalence of abnormal ECGs, higher vital capacity, and less dyspnea on exertion. These differences make interpretation of the effect of

stopping smoking difficult. Therefore, the real benefit associated with smoking cessation is best ascertained in clinical trials.

Several epidemiological studies have shown that patients who quit smoking within months of an acute myocardial infarction have a much better long-term prognosis than patients who continue to smoke. The same methodological problems pertain, but few would dispute the overall benefit of smoking cessation following a coronary event.

Randomized clinical trials The results from three clinical trials have been reported. Only one, the Whitehall study, was a single-factor intervention study. A second trial from Oslo tested the effect of combined life-style intervention, smoking cessation, and diet on the incidence of CHD. The MRFIT, the third trial, examined a multiple factor intervention which involved primarily pharmacological treatment of hypertension, dietary planning, and smoking cessation. In any clinical trial involving two or more combined treatments, it is difficult to determine the contribution of each individual one.

In the Whitehall study, a 25 percent reduction in cigarette consumption led to an 18 percent lower CHD mortality in the intervention group compared to the control group. The incidence of lung cancer was 23 percent lower. However, these differences were not statistically significant. The intervention group also experienced fewer symptoms of pulmonary disease and of loss of ventilatory function. A disturbing and as yet unexplained finding was a higher incidence of nonlung cancer in the intervention group over the 10 years of follow-up. By correcting for the dilution effect of those in the intervention group who continued to smoke, the investigators have estimated that smoking cessation reduced smoking-related mortality by approximately 30 percent over a decade. Observational studies indicate that the decrease in risk of CHD and lung cancer mortality continues for 20 years, at which time the rates for ex-smokers are similar to those of nonsmokers.

In the Oslo trial, a 5-year randomized controlled study of 1232 high-risk men, lowering of serum cholesterol and smoking cessation reduced the CHD by 47 percent. The investigators have estimated that, at most, one-quarter of the observed benefit in the intervention group can be explained by the 45 percent differences in tobacco consumption between the study groups. The smoking quit rates at the end of the 5-year study were 25 and 17 percent, respectively.

The impact of the successful smoking-cessation program on CHD mortality cannot be ascertained in MRFIT. The overall difference (7.1 percent) in CHD mortality between the SI and UC groups was not statistically significant. It is of special interest that in an "Oslo-like" cohort within MRFIT (excluding all hypertensives) the difference (48 percent) in CHD mortality between the SI and UC groups favored the SI group. This subgroup finding supports the results of the Oslo trial and the view that changes in life-style (smoking and diet) reduce the risk of CHD.

In summary, although no clinical trial has convincingly demonstrated that smoking cessation prolongs life and reduces CHD risk, the evidence points to some benefit which is difficult to quantify. It is possible that the full value of smoking cessation takes 10 to 20 years to substantiate. This would further emphasize the importance of programs aimed at preventing children and adolescents from ever starting to smoke.

RECOMMENDATIONS FOR THE PRIMARY PREVENTION OF CHD

The information just presented provides considerable justification for the identification and treatment of people at risk for developing CHD. Many official bodies in various parts of the world have regarded it as a basis for a variety of recommendations to the practitioner and the general public. Most recently, an expert committee of the World Health Organization has provided a detailed comprehensive series of recommendations in a report on the prevention of CHD which reflects a growing consensus on this matter.

We have recently been reminded of the potential for reducing CHD mortality. Over the past 15 years or so there has been a marked and unprecedented decline in cardiovascular disease mortality in the United States (Fig. 5). This has been observed in all age, sex, and race groups and does not appear to be merely a product of altered classifications of cause of death. Other

countries such as Australia and Finland have also experienced a decline. Although the secondary prevention of CHD through acute coronary care units, coronary artery bypass procedures, improved medical care, and noninvasive diagnostic methods for earlier disease detection have undoubtedly been responsible for some of the decline in CHD mortality, primary prevention measures related to increasing awareness of CHD risk factors and their modifications are also thought to have played an important role. There is suggestive evidence that total plasma cholesterol levels have dropped in the United States, possibly related to a coincident decline in the intake of dietary cholesterol and saturated fat and an increase in the intake of polyunsaturated fat. Cigarette smoking has declined in middle-aged males, and the detection, treatment, and control of high blood pressure has improved greatly. Whatever the precise explanation for the decline in coronary mortality, it is obvious that a high annual toll of life from CHD is not inevitable and that measures for the primary prevention of CHD are likely to be attended with success.

The major risk factors for CHD are susceptible to change. Cholesterol (and LDL levels) frequently have been reduced by 10 to 15 percent in large groups of subjects by dietary change. Single- or combination-drug therapy can substantially reduce this further in selected subjects. Impressive reductions in blood pressure can also be achieved in large numbers of subjects through stepped-care therapy. Nonpharmacological approaches such as weight reduction offer considerable potential. Cigarette smoking is declining markedly in certain age groups in many countries. The potential to raise HDL levels substantially through appropriate life-style alterations has been illustrated above.

Relatively small changes in CHD risk factors might produce considerable reductions in CHD risk. For example, in populations it has been calculated that average declines in serum cholesterol of 5 mg/dl, in DBP of 2 mmHg, and in the proportion of cigarette smoking of 20 percent could, in combination, result in a 21.8 percent reduction in the CHD death rate and a 15.6 percent reduction in the total death rate (Fig. 6).

The primary prevention measures should be

**Percent Change
from 1950 Rates***

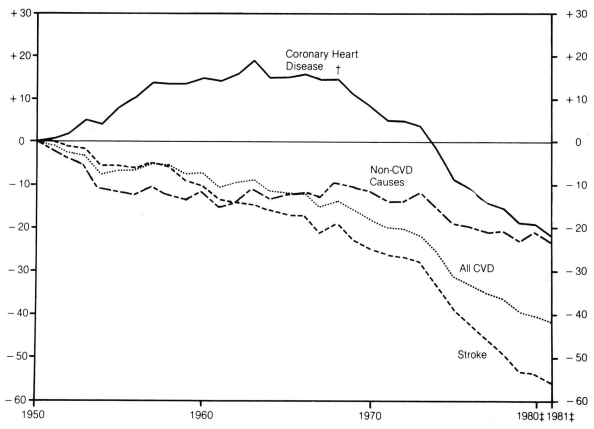

FIGURE 5

Trends in mortality for cardiovascular diseases (CVD) (and major components) and noncardiovascular

causes of death in the United States from 1950 to 1981. Rates shown are percent changes from the 1950 base line.

directed not only at high-risk individuals with very high levels of given risk factors (the traditional focus of attention of the practicing physician) but also at the population as a whole. Most people in industrialized countries have higher than optimum levels of CHD risk factors. The majority of subjects who develop CHD come from the much greater number of subjects whose risk-factor levels are not at the very top end of the distribution curve. Reduction of the major risk factors, especially by nonpharmacological means, appears to be achievable with safety, especially when the large number of subjects who are eligible for such measures are considered.

It is important to correct all relevant risk fac-

tors and not to concentrate on any one to the exclusion of the others. It makes little sense to set about reducing cholesterol (even in the hypercholesterolemic subject) without ensuring that, for example, high levels of cigarette smoking and hypertension are also addressed. Other, albeit sometimes less powerful, risk factors should also be considered, such as coincident diabetes and increased alcohol intake and its attendant risk of hypertension and CHD. Obesity probably has been underestimated as a risk factor in its own right and also as a determinant of other risk factors such as hypertension, increased serum lipids, decreased HDL, and reduced levels of exercise.

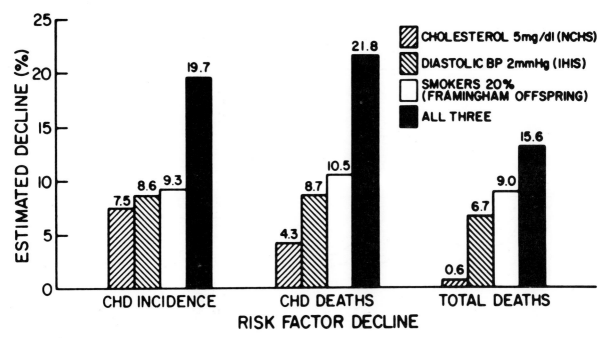

FIGURE 6
Relationship between estimated decline in a population's death rate and average declines in coronary heart disease (CHD) risk factors.

Ideally, preventive measures that have been proved to be beneficial should be instituted as early in life as possible, both to minimize the effect that the risk factor(s) can have on the development of atherosclerosis and its consequences and to counter the behaviors that lead to the development of the risk factors in the first place. Indeed, prevention should start in childhood.

With these considerations in mind, the specific preventive objectives in relation to each of the risk factors are presented below.

Serum and LDL cholesterol In general, subjects should be encouraged to reduce their fat intake from more than 40 percent of total calories to about 30 percent. Saturated fat intake should be restricted to provide not more than 10 percent of these calories, and the polyunsaturated fat intake could be increased to provide 10 percent. The P/S ratio should equal or exceed 1.0. Also, dietary cholesterol intake should be reduced to 250 mg or less per day. The substitution of animal fat by vegetable fat is the key element in achieving these changes. The decrease in dietary fat can be compensated by increasing the percentage of calories derived from carbohydrate, especially from so-called complex (high-fiber) sources. The aim should be to reduce the cholesterol level to between 180 to 200 mg/dl. Obese subjects should reduce weight since weight reduction produces additional falls in serum cholesterol levels.

Drug therapy should be reserved for subjects with high initial blood cholesterol levels in whom dietary measures fail to produce substantial reductions. Drug therapy should be tailored to the type of hyperlipidemia. Few subjects with hypertriglyceridemia without hypercholesterolemia require drug therapy.

Hypertension The beneficial effects of drug therapy are compelling in subjects with a DBP in excess of 100 mmHg. In subjects with DBPs between 90 and 99 mmHg, treatment is also advised but here there may be alternatives to drug intervention. These include weight reduction in obese subjects, perhaps salt restriction, and reduction in alcohol intake; whether one of the diuretics or beta-adrenergic blockers is preferred over the other is a subject of active investigation.

Smoking   The health implications of cigarette smoking are well known; whether cessation reduces CHD risk has not been convincingly demonstrated. However, other evidence requires us to provide strong advice to smokers to quit, and, of even more importance to nonsmokers, never to start. These measures will produce benefits on general health as well as the cardiovascular system.

References

BERTRAND E et al: Prevention of coronary heart disease: Report of a WHO expert committee. WHO Tech Rep Ser 678, 1982

CORNFIELD J, MITCHELL S: Selected risk factors in coronary disease: Possible intervention effects. Arch Environ Health 19:382, 1969

FEINLEIB M: Summary of a workshop on cholesterol and noncardiovascular disease mortality. Prev Med 11:360, 1982

GORDON T et al: High density lipoprotein as a predictive factor against coronary heart disease: The Framingham Study. Am J Med 62:707, 1977

GRUNDY SM: Dietary fats and sterols, in *Nutrition, Lipids, and Coronary Heart Disease: A Global Overview,* RI Levy et al (eds). New York, Raven Press, 1979, pp 89–118

HEISS G et al: The epidemiology of plasma high-density lipoprotein cholesterol levels: The Lipid Research Clinics Program Prevalence Study. Circulation 62 (Suppl IV):116, 1980

HJERMANN I et al: Effect of diet and smoking intervention on the incidence of coronary heart disease: Report from the Oslo Study Group of a randomized trial in healthy men. Lancet 2:1303, 1981

Hypertension Detection and Follow-up Program Cooperative Group: The effect of treatment on mortality in "mild" hypertension: Results of the Hypertension Detection and Follow-up Program. N Engl J Med 307:976, 1982

KANNEL WB et al: Serum cholesterol, lipoproteins, and the risk of coronary heart disease: The Framingham Study. Ann Intern Med 74:1, 1971

LEVY RI: Review: Declining mortality in coronary heart disease. Arteriosclerosis 1:312, 1981

Multiple Risk Factor Intervention Trial Research Group: Multiple risk factor intervention trial: Risk factor changes and mortality results. JAMA 248:1465, 1982

Report from the Committee of Principal Investigators: A cooperative trial in the primary prevention of ischaemic heart disease using clofibrate. Br Heart J 40:1069, 1978

ROSE G ET AL: A randomized controlled trial of antismoking advice: 10-year results. J Epidemiol Community Health 36:102, 1982

STAMLER J: Population Studies, in *Nutrition, Lipids, and Coronary Heart Disease: A Global Overview,* RI Levy et al (eds). New York, Raven Press, 1979, pp 25–88

THERAPEUTIC PLASMAPHERESIS AND RELATED APHERESIS TECHNIQUES

DAVID WARD

Therapeutic plasmapheresis has become popular within the last few years. One estimate is that 140,000 procedures were done between 1979 and early 1983 in the United States, Britain, France, and Canada. The widespread availability of automated cell-separator centrifuges, and to a lesser extent membrane-filtration machines, probably has been both a result and a cause of this remarkable upsurge of interest. Plasmapheresis or other apheresis techniques are being applied to the treatment of a large variety of diseases in which immunological derangement or abnormal plasma biochemistry occurs. Clinical use was accelerated by initial reports of dramatic successes, though the theoretical justification for the procedure is tenuous for some diseases, and justification in terms of demonstrated efficacy in clinical trials has often lagged far behind empirical use. Nevertheless, investigational interest has been intense during the last 3 years, and data are now accumulating to evaluate some of the more prominent uses of apheresis. These data permit a preliminary assessment of the current and potential place in medical therapeutics of this costly and not hazard-free procedure. Therapeutic cytapheresis, using centrifugal cell-separators for white cell removal or red cell exchange, is also being actively pursued and is included in this discussion.

HISTORICAL PERSPECTIVE

The origins of plasmapheresis

The term *plasmapheresis* was introduced in 1914 by J. J. Abel and his colleagues in a remarkable account of their animal experiments at Johns Hopkins University (Fig. 1). Similar methods for selective plasma removal had previously been employed in France: in animals in 1902 and in a patient with renal failure in 1909. These pioneering attempts succeeded in removing large quantities of plasma by repeated phlebotomy and sequential reinfusion of separated red cells in a replacement salt solution. Conservation of red cell mass and intravascular volume in this way permitted the procedure to be repeated multiple times.

From the outset, therefore, plasmapheresis overcame the major limitations of its time-honored predecessor, bloodletting. However, the intuitive rationale was the same. Indeed, the concepts of removal of toxins and restoration of humoral balance by bloodletting can be traced back to ancient Egyptian times. In many other cultures, from ancient Hindu medicine to the healing magic of some primitive South American tribes, bloodletting was performed for the treatment of disease. Hippocrates (ca. 460 to 377 B.C.) from his own experience recommended the use of bleeding for conditions ranging from acute pleurisy to headache. Bleeding became widespread among the followers of Eristratus (died 304 B.C.) whose theories ascribed many illnesses to "plethora," or surfeit of blood. The balance of the four humors (blood, phlegm, yellow bile, and black bile) as the determinant of temperament was proposed by Galen (ca. 130 to 200 A.D.), who also recorded criteria for the utilization of phlebotomy. Thereafter, bloodletting was a regular practice in European cultures and reached its zenith in the sixteenth and seven-

PLASMA REMOVAL WITH RETURN OF CORPUSCLES
(PLASMAPHAERESIS)

FIRST PAPER

JOHN J. ABEL, L. G. ROWNTREE AND B. B. TURNER

From the Pharmacological Laboratory of the Johns Hopkins University

Received for publication, July 16, 1914

I. In connection with our experiments on vividiffusion[1] with a view to the ultimate use of the method for the relief of toxaemia the idea suggested itself to try the effects of the repeated removal of considerable quantities of blood, replacing the plasma by Locke's solution and reinjecting this together with the sedimented corpuscles.

FIGURE 1

The first published description of plasmapheresis ("plasmaphaeresis"). (Reproduced from J Pharmacol Exp Ther, 5:625, 1914 with permission of the publisher.)

teenth centuries. Even well into the nineteenth century, leeches and phlebotomy enjoyed acceptance in the treatment of many diseases. However, by then the hazards and abuses of excessive bleeding had increasingly overshadowed and obscured any merits of the procedure. In Philadelphia, for instance, the unusually high mortality rate of the yellow fever epidemic of 1793 was linked to the aggressive bloodletting practices of Benjamin Rush, a figure of medical and political prominence. Bloodletting probably also hastened the death of George Washington. Bleeding of patients three or four times daily for days on end was practiced in Europe until the 1880s, when with the death of Bouillaud, "the last of the great bleeders," the era of indiscriminate bloodletting came to an end.

Abel, circumventing the principal drawbacks of bloodletting but expecting to find "some basis of truth" in "an empirical method so universally practiced since prehippocratic days," pursued evaluation of plasmapheresis in animals and

showed that the "toxemia" following bilateral nephrectomy was relieved by this procedure. From 1920 to 1940, Whipple and others established the safety of frequent plasmapheresis in animals. The use of manual plasmapheresis in human volunteers was reported in 1944 as a means of obtaining plasma for transfusion, a military need in wartime. In the 1950s and 1960s, this was developed as a practical and efficient means of supplying plasma. In contrast, plasmapheresis for therapeutic purposes, when done manually, is time-consuming and cumbersome, since it requires numerous cycles of phlebotomy, centrifugation, and reinfusion of the packed cells and replacement volume. In 1955, its use was first described for the treatment of autoimmune hemolytic anemia; in 1960, for Waldenström's macroglobulinemia.

The development of automated apheresis

Efficient large-volume plasmapheresis using automated equipment and on-line extracorporeal blood flow became possible with the advent of blood cell separators in the late 1960s.

One lineage of technical development can be

traced back to 1878 with the invention in Sweden of the DeLaval cream separator, a centrifuge device which revolutionized the dairy industry. Using the principle of centrifugal separation, the Cohn fractionator was developed in the 1940s for the in vitro separation of plasma from whole blood. In 1961 Bierman modified this for on-line leukocyte depletion, mainly to study the kinetics of cell populations. Further development of the centrifuge bowl by Latham led to production in 1970 of the Little/Abbott Model 10 and in 1973 of the Haemonetics Model 30 centrifuge, which is a single-speed discontinuous-flow machine still widely used for harvesting platelets and granulocytes and for plasma-exchange therapy (Fig. 2A).

The main stimulus to the development of blood-cell-separator machines in the 1960s was the collaboration of E. J. Freireich of the National Cancer Institute (NCI) and G. Judson of the International Business Machine Corporation (IBM), whose interest in white cell removal therapy for the treatment of leukemia led to the development of the NCI-IBM experimental blood cell separator (IBM model 2990-6) in 1965. This was the first production model of an on-line blood centrifuge, and it utilized two concentric rotating seals to overcome the difficult technical problem of simultaneously passing blood and various blood components into and out of the rotating centrifuge bowl. The Aminco Celltrifuge, a further development of the same design, was the dominant continuous-flow machine from its introduction in 1970 until 1978. The NCI-IBM and Aminco machines had reusable bowls that had to be cleaned and sterilized for each use.

CONTEMPORARY APHERESIS MACHINES

Contemporary centrifuge machines all have sterile, disposable, closed circuits for the blood. Though there are many different configurations and designs, the basic principles are the same as those employed in the prototypes described above. In all models, the blood is layered into packed red cells at the bottom, above which is the buffy coat, and then the plasma at the top. Any of these three components can be removed selectively with appropriately placed sampling

ports. Within the buffy coat, the granulocytes, lymphocytes, and platelets also achieve some degree of separation. The modern continuous-flow machines employ a variable-speed centrifuge, allowing additional control over the degree of separation of different components. For instance, at a lower g force, a platelet-rich plasma is formed and a highly selected white cell product can be removed from the buffy coat without losing platelets.

Among the continuous-flow centrifuge machines, the IBM 2997, introduced in 1978, incorporates radically different design features, notably a separation channel of narrow cross-sectional area which forms a closed loop around a large flywheel; it is versatile and efficient in all types of therapeutic and harvesting techniques (Fig. 2B). The Fenwal Centrifuge II is a derivative of the Aminco Celltrifuge. The Fenwal CS-3000 has a unique sealless system, including collection bags within the centrifuge and microprocessor-controlled programs; thus it is most suited for the purpose of efficient blood-product harvesting from donors (Fig. 2C). Other continuous-flow machines include one by the Dideco Company of Italy.

Contemporary discontinuous-flow machines include the still-popular Haemonetics 30 and the newer models by Haemonetics and other manufacturers. In these, while the centrifuge bowl continues to fill, plasma, platelets, and white cells are pumped out in succession. The centrifuge is then stopped, and the packed red cells are returned to the patient or to a reservoir before the cycle is repeated.

Centrifugal cell-separators have virtually superseded the technique of filtration leukapheresis, a method of harvesting granulocytes by adherence to nylon fibers. This system was developed by Djerassi and marketed by Fenwal. It allowed efficient collection of granulocytes from a single donor on a continuous-flow basis.

A second-generation technique consists of membrane filters for the separation of plasma from whole blood. Several manufacturers have developed hollow-fiber filters with configurations similar to modern hemodialyzers. The pore sizes are 0.2 μm or larger, allowing sieving of all but the cellular elements of the blood. The Cobe therapeutic plasma-exchange machine utilizes a plasma-permeable membrane in a flat-layer con-

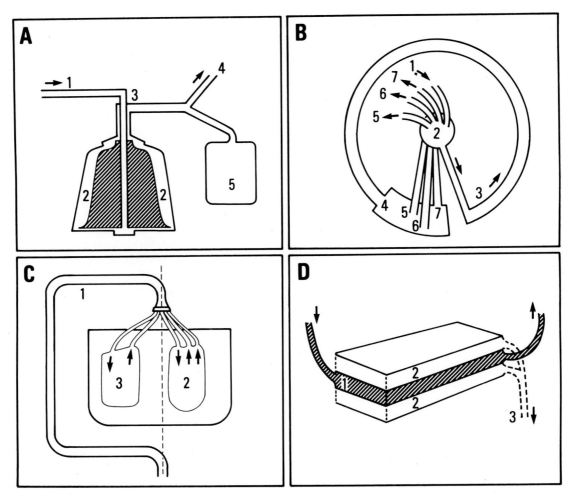

FIGURE 2

A. Side view of the Latham bowl of the Haemonetics discontinuous-flow centrifuge machine. Whole blood entering (1) is centrifuged (2), and the plasma, platelets, and white cells are removed sequentially through the coaxial exit port (3) and then either returned to the patient (4) or diverted to waste (collection) (5). B. Vertical view of the centrifuge insert of the IBM 2997 continuous-flow machine. Whole blood (1) entering through the rotating seal (2) enters the centrifugation channel (3) and is layered by the time it reaches the collection chamber (4), where ports at different levels remove the buffy coat (5), packed red cells (6), and remaining plasma (7), which are pumped out via the rotating seal (2) to be selectively removed or returned to the patient. C. Side view of the centrifuge of the Fenwal CS 3000 continuous-flow machine. Whole
blood enters the centrifuge via a unique sealless multiple lumen tube (1) and enters the separation bag (2) where it separates into packed red cells and platelet-rich plasma. These are then pumped out separately (1), and the component-rich plasma is then pumped in again (1) to the collection bag (3), which is further from the axis of rotation and, therefore, experiencing higher g force. The platelets collect in the bag (3) throughout the run, and the platelet-free plasma is pumped out and discarded. In therapeutic plasmapheresis, the platelet bag is reinfused to the patient after the run is completed. D. Schematic representation of a flat-plate membrane plasma-separator as in the Cobe machine. Whole blood (1) runs between alternate layers of semipermeable membranes, and the plasma is filtered through (2) and is extracted (3).

figuration (Fig. 2D). Centrifugal plasmapheresis has been the predominant method employed, especially in North America, whereas membrane plasmapheresis was pioneered in Europe and Japan.

APHERESIS MODALITIES AND TERMINOLOGY

Apheresis is derived from the Greek αφαιρειν, which means "to remove" or "to take away by force'' (quite different from the derivation of *electrophoresis*). Contraction of the word *apheresis* to *pheresis* is not justifiable. The proliferation of composite words such as lymphoplasmapheresis is probably acceptable, provided that an ''o'' is never allowed to replace the ''a.'' The terms *thrombocytapheresis* or *thrombapheresis* are correct, but ''thrombocytopheresis'' and ''thrombopheresis'' are unacceptable misspellings. *Hemapheresis* is now used synonymously with apheresis as a general term encompassing all procedures for the selective removal of any fraction of .the blood, either as therapy for a disease or as a means for harvesting blood products from healthy donors. Similarly, *cytapheresis* refers to removal of any cellular fraction of the blood in any setting. Donor apheresis applications include collection of plasma, platelets, white cells, or neocytes (the youngest, least dense, red cells); donor procedures will not be discussed further.

Plasmapheresis

Therapeutic plasmapheresis is now rarely done manually and is usually accomplished with either a centrifuge machine or a membrane plasma-separator. The term *plasma exchange* has been proposed as more descriptive when amounts of the order of 1.0 volume of plasma are removed. However, plasma is often not exchanged for plasma, because the replacement volume more commonly consists of an albumin solution. Nevertheless, *therapeutic plasmapheresis* and *therapeutic plasma exchange* are used virtually interchangeably, and either term can refer to any therapeutic plasma-removal procedure of whatever volume, regardless of the type of replacement solution used.

At a time when the mechanism of action and efficacy of even whole-plasma removal remain debatable, there is only a limited clinical role for methods where most of the plasma is returned to the patient after it has been selectively ''purified'' by the specific depletion of putative pathogenic factors. However, research is well-developed using several plasma-processing techniques, including plasmaperfusion columns, cascade plasma separation, and cryogelation (see below). The discussion given below of the clinical use of plasmapheresis in specific diseases refers only to whole-plasma removal, except

where specifically stated. It is assumed that the results obtained for centrifugal plasmapheresis will pertain also to membrane plasmapheresis (i.e., that any differences in the handling of large macromolecules will always be too subtle to be of clinical significance).

Leukapheresis

Cytapheresis, using centrifugal machines of either discontinuous- or continuous-flow type, can be tailored for the removal of any specific type of circulating white blood cell (*leukapheresis*). However, the efficiency and selectivity differ depending on the system used. Leukemic cells, be they abnormal lymphocytes, mature granulocytes, or blast cells, can be selectively removed from leukemic patients with high white cell counts; these forms of leukapheresis are also known as ''therapeutic white cell reduction.'' Leukapheresis for lymphocytes (*lymphocytapheresis*) has been used for some immunological diseases; lymphocytapheresis has often been used together with plasmapheresis, as described in the next section. Leukapheresis techniques can be adjusted to achieve removal of large numbers of eosinophils from patients with eosinophilia, but this appears to be of no value in the control of hypereosinophilic syndromes.

Lymphoplasmapheresis

The combination of lymphocytapheresis and plasmapheresis (*lymphoplasmapheresis*) is employed to interrupt the cell-mediated as well as the humoral components of immunity in some immunological diseases. Most centrifugal machines can isolate a lymphocyte-rich layer from the buffy coat, though in some systems a choice must be made of either a sequential removal first of lymphocytes and then of platelet-free plasma or a more rapid simultaneous removal in which platelets must also be sacrificed. A large yield of lymphocytes is usually obtained, though the quantity and purity vary in different systems.

Thrombocytapheresis

Cytapheresis for platelets can be readily applied as a therapeutic procedure (''therapeutic platelet reduction'') in cases of severe thrombocythemia, which occurs usually in the context of leukemia.

Techniques using all types of centrifugal machines have been perfected based on their frequent use in donor (harvesting) work.

Erythrocytapheresis

Therapeutic red cell exchange (*erythrocytapheresis*), which has found an established place at least in the management of sickle cell disease, can be achieved very elegantly using some of the modern continuous-flow centrifuge machines. The packed red cell layer is discarded and replaced by donor packed cells. Except in infants and small children, the ease and efficiency of this procedure usually makes it preferable to manual exchange transfusion.

PERFORMANCE OF THERAPEUTIC PLASMAPHERESIS

Therapeutic plasmapheresis can now be performed safely and efficiently in the great majority of patients. The key ingredients are state-of-the-art equipment and a highly trained and experienced nurse-operator. Plasmapheresis has been tolerated well by patients of all ages and by pregnant patients. It has become feasible even in small infants, though it is necessary to use a continuous-flow centrifuge and to devote special skill and attention to the appropriate priming of the blood circuit and to the very accurate maintenance of intravascular volume. Most authorities are agreed that therapeutic apheresis should be carried out only in a hospital setting. A physician with special knowledge and experience of apheresis should be responsible for supervision of each procedure and for making appropriate choices regarding the medical practicalities.

Medical practicalities

A whole-blood flow rate between 30 and 90 ml/min is desirable with centrifugal apheresis equipment. Membrane plasmapheresis machines handle a higher flow rate if this can be achieved. In the majority of adult patients, the extracorporeal blood circuit runs from one antecubital vein to the other, and needles are placed at the start and removed at the end of each procedure. If necessary, outflow can be aided by a tourniquet to produce venous distention. Single-needle access is feasible with some machines, but two needles are usually preferred for therapeutic procedures, particularly in children where volume shifts are proportionately larger. In adults with tenuous veins, and in children, some type of indwelling vascular access is usually needed and can avert repeated painful venipunctures when a course of several procedures is planned. Semirigid subclavian vein catheters, either single-lumen or double-lumen, as developed for hemodialysis use, are effective for hemapheresis. They can be kept free of thrombosis and infection for long periods if handled correctly and can even be maintained in outpatients. Ordinary subclavian vein catheters collapse with negative pressure and are useless for drawing blood. Hickman catheters and some other large central lines can be used as the draw line. Occasionally, a femoral vein catheter, a Scribner shunt, or even a permanent arteriovenous fistula is needed, but thrombosis and infection may be troublesome.

Anticoagulation   Citrate, usually in a standard blood-banking formulation, is the most commonly employed anticoagulant. It is infused into the extracorporeal circuit close to the draw-line needle, and because it chelates all calcium it ensures complete extracorporeal anticoagulation, even if the blood flow has to be discontinued for a period. On reentering the patient, the citrate is immediately neutralized by excess blood calcium and is then metabolized, though the patient must be monitored for the hypocalcemic symptoms of citrate toxicity. Supplemental calcium may be given prophylactically in unstable patients. Heparin is preferred in membrane plasmapheresis systems and may also be used in centrifugal machines. Systemic heparinization (with its usual risks) of course occurs, and the platelet effects of heparin may be undesirable. However, at least some heparin should be used in addition to citrate when the outflow line is a Hickman catheter or other long line that would otherwise not be anticoagulated throughout its length.

Therapeutic regimens   The volume of plasma to remove in a single procedure should usually be 1.0 to 1.5 times the calculated plasma volume. A 1.0-volume exchange will remove 63 percent of native plasma, and a 1.5-volume exchange will increase this to 78 percent. Because of the semilogarithmic relationship (Fig. 3), progressive prolongation of the procedure is of decreasing benefit. The plasma volume of an adult is approximately 40 ml/kg; therefore, a typical plasma exchange is in the range of 2.5 to 4.5 liters.

The frequency at which plasmapheresis procedures should be repeated depends on the disease being treated or, theoretically, on the rate of reappearance in the plasma of the putative noxious material that is to be removed. After the end of a plasmapheresis, the rate of reappearance in the plasma of various materials differs widely, depending on whether there is rapid reequilibration from extravascular sites and on the rate of resynthesis. In hyperviscosity syndrome, for example, an IgM paraprotein can be largely depleted in one or two standard runs because IgM is predominantly confined to the vascular space and the rate of resynthesis may be slow. In contrast, an IgG autoantibody will reappear rapidly by reequilibration from the rest of the extracellular fluid space, and its resynthesis may be difficult to suppress (Fig. 4). In many such conditions, a regimen of intensive plasmapheresis is employed, commencing with alternate-day, or even daily, procedures and continuing as often as three times per week for 3 weeks or longer. In diseases due to a single abnormal

KINETICS OF PLASMA REMOVAL

FIGURE 3

For a plasma constituent that is not augmented from the extravascular space by reequilibration or resynthesis during continuous-flow plasmapheresis, the fraction remaining ("y") in the plasma after "x" plasma volumes have been exchanged is given by the equation $y = e^{-x}$. Thus, after 1.5 volumes of plasma have been exchanged, 0.22 of the original constituents remain (78 percent removal).

plasma constituent that can be accurately measured, monitoring of serial plasma levels can guide the duration and intensity of plasmapheresis treatment. On the other hand, an arbitrary

FIGURE 4

Life-threatening hyperviscosity caused by an IgM para(cryo)protein was corrected very efficiently (A) by two 3-liter plasmapheresis exchanges (↑) reflecting the fact that IgM is mostly intravascular and that paraproteins are usually synthesized slowly. The patient had no more symptoms and responded well to cytotoxic drug treatment of an underlying lymphocytic lymphoma. In contrast, an IgG autoantibody causing

very severe pemphigus vulgaris continued to be synthesized despite immunosuppressive therapy, and the plasma levels rebounded after each of several 3.5-liter plasmapheresis exchanges (B) because of extravascular IgG pools. This patient's skin was greatly improved for several months, but autoantibody levels could not be contained by immunosuppression alone, and he later died of uncontrollable skin breakdown and infection.

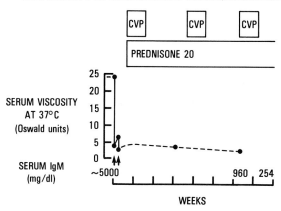

PLASMAPHERESIS FOR WALDENSTROM'S MACROGLOBULINEMIA

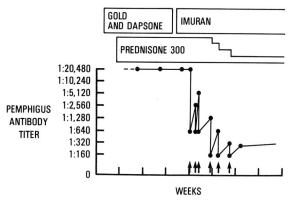

PLASMAPHERESIS FOR SEVERE PEMPHIGUS VULGARIS

approach is necessary if no marker is available, or in so-called immune-complex diseases, where measurements of circulating immune complexes may not directly reflect the activity of the underlying disease process.

Replacement fluids The plasma removed during plasmapheresis must be matched by a similar volume of replacement solution. Commonly, the first one-third is given as isotonic saline and the remaining two-thirds as 5% albumin solution or 4% plasma-protein solution. Albumin solutions are well tolerated and are free of viral particles; most preparations have a suitable electrolyte composition, though a few should not be used for large-volume infusion because of their low chloride and high acetate or citrate content that will cause metabolic alkalosis. Plasma protein fraction (PPF) is also hepatitis-free, but may contain more aggregated protein than pure albumin solutions and may cause hypotension due to the presence of activated kinin precursors. A balanced salt solution may be used instead of saline, or calcium, magnesium, and potassium may be added to the replacement fluids on an individualized basis. Salt solutions should be given at a rate slightly faster than the rate of plasma removal, in order to conserve circulating volume in the face of falling plasma oncotic pressure. Fresh frozen plasma (FFP) replacement has also been used widely in plasmapheresis. FFP is specifically indicated in disorders such as thrombotic thrombocytopenic purpura, where factor replenishment is thought to be of crucial importance to therapy. When an intensive plasmapheresis regimen is being pursued using albumin replacement, the addition of some FFP can help correct cumulative depletion of clotting factors, though this must be balanced against the risk of hepatitis from FFP. Dextrans, hydroxyethyl starch, modified fluid gelatin, and other artificial colloids are cheaper but may have unphysiological effects when used as replacement fluids.

Risks and complications

Therapeutic plasmapheresis is usually well tolerated, though transient side effects are seen in 15 percent or more of patients. Paresthesiae around the mouth or in the extremities, or a feeling of tension or vibration, can occur due to citrate-induced hypocalcemia but will usually respond to stopping the citrate temporarily or to infusion of 10% calcium chloride. Left untreated, citrate toxicity can progress to nausea, vomiting, twitching, chills, spasms, syncope, or various arrhythmias. Other electrolyte changes, including reduction of magnesium or potassium, are usually self-limited but potentially could also precipitate symptoms. Hemodynamic imbalance due to volume mismatching may also occur, despite the sophisticated monitors and calibrated pumps of modern machines. Moreover, careful clinical assessment is mandatory to determine unexpected volume shifts into and out of the intravascular space due to increased or depleted plasma colloid. For reasons that are unclear, hypotension or hypertension may occasionally occur even when plasma volume and plasma oncotic pressure appear to have been accurately conserved. A few patients who have no symptoms during plasmapheresis report ill-defined tiredness for several hours after the procedure is over.

The risk of life-threatening emergencies during apheresis procedures is low, but the incidence varies greatly among different surveys. Overall, fatalities during or immediately following therapeutic plasmapheresis have been estimated at about 3 per 10,000 procedures. However, a disproportionate number of the unexpected deaths appear to have occurred during FFP replacement. Many were ascribed to cardiac events or to acute pulmonary edema not due to volume overload but heralded by coughing and dyspnea. A few were recognized as anaphylactic in type, and leukoagglutinins (not anti-histocompatibility leukocyte antigen) have been postulated as the cause in at least one fatal case. The incidence of urticaria, fevers, and other possibly allergic events is also quite different in reports from different countries. It has not been determined whether this reflects known differences in local preference for various types and sources of replacement colloids. Severe, even fatal, cardiac arrhythmias have been recorded during apheresis in the absence of overt citrate toxicity or electrolyte imbalance. One avoidable cause is the rapid return of cold or citrated blood via a long central line too close to the heart.

A common practical difficulty in performing apheresis is inadequacy of blood flow from peripheral vein needles. Indwelling catheters in large veins can also cause problems, including perforation of the vessel, thrombosis, infection, and pneumothorax (during the insertion of subclavian lines). Blood leaks in the extracorporeal circuit are unusual and are easily controlled. Clotting within the machine occurs occasionally, but clot traps in the return line provide considerable protection. Modern machines are equipped with bubble traps and air-foam detectors, which eliminate the risk of air embolism. In treating patients with mixed cryoglobulins, cryoprecipitable paraproteins, or cold agglutinins, there is a risk of gelation of the blood in the extracorporeal circuit due to cooling. This can usually be prevented only by heating ambient air in the treatment room to body temperature.

Hemolysis is not a problem in centrifuge machines, and membrane machines have hydraulic systems to limit the transmembrane pressure so that shear forces on cells near the membrane surface remain insufficient to cause hemolysis. Membrane filters show progressive loss of the sieving coefficient for larger molecules, due to the accumulation of proteins within the membrane pores, but this tendency has been reduced to acceptable levels in modern designs. Some loss of platelets occurs with every plasmapheresis but is of clinical importance only if there is preexisting thrombocytopenia. Cumulative anemia during intensive plasmapheresis is recognized occasionally and has not been fully explained. Overenthusiastic blood sampling may sometimes contribute to anemia, but red cell trapping in the machine appears to be only a minor or a negligible factor in most cases. Oral iron and folic acid appear to help prevent this syndrome.

Intensive plasmapheresis with only albumin-saline replacement depletes clotting factors, and clinically troublesome hemorrhagic states have occurred even in patients who did not receive heparin. The rate of reappearance is different for different blood proteins, and indeed, plasmapheresis has afforded an opportunity for interesting observations concerning coagulation factors. For example, fibrinogen and factors XI and XIII tend to recover slowest. Also, antithrombin factor III tends to become depleted, though it is unclear how much this contributes to thrombotic events. These have included stroke, peripheral gangrene, and avascular necrosis of bone. Plasma cholinesterase depletion has been described, presenting clinically as a prolonged suxamethonium-apnea syndrome. The possibility of other unexpected events being due to deficiency or imbalance of other plasma factors must also be considered. For instance, rare cases of altered vascular tone, seizures, and disseminated intravascular coagulation are currently unexplained, and other complications will likely be described. Dilution of blood-group antibody titers, especially if compounded by transient acquisition of others from FFP replacement, may cause difficulty in cross matching the patient for transfusions. Also there is temporary lowering of transaminases and other enzymes which are used as diagnostic tests.

Alterations in drug kinetics have now been quantitated in some instances. Protein-bound drugs, such as corticosteroids, are most prone to being depleted. Indeed, after plasmapheresis some steroid-treated patients have developed volume-unresponsive hypotension that has only been corrected when intravenous steroids were given.

Infection related to plasmapheresis takes two forms. First, the commonest applications of therapeutic plasmapheresis are now in patients with diseases already being treated with corticosteroids or other immunosuppressive drugs, which can be expected to increase the risk of opportunistic infection. Also, indwelling vascular lines are a ready portal for bacterial entry in these patients. However, it is debated whether there is an increased incidence of septicemias, pneumonias, and other infections with plasmapheresis compared to patients with the same diagnoses that are treated only with corticosteroids and other immunosuppressives. Avoidance of immunoglobulin depletion below 25 percent of normal by the administration of FFP or intravenous immunoglobulin during plasmapheresis has been recommended to help prevent infection, but the balance of risks and benefits has not been evaluated in this circumstance. The second category of infectious risk is viral transmission from blood products. This does not occur with most protein solutions but is a prominent reason for caution in the use of FFP. Now that hepatitis B can be avoided routinely, non-A, non-B hepatitis is the commoner problem and constitutes a major risk when 15 or 20 units of FFP are used each time for frequently repeated plasmapheresis procedures. Though not yet reported in this setting, transmission of acquired immunodeficiency syndrome (AIDS) by FFP must be considered a possibility.

THERAPEUTIC USES OF PLASMAPHERESIS AND LYMPHOCYTAPHERESIS

Potential rationales

Plasmapheresis therapy has been applied to over 100 different diseases (Table 1). So far, in only a few of these is there convincing evidence of worthwhile therapeutic benefit. The need for more controlled trials is widely recognized, and many are in progress. The caveats against recommending treatment based only on belief or anecdotal evidence are germane, though many of the diseases in question are capricious and notoriously difficult to study.

For most potential indications for plasmapheresis, the theoretical rationale is the removal of either demonstrable or putative pathogenic materials from the bloodstream. Most such materials presumably are proteins, protein-bound, or otherwise large enough to be nondialyzable. Those that are known include paraproteins, excess lipids or lipoproteins, abnormal metabolites, excess hormones, exogenous poisons and drugs, autoantibodies and alloantibodies of many types, and circulating immune complexes and other potentially harmful products of humoral immune reactions. Circulating immune complexes (CIC), meaning antigen-antibody complexes, have been implicated not only because of their apparent ability to induce inflammatory damage where they are deposited but possibly because of potential interference with other immune mechanisms. For instance, evidence has been offered that reticuloendothelial blockade, specifically involving immune-mediated phagocytosis, occurs in systemic lupus erythematosus and related diseases, and that CIC removal by plasmapheresis

may relieve this blockade and thus allow resumption of endogenous removal of CIC. Other speculations concerning the potential benefits of plasmapheresis therapy include the removal of possible blocking factors of cell-mediated and tumoricidal immunity. In some diseases where CIC are found, it is unclear whether it is the removal of CIC themselves that is of importance. Indeed, much of the time CIC may be relatively innocuous and may be merely by-products of other, more important immunological events. Although claims have been made in several diseases that the response to plasmapheresis has been more favorable in patients with high levels of CIC than in those without, this observation has often been disputed.

Inferring the success of plasmapheresis therapy by following serial blood tests may be misleading. Some epiphenomena traditionally useful in monitoring the activity of inflammatory diseases may be artificially altered by plasma exchange. For instance, an elevated erythrocyte sedimentation rate (ESR) or gamma globulin is very often improved by intensive plasmapheresis, irrespective of whether or not the underlying disease is affected. In contrast, if an abnormal plasma constituent, such as a specific autoantibody, is known to actually cause a disease, demonstration of its depletion by plasmapheresis may be predictive of clinical benefit. However, in the majority of autoantibody-induced or immune-complex-type diseases, concurrent treatment with corticosteroids, often plus azathioprine or cyclophosphamide, is necessary to effect serial depletion of antibodies. Otherwise "rebound" antibody resynthesis will occur. Evidence that a stimulus to antibody production is a low plasma immunoglobulin level has been quoted as a theoretical reason to favor preventing immunoglobulin depletion in these diseases, either by FFP replacement or by the parenteral administration of a human IgG preparation after each plasmapheresis. Indeed, loss of feedback inhibition of antibody production has been suggested as a reason for caution in performing plasmapheresis during acute immune responses.

For a few diseases the rationale of plasmapheresis is quite different; rather than removing abnormal materials, the benefit appears to be due to replacing missing factors present in normal plasma. In these instances, the volume of FFP required is greater than can be given without plasma exchange. As well as providing unidentified plasma factors important in the treatment of thrombotic thrombocytopenic purpura and perhaps hemolytic-uremic syndrome, massive plasma exchange has been used to replace congenitally missing enzymes (e.g., Hunter's syndrome) and potentially could work to take up and remove excesses of protein-bindable hormones.

The use of lymphocytapheresis and lymphoplasmapheresis is discussed together with plasmapheresis because these modalities have been used almost interchangeably in several inflammatory and immunological diseases. Lymphocytapheresis has been shown capable of achieving prolonged lymphocyte depletion and immunological changes comparable to those recorded with thoracic duct drainage but with greater simplicity and safety. Therefore, the conditions to which it has been applied include rheumatoid arthritis and renal transplantation, in both of which a beneficial effect of thoracic duct drainage has previously been described.

Hematological diseases

Hyperviscosity syndrome The hyperviscosity syndrome is one of the few diseases in which plasmapheresis is of undisputed therapeutic value. Waldenström's macroglobulinemia, in which IgM paraprotein (monoclonal immunoglobulin) is overproduced by proliferating neoplastic B lymphocytes or plasma cells, is typified by fatigue, cerebral dysfunction, congestive retinopathy, mucous membrane bleeding, and congestive cardiac dysfunction. These clinical features are due to an increase in plasma viscosity and an expansion of plasma volume. Sometimes the paraprotein is cryoprecipitable, which may cause cold urticaria or livedo reticularis. Because the IgM paraprotein is 80 percent intravascular, most of it can be removed in one or two plasmapheresis procedures (Fig. 4A). Plasmapheresis is indicated at the time of presentation if the patient is symptomatic or if plasma viscosity is elevated above about 5 Oswald

units.[1] Plasmapheresis usually produces immediate symptomatic relief from hyperviscosity, and reduction of hypervolemia can also be achieved during the procedure by giving only partial volume replacement. Anemia in this syndrome is usually part dilutional and part real, and red cell transfusion is safe once some reduction in viscosity and hypervolemia has been obtained. Chemotherapy commenced simultaneously is effective in controlling paraprotein production in most cases, and only a few patients need repeated plasmapheresis at intervals of weeks or months. IgG or IgA paraproteins, usually associated with multiple myeloma or lymphocytic lymphoma, may cause similar hyperviscosity problems. In the initial treatment, plasmapheresis may be needed several times because typically only 40 percent of these smaller paraproteins is in the vascular compartment. Serial measurements of viscosity or immunoglobulin quantitations are an excellent guide to determining the need for subsequent plasmapheresis.

Thrombotic thrombocytopenic purpura (TTP)

TTP is a rare disorder of unknown cause in which thrombocytopenia, microangiopathic hemolytic anemia, fever, neurological dysfunction. and other organ involvement fluctuate repeatedly during a course that may last from a few weeks to many months. While in the past the disease was usually fatal, modern therapy now achieves a survival rate estimated at 60 to 80 percent. This is attributable to the effects of plasmapheresis with plasma infusion, employed usually in conjunction with antiplatelet agents.[2] Plasma exchange was the natural successor to promising results with whole-blood exchange, but benefit from other treatments, including steroids, heparin, aspirin, and splenectomy, is much less consistent. Reported successes with plasma infusion alone make it unclear whether plasma removal is important or whether it is the replenishment of a missing plasma factor that produces the improvement. Controlled trials to try to answer this

[1] *See the tenth edition of* Harrison's Principles of Internal Medicine, *chap. 65.*

[2] *See the tenth edition of* Harrison's Principles of Internal Medicine, *chap. 329.*

TABLE 1
Diseases treated by apheresis

	Accepted therapy	Prospective randomized controlled trials in progress	Case reports or series only
*Plasmapheresis (and lympho-cytapheresis)**			
Hematological diseases	Hyperviscosity syndrome (Waldenström's syndrome and others)	Thrombotic thrombcytopenic purpura† Idiopathic thrombocytopenic purpura Rhesus hemolytic disease	Autoimmune hemolytic anemia Evans' syndrome Paroxysmal cold hemoglobinuria Paroxysmal nocturnal hemoglobulinuria Gardner-Diamond syndrome Aplastic anemia (autoimmune) Factor VIII inhibitor Posttransfusion purpura Incompatible transfusion Factor IX deficiency Vasoocclusive crises (sickle) Granulopoiesis and macrophage inhibitors Marrow transplant rejection
Rheumatological diseases		Systemic lupus erythematosus (SLE) nephritis SLE arthritis Rheumatoid (arthritis)*§ Scleroderma	SLE complications* Rheumatoid (complications)* Systemic vasculitis (polyarteritis, Wegener's syndrome, and others) Polymyositis (and dermatomyositis)* Juvenile rheumatoid arthritis Psoriatic arthritis Sjögren's syndrome (primary) Mixed connective-tissue disease Behçet's syndrome Raynaud's disease Cryoglobulinemia
Neurological diseases	Myasthenia gravis	Guillain-Barré syndrome§ Chronic progressive polyneuropathy§ Multiple sclerosis*§ Schizophrenia [Excluded: Amyotrophic lateral sclerosis (motor neuron disease)—several published trials negative]	Chronic relapsing polyneuropathy Paraprotein neuropathy Miller-Fisher syndrome Eaton-Lambert syndrome Acute myelitis Acute encephalomyelitis Subacute sclerosing panencephalitis Parkinson's disease (Refsum's disease—see Metabolic Diseases below) (Hunter's syndrome—see Metabolic Diseases below)
Renal diseases	Antiglomerular basement membrane nephritis (including Goodpasture's syndrome)	Rapidly progressive (crescentic) glomerulonephritis (GN)† (SLE nephritis—see Rheumatological Diseases above) Hemolytic uremic syndrome Myeloma acute renal failure Kidney transplant rejection*§	Henoch-Schönlein nephritis Subacute bacterial endocarditis (SBE) nephritis Focal glomerulosclerosis Membranoproliferative GN (MPGN) type I MPGN type II (dense deposit disease) Mesangial IgA GN Mesangial proliferative GN Kappa-chain nodular glomerulopathy Rhabdomyolysis ABO-incompatible transplant Preeclampsia Hypertension (Renal vasculitis—see Rheumatological Diseases above)

TABLE 1
Diseases treated by apheresis (Cont.)

	Accepted therapy	Prospective randomized controlled trials in progress	Case reports or series only
Metabolic Diseases	Familial hypercholesterol-emia (homozygous type II)		Refsum's disease Fabry's disease Hunter's syndrome Primary biliary cirrhosis Hepatic encephalopathy Reye's syndrome Hypertriglyceridemia Anti-islet-cell Ab Anti-insulin-receptor Ab Thyroid storm Graves' exophthalmos Homocystinuria Hypercholesterolemia (heterozygous type II)
Miscellaneous diseases		*Pemphigus vulgaris†* Bullous pemphigoid Psoriasis§	Porphyrias Herpes gestationis Dermatitis herpetiformis Pyoderma gangrenosum Hyperglobulinemic purpura Neoplasia (various) Pruritus and night sweats (associated with malignant disease) Acquired immunodeficiency syndrome (AIDS) Hyper-IgE syndromes Hypereosinophilic syndromes Hereditary angioneurotic edema Familial erythrophagocytic lymphohistiocytosis Angioimmunoblastic lymphadenopathy Hypogammaglobulinemia Crohn's disease Weber-Christian disease Rheumatic fever Asthma Lepromatous leprosy Congenital herpes Leptospirosis Meningococcemia Heart transplant rejection *Amanita* mushroom poisoning Paraquat poisoning Phenylbutazone overdose Dextran overdose Aluminum intoxication Other poisonings
Therapeutic white-cell reduction	Hyperleukocytosis (acute myeloid leukemic blasts)		Hyperleukocytosis (chronic myeloid leukemia, acute lymphocytic leukemia) Chronic lymphocytic leukemia Sézary syndrome Hairy-cell leukemia
Therapeutic platelet reduction			Thrombocythemia
Red-cell exchange (erythrocyta-pheresis)	Sickle cell disease (cholestasis, priapism, presurgery)		Sickle-cell disease (pregnancy, ulcers, others) Thalassemias Polycythemias

* Lymphocytapheresis or lymphoplasmapheresis also used.   † *Preliminary results of controlled trials are positive.*
§ *Equivocal or negative results in controlled trials, but other trials are continuing.*

question are in progress. The suggestion that the missing factor may be related to prostacyclin is uncertain. There are also isolated reports of benefit from plasmapheresis with only albumin replacement. However, most authorities currently treat this condition using plasmapheresis with FFP infusion, persevering aggressively for months if necessary, and using recovery of the platelet count as the criterion for cessation of therapy. In some centers, intensive plasmapheresis is used in the severe stage of the disease and FFP infusions alone are continued thereafter until the platelet count has normalized. Dipyridamole is the most frequently used adjunctive therapy. A relapse of thrombocytopenia usually responds to repeated treatment, unless it is due to folate deficiency. For this reason, prophylactic folic acid is an important adjunct to treatment.

The hemolytic-uremic syndromes, which are related to TTP, are discussed below under "Renal Diseases." Though disseminated intravascular coagulation has been treated by plasmapheresis, this is not usually recommended.

Idiopathic thrombocytopenic purpura (ITP)
In ITP, the apparent autoimmune basis of the thrombocytopenia provides a rational reason to consider plasma-exchange therapy, but experience has been discouraging. Patients with chronic disease who remain thrombocytopenic for more than 6 months despite steroids, immunosuppressives, and splenectomy have not been improved by plasmapheresis, though the effects of an intensive course of more than three procedures has not been adequately assessed. Acute ITP is usually transient in children, but in adults it responds to steroids in only about 50 percent of cases.[3] Intervention with plasmapheresis after 1 to 8 weeks of prednisone has been followed by a sustained recovery of the platelet count in some patients, though there are no controlled data to indicate how many might have shown a late response to steroids alone. Adults with acute ITP who show no benefit from plasmapheresis may still respond to subsequent splenectomy.

Moreover, "responses" to plasmapheresis have occurred only with FFP replacement, not when albumin was used. Plasmapheresis has not been compared with high-dose gamma globulin infusion, which can normalize the platelet count transiently (permanently in some childhood cases), apparently by decreasing platelet destruction. The mechanism is not clear but may be related to blocking of immune-mediated reticuloendothelial phagocytosis by the gamma globulin.

To sum up, it is not yet established whether plasmapheresis with FFP replacement has a place as an alternative treatment for steroid-unresponsive acute ITP in cases where splenectomy or immunosuppressives are relatively contraindicated.

Autoimmune hemolytic anemia (AIHA) In "cold agglutinin" AIHA, red cell destruction is initiated by IgM-class autoantibodies which bind to red cells increasingly as the temperature is reduced below 32°C.[4] Plasmapheresis can deplete the IgM antibody, if the technical requirements for doing the procedure at adequate temperature can be met. Red cell survival can be improved, but the IgM is usually rapidly resynthesized even when steroids and cyclophosphamide are used. At best, therefore, plasmapheresis may achieve short-term clinical benefit; there is no evidence that prolonged intensive plasmapheresis regimens are of value in this usually chronic disease. Paroxysmal cold hemoglobinuria, due to cold-reacting IgG antibodies of Donath-Landsteiner type, has been treated with plasmapheresis, but with doubtful benefit.

The commonest kinds of AIHA and Evans syndrome (AIHA plus ITP) are due to warm-reacting IgG antibodies (occasionally IgA). In patients who do poorly despite drug therapy and splenectomy, or who present with life-threatening fulminant hemolysis, there are anecdotal reports of occasional rapid recovery following plasmapheresis. However, most patients show no improvement at all, and it is not yet known whether plasmapheresis has any role in warm-antibody-mediated AIHA.

Factor VIII inhibitor Between 5 and 20 percent of hemophiliacs develop factor VIII inhibitors, which are usually IgG antibodies. These can negate the effect of factor VIII supplements and

---

[3] *See* Update II, *p. 85.*

[4] *See the tenth edition of* Harrison's Principles of Internal Medicine, *chap. 329.*

can create extreme difficulties if uncontrollable hemorrhage occurs or if surgery is needed. Immunosuppressive therapy may be useful in diminishing antibody production, and "activated" prothrombin complexes have been advocated, but these measures are frequently insufficient. Plasmapheresis with FFP replacement has been effective and is cheaper than massive use of factor concentrates. It should be considered in life-threatening situations, though sometimes even intensive exchanges with immunosuppression have been insufficient to lower the antibody level adequately. Factor VIII inhibitors may also be acquired by nonhemophiliacs, usually in the elderly in association with a systemic disease or in women after childbirth. Plasmapheresis may be lifesaving in severe situations.

Rhesus hemolytic disease Despite the success of immune-globulin injection as prophylaxis against Rhesus (Rh) immunization in Rh-negative women, pregnancies complicated by Rh hemolytic disease continue to occur. Intrauterine transfusion is helpful but risky, and intensive plasmapheresis has been under assessment as an alternative treatment since 1968. Maternal blood levels of anti-D can be measured either as the hemolytic titer or by quantitation of specific IgG (only IgG antibodies can cross the placenta). Intensive plasmapheresis usually reduces these levels, and benefit to the fetus can be inferred from improvement of the optical density at 450 nm wavelength (OD_{450}) of the amniotic fluid. In several centers fetal survival in the high-risk group appears to have improved since the introduction of plasmapheresis, compared to historical controls. Complications from plasmapheresis procedures during pregnancy are few. However, worsening of anti-D levels has been described on occasion, and conjectural explanations include feedback enhancement of antibody synthesis due to plasma immunoglobulin depletion and antigenic stimulation either from fetal-maternal bleeding (for instance during amniocentesis) or from red cell remnants in FFP that was not obtained from Rh-negative donors.

Although clinical results have varied and no prospective controlled trials have been performed, some advocates recommend weekly plasmapheresis from the second trimester onward for problem cases. The advocates claim that good results are likely if the mean maternal anti-D level can be maintained below 4 mg/liter (15 IU/ml). However, in many centers intrauterine transfusion remains the treatment of choice, and the role of plasmapheresis therapy is regarded as uncertain or very limited.

Plasmapheresis has also been used in pregnancy to remove anti-M antibodies that can cause hemolysis in the fetus.

Marrow transplantation Plasma exchange has become a standard method to prepare bone marrow transplant recipients for the infusion of ABO-incompatible marrow. Depletion of anti-A and anti-B successfully avoids acute hemolysis, and allows marrow transplantation across ABO barriers with no impairment of overall results.

Other hematological conditions Plasmapheresis has been used with anecdotal success for numerous other purposes in hematology, including antibody removal before or after incompatible blood transfusion, treatment of posttransfusion purpura, treatment of a type of aplastic anemia apparently due to autoantibodies against stem cells, and treatment of a few cases of autoerythrocyte sensitization syndrome (Gardner-Diamond syndrome).

Rheumatological diseases

Systemic lupus erythematosus (SLE) SLE is often regarded as the archetype of immunologically mediated disease. The inflammatory damage in multiple organ systems is typified by deposition of various autoantibodies and immune complexes, and these usually are also demonstrable in the plasma. Plasmapheresis is theoretically attractive as a means of removing these materials from the circulation and, potentially, even from the tissues. However, the basic immunologic defect in SLE remains obscure, and the multiplicity of humoral and cellular immune derangements is perplexing. "Unblocking" of reticuloendothelial phagocytosis has been demonstrated with plasmapheresis therapy in SLE, but the relative importance of this and other potential mechanisms that might be beneficial is unknown.

More than 100 instances of plasmapheresis therapy for SLE have been reported, and lymphocytapheresis has also been used. Most plasmapheresis has been in conjunction with major steroid and immunosuppressive treatment for severe complications or life-threatening exacerbations. These indications have included severe nephritis (ranging from nephrotic syndrome to acute oliguria), cerebritis, vasculitis, serositis, carditis, pneumonitis, arthritis, aplastic anemia, thrombocytopenia, and sudden deafness. Major improvement has been the most frequent outcome, though rarely can the independent contribution of plasmapheresis be clearly distinguished.[5] Claims that plasmapheresis is effective in patients with plentiful CIC and not in those without them have been made, only to be retracted later. Indeed, benefit has been seen when CIC could not be detected. Plasmapheresis without concomitant immunosuppressive or steroid therapy is not beneficial in SLE and may even make matters worse.

Randomized trials of plasmapheresis are costly and are particularly difficult to apply to the treatment of SLE crises, which are unpredictable and involve different manifestations in various combinations. For patients with active but relatively stable disease, a few short-term prospective studies have been completed. When sham-plasmapheresis has been used as a control, the overt symptoms and physical signs of active SLE have not been helped by short-term intensive plasmapheresis. Tests for CIC and for anti-DNA antibodies have shown improvement, which has been extremely transient in some patients and quite long-lasting in others. Long-term trials are in progress specifically to study the progression of lupus glomerulonephritis of the diffuse proliferative type, which is the leading cause of mortality in SLE patients.[6] Interim assessment of one ongoing controlled study has suggested that monthly plasmapheresis added to a normal steroid regimen does indeed result in better preservation of renal function; however, confirmation by other studies is needed. In the treatment of fulminant organ damage that cannot be suppressed by maximized standard therapy, there is uncontrolled evidence that there may be additive benefit from the combination of intensive plasmapheresis and cyclophosphamide, but the limitations of anecdotal experiences must be clearly recognized. The unpredictable nature of this disease may make the task of defining the role of plasmapheresis even more difficult than has been obtaining proof that steroids and cytotoxic drugs are effective.

Systemic vasculitis Plasmapheresis has been used to treat patients with polyarteritis nodosa and related syndromes. The clinical features described in these cases include various combinations of fever, weight loss, arthralgia, myalgia, cutaneous vasculitis (palpable purpura or ulceration), small-bowel necrosis, renal involvement, cerebral vasculitis, peripheral neuropathy (often mononeuritis multiplex), or digital gangrene. Frequently aneurysmal visceral arteries have been shown by angiography, or skin biopsy has demonstrated leukocytoclastic vasculitis. Mixed cryoglobulinemia was a prominent feature in several cases, and another overlapping subset had hepatitis B antigenemia (HBsAg). Abnormal levels of CIC are frequently demonstrated in these syndromes, but they often correlate poorly with disease activity. However, in the great majority of reported cases where intensive plasmapheresis has been used, unmistakable clinical improvement has been claimed. Prednisone or cyclophosphamide was used concurrently in most cases, though sometimes they had been judged inadequate before plasmapheresis was added. In a few cases, including some with cryoglobulins, some with HBsAg, and some with neither, no steroids or cytotoxic agents were used, yet improvement with plasmapheresis still appeared to occur. Given the apparent efficacy of cyclophosphamide in polyarteritis, and the self-limiting course in some patients, further detailed studies will be needed to determine in what clinical situations this encouraging though limited experience with plasmapheresis represents a real advantage over the standard drug regimen alone.

There is little experience with plasmapheresis in other vasculitic illnesses, except some anecdotal success with Wegener's granulomatosis.

Rheumatoid arthritis (RA) In about one-third of patients with rheumatoid disease, the arthritis is progressive and requires more than salicylate,

---

[5] *See the tenth edition of* Harrison's Principles of Internal Medicine, *chap. 70.*

[6] *See the tenth edition of* Harrison's Principles of Internal Medicine, *chap. 295.*

chloroquine, or low-dose steroid therapy; about 10 percent do not respond adequately even to powerful but toxic remission-producing agents such as D-penicillamine and gold. Because most patients are women of childbearing age, alternative therapies with azathioprine, cyclophosphamide, or total lymphoid irradiation may be viewed as a last resort. The removal of plasma factors such as immunoglobulins, CIC, or rheumatoid factor, is a potential rationale for using plasmapheresis in RA, while lymphocytapheresis has been predicated on evidence of benefit from thoracic duct drainage.

In a disease as prevalent as RA, randomized prospective trials, even if restricted to severe cases, are possible. However, difficulties arise because costs limit the scope and duration of studies, because spontaneous exacerbations and remissions may obscure the effects of therapy when small groups of patients are used, and because placebo effects may be prominent when assessing pain, stiffness, walking speed, and other parameters of clinical activity. Therefore, double-blind, sometimes crossover protocols using sham-apheresis as the control have been necessary, and have usually studied small groups of patients treated two or three times weekly for 3 to 5 weeks. Though plasmapheresis always produces improvement in serological markers and had seemed clinically promising in uncontrolled series, prospective studies reveal only marginal benefit compared to controls receiving drug therapy alone, and no clinical efficacy has been demonstrated when compared to sham plasmapheresis controls.

Patients whose arthritis is thought to be most appropriate for such therapeutic trials are those with seropositive erosive disease that is still actively inflamed, who have not responded to remittive or cytotoxic drugs, but who can continue to take them during intensive apheresis. Such patients treated with lymphocytapheresis or lymphoplasmapheresis have shown reduced lymphocyte counts and changes in other blood tests but only small or equivocal improvement in indexes of joint activity and joint swelling, compared to sham-treated controls. In patients who appear to respond, the benefit may last 3 months or longer. The interpretation of these trials has been controversial, and it remains unknown whether more prolonged lymphocytapheresis or lympho-

plasmapheresis may turn out to have a place in the treatment of severe unremitting joint disease.[7]

Life-threatening extraarticular complications of RA, such as cryoglobulinemic vasculitis and hyperviscosity syndrome, are rare, but they usually show a promising response to plasmapheresis, which is probably justifiable when other therapies have failed or when the problem is acute and severe.

Scleroderma (progressive systemic sclerosis) (PSS) As well as causing thickening of skin, joints, and digital arteries, scleroderma may involve the heart, lungs, intestinal tract, and kidneys. Uncontrolled experience with intensive plasmapheresis together with prednisone and cyclophosphamide has suggested improvement of some manifestations of PSS, particularly loosening of skin and sometimes dramatic improvement of severe intestinal symptoms. It appears that highly active, evolving lesions may be more treatable than long-standing or slowly progressing disease. Antinuclear antibody titers may be improved by plasmapheresis, but the nature of the putative immunologic basis of scleroderma remains unknown. More information on the value of plasmapheresis must await results of a prospective double-blind trial now in progress.

Polymyositis and dermatomyositis Idiopathic polymyositis usually affects adults. Dermatomyositis, which combines the same inflammatory disease of skeletal muscle with an erythematous rash that may herald malignancy, occurs both in adults and children. Standard treatment consists of steroids, and for troublesome cases methotrexate may be of some value. Intensive plasmapheresis together with cyclophosphamide or chlorambucil appears to benefit muscle strength and inflammation in some patients, particularly those with active acute disease and markedly elevated creatine phosphokinase (CPK) levels. CPK is a good barometer of disease activity, except that it is removed by plasmapheresis and remains artificially low for several days. A prominent feature of the muscle

---

[7] *See the tenth edition of* Harrison's Principles of Internal Medicine, *chap. 346.*

pathology is lymphocytic infiltration. Lympho-plasmapheresis used without other medications has been reported to be of value in otherwise terminally ill patients.

Other rheumatological conditions Juvenile rheumatoid arthritis and psoriatic arthritis have been treated with plasmapheresis with occasional apparent benefit. Experience with primary Sjögren's syndrome, mixed connective-tissue disease, and Behçet's syndrome is very limited. Raynaud's phenomenon, either primary or in association with other rheumatological disease, appears often to respond to plasmapheresis. The effect may depend on fibrinogen depletion and reduction of blood viscosity, or, in some patients, mechanisms involving immunologic factors may be important. Appropriate use of plasmapheresis for this usually benign symptom must presumably be limited to extreme cases.

Neurological diseases

Myasthenia gravis Acquired myasthenia gravis is caused by autoantibodies directed against the nicotinic acetylcholine receptor (AChR) of skeletal muscle. These antibodies (anti-AChR Ab) are detectable in 80 to 95 percent of patients and are usually of the IgG class. They act by impairing neuromuscular conduction, and they cause weakness and easy fatigability. Most patients respond well to anticholinergic drugs, steroids, or thymectomy. However, for the refractory or emergency case, plasmapheresis, presumably by removing anti-AChR Ab, can be effective and has established an important role in management.[8] Intensive plasmapheresis, starting with daily treatments, can induce improvements in objective neuromuscular tests as early as 24 or 36 h after the first treatment, but demonstrable improvement in muscle strength usually takes at least 3 to 7 days. Reports of dramatic clinical recovery within hours are rare and unexplained. Most patients undergoing plasmapheresis are treated also with prednisone and either azathioprine or cyclophosphamide, though often these are not started until several days of plasmapheresis have been completed. As in

other diseases, these drugs appear to reduce antibody synthesis over the long term, but in myasthenia there is controversy over whether they are needed to prevent immediate antibody rebound after plasmapheresis. Depletion of serum anti-AChR levels usually parallels the clinical response to plasmapheresis. Occasionally, however, major reduction of anti-AChR has been attained without clinical improvement. Also, patients with myasthenia gravis but without anti-AChR Ab may respond to plasmapheresis. Speculations include that the removal of other factors may be important or that some cases are due to an antibody of somewhat different specificity.

Plasmapheresis is now justified for the short-term control of severe or deteriorating symptoms in patients with generalized myasthenia gravis classified as moderate, acute severe, or chronic severe (Osserman grades IIB, III, and IV, respectively). Even some patients who were respirator-dependent and had failed thymectomy and prednisone treatment have attained remarkable remissions. Though some patients appear to remain well for many months after a course of plasmapheresis and are able to reduce their steroid and anticholinesterase dosages, this persistent benefit appears more likely to be the consequence of the concomitant use of immunosuppressive drugs. Relapses can be treated by repeat courses of plasmapheresis, though the response may be slower or less complete on second or subsequent occasions.

Guillain-Barré syndrome (GBS) The acute form of inflammatory demyelinating polyradiculoneuropathy is best known as Guillain-Barré syndrome. It appears to be an autoimmune disease of the peripheral nerves, often triggered by a viral infection or other stimulus. The pathogenesis remains unclear, though a serum factor which is toxic to myelin in tissue culture now seems a more plausible mechanism than cell-mediated immune damage. The evidence incriminating various different proteases and antibodies is conflicting. It is possible that more than one different disease exists within this very heterogeneous group of patients. Clinical variability makes it difficult to distinguish medically induced benefit from spontaneous recovery. Though only 5 percent of patients die, 20 percent require assisted ventilation during their illness,

---

[8] *See the tenth edition of* Harrison's Principles of Internal Medicine, *chap. 372; and* Update III, *pp. 232–233.*

and while steroids had been favored because they induced early improvement in 75 percent of patients, it turns out that 70 percent of untreated patients make a complete recovery. One carefully controlled trial has shown that steroid-treated patients have a worse outcome.

Reports of dramatic cures using intensive plasmapheresis are similarly suspect; about two-thirds of more than 70 cases in the literature improved with plasmapheresis. A randomized trial in Britain comparing plasmapheresis versus no treatment (steroids were not used) showed slight benefit after 20 patients had been entered, but no lasting difference was demonstrated after 30 patients had been analyzed. Nevertheless, as in other diseases, occasional patients appear to respond and to relapse when plasmapheresis is withdrawn, only to respond again to retreatment. In some uncontrolled series, apparent response has been linked to the presence of a particular antibody. Experience with the Miller-Fisher variant of GBS is equally uninterpretable. A larger controlled study is underway in this country, but at present the evidence is lacking that would support the efficacy of plasmapheresis in early acute GBS. Because of autonomic instability in GBS patients, hypotension may be troublesome during plasmapheresis procedures.

Chronic demyelinating polyneuropathies
The chronic, progressive form of demyelinating polyradiculoneuropathy starts more slowly and behaves differently than GBS. Prednisone is probably preferable to no treatment but must be used over long periods, entailing the hazard of major side effects. Apparent improvements have occurred using plasmapheresis, though a double-blind trial comparing 3 weeks' plasmapheresis to sham-apheresis controls is in progress and has not yet shown a difference.

The chronic relapsing form comprises the 20 percent of GBS patients who have recurrent attacks. Steroids and immunosuppressives are beneficial, and improvement with plasmapheresis has been sufficiently frequent to warrant further controlled studies or to justify a trial of therapy in cases where drug therapy proves inadequate. However, the question whether the addition of plasmapheresis has any advantage over treatment with just steroids and immunosuppressives has not been answered.

A specific polyneuropathy associated with benign monoclonal gammopathy (often IgM paraprotein of kappa light-chain type) has been treated with prednisone, melphalan, and plasmapheresis. Plasmapheresis, even by itself, appears to have a marked beneficial effect in many cases.

Multiple sclerosis (MS)
Purported treatments for multiple sclerosis abound, but very few have been shown conclusively to have merit. Adrenocorticotropic hormone (ACTH) and steroids ameliorate acute attacks but seem to confer no long-term benefit. Evidence of an immunologic component in MS has spurred trials of azathioprine, cyclophosphamide, antilymphocyte serum, plasmapheresis, and lymphocytapheresis.[9]

Following early enthusiastic reports, MS patients have been treated with plasmapheresis in numerous centers in North America. Some controlled trials are underway and two have been reported. From these it appears that patients treated with azathioprine plus plasmapheresis (three or four initial treatments, then monthly for a year) fare no better than comparable patients treated with azathioprine alone; patients receiving plasmapheresis plus low-dose cyclophosphamide and ACTH do somewhat better than patients receiving ACTH alone but not nearly as well as patients receiving high-dose cyclophosphamide and ACTH. These results have naturally kindled interest in cyclophosphamide but add to the growing impression that plasmapheresis is of no merit in MS.

Lymphocytapheresis has also been pursued vigorously, probably now in more than 200 MS patients. Despite the likely impact of placebo effects, few patients show more than equivocal improvement. Patients with rapidly progressive disease certainly do not seem to benefit, and those with slower declines are extremely hard to evaluate. Until randomized trials have been completed, there is danger of raising false hopes. It appears at the present time that lymphocytapheresis for MS cannot be justified, except as part of carefully conducted and properly controlled experiments.

---

[9] *See the tenth edition of* Harrison's Principles of Internal Medicine, *chap. 361.*

Other neurological conditions Amyotrophic lateral sclerosis (motor neuron disease) was the first major disease in which adequate studies from several centers agreed in returning a verdict that plasmapheresis is of no value in treatment.

Plasmapheresis has been used with apparent benefit in several cases of Eaton-Lambert syndrome and in some patients with transverse myelitis, encephalitis, or polyradiculitis associated with *Mycoplasma pneumoniae* infection. Plasmapheresis has also been used to attempt to treat other diseases of the nervous system including subacute sclerosing panencephalitis, Parkinson's disease, and schizophrenia. Refsum's disease and hepatic encephalopathy (and Reye's syndrome) are discussed below under "Metabolic Diseases."

Renal diseases

Anti-GBM nephritis and Goodpasture's syndrome
Antibodies reactive with glomerular basement membrane (anti-GBM Ab) may also sometimes cross react with alveolar basement membrane. The glomerulonephritis that is caused is usually severe, typified histologically by extracapillary crescent formation in a majority of glomeruli (crescentic glomerulonephritis) and clinically by a rapidly progressive nephritis leading to renal failure. When the lungs are also affected, the dominant pulmonary feature is hemorrhage, which can be fatal. Either renal or lung disease may occur first or in isolation; when both coincide the term Goodpasture's syndrome is used.

Plasmapheresis together with steroids and immunosuppressives has been used widely for this devastating illness, because the precise knowledge of the pathogenesis provides a clear rationale and because other therapies have not been helpful.[10] Evidence that this treatment yields better results than historical controls has now been confirmed in a prospective, randomized, controlled trial. Accurate measurement of anti-GBM Ab in the serum by radioimmunoassay has shown that the rate of disappearance is linear over a long period of treatment and is more rapid in patients receiving plasmapheresis every third day with prednisone and cyclophosphamide treatment than in those receiving equal doses of prednisone and cyclophosphamide alone. The immunosuppression appears necessary to prevent rebound antibody synthesis, and plasmapheresis must be intensive and continued for many weeks to eliminate anti-GBM Ab effectively. Patients with very severe renal histology who are already in oliguric renal failure may be unsalvageable, whereas those with mild disease do equally well with only prednisone and cyclophosphamide. Patients with moderate or severe disease who begin treatment early, before renal damage is intense, are the ones in whom plasmapheresis is most efficacious. For this reason, rapid investigation and early intervention are essential. Though in many uncontrolled series lung hemorrhage appeared to respond rapidly to plasmapheresis therapy, more recent experience leaves uncertain whether plasmapheresis is truly helpful for the pulmonary component of this disease.[11]

Plasmapheresis is effective for anti-GBM disease when FFP replacement is used (indicating at least that the effect is not due to fibrinogen depletion). Replacement with albumin alone, which in intensive plasmapheresis reduces levels of coagulation factors, might (together with a platelet defect if the patient is uremic) theoretically increase the risk of lung hemorrhage in Goodpasture's syndrome. In patients with total renal failure, plasmapheresis may cause metabolic alkalosis because citrate is metabolized to bicarbonate that cannot be excreted.

Other forms of crescentic glomerulonephritis
Most patients with rapidly progressive glomerulonephritis with glomerular crescents on renal biopsy do not have anti-GBM disease. Mechanisms involving immune complexes or other unknown factors are implicated. Many cases are idiopathic, but some represent extreme forms of renal involvement of known systemic diseases, including vasculitis, SLE, Henoch-Schönlein purpura, and subacute endocarditis with nephritis. When treatment of the underlying disease is inadequate or does not exist, plasmapheresis plus steroids and other immunosuppressive drugs have been used in patients with each of

---

[10] *See the tenth edition of* Harrison's Principles of Internal Medicine, *chap. 295.*

[11] *See the tenth edition of* Harrison's Principles of Internal Medicine, *chap. 280.*

these types of nephritis. It is unclear whether it is the removal of immunoglobulins, fibrinogen, inflammatory mediators, or other factors that is important, but clinical results with this treatment modality have appeared very encouraging, especially when treatment is instituted early.[12] Interpretation is difficult because of the unpredictability of these diseases, including some cases that recover spontaneously. Reduction of CIC levels can be hastened by plasmapheresis in some cases, including IgA-class CIC in patients with Henoch-Schönlein disease, but apparent response has also been documented when CIC were undetectable. Pulse methylprednisolone has been advocated as an adjunct to immunosuppression, but one randomized prospective study from France suggests that plasmapheresis-treated patients did slightly better. Though several prospective controlled studies have been initiated, it may take some time to acquire adequate data regarding the efficacy of plasmapheresis in these conditions.

Primary glomerulonephritis (GN)   Failure to detect CIC in many of the forms of primary GN has coincided with several successes in defining possible alternative pathogenic mechanisms that do not involve CIC. In addition, at least two diseases, focal glomerulosclerosis (FGS) and membranoproliferative GN type II ("dense deposit disease"), appear to depend on glomerular accumulation of materials that do not primarily react with immunoglobulins. Both these diseases recur in transplants, suggesting that the abnormal material gets to the kidney via the circulation; also, membranoproliferative GN (MPGN) type II may be capable of maternal-fetal transmission. These observations provide a rationale for plasmapheresis in these diseases, as well as in those in which immune-complex deposition appears important.

Apparent benefit from plasmapheresis has been reported in a few cases of noncrescentic immune-complex-type GN. These have included patients with MPGN type I and patients with diffuse mesangial proliferative GN (including mesangial IgA nephritis and mesangial IgM nephritis). Limited experience (including one pregnant patient) with plasmapheresis for MPGN type II (dense deposit disease) has shown the procedure to be helpful. At present there are insufficient data to comment further on the efficacy of plasmapheresis in any of these diseases.

Hemolytic-uremic syndromes (HUS)   There is considerable similarity between HUS and TTP. The rationale for plasmapheresis in HUS is the same as already described for TTP, and FFP replacement is recommended. Several case reports show plasmapheresis to be useful even in oliguric patients, not only in children where the chances of spontaneous recovery are likely if oliguria is of short duration but also in adults where the prognosis is poor in any case and worse when the patient is oliguric. This experience has been recorded in the idiopathic form of HUS, in HUS following infectious diarrhea, and in the postpartum form of HUS. Patients with TTP occurring during pregnancy and in association with severe preeclampsia also appear to have derived some benefit from plasmapheresis.

Kidney transplantation   Kidney transplant rejection involves a mixture of cell-mediated and humoral mechanisms. Although the former are more prevalent in early acute rejection and the latter in episodes occurring after several weeks, both may coexist. Trials of plasmapheresis as an adjunct to other standard and experimental antirejection measures have been largely disappointing, though some centers offer evidence of efficacy in certain specific subsets of patients, and some controlled series report apparently better graft-survival statistics in patients who have undergone plasmapheresis.

Lymphocytapheresis, predicated on the known though mild beneficial effects of lymphocyte depletion by thoracic duct drainage in transplant recipients and on the intense lymphocytic infiltration that occurs with acute cellular rejection, has been investigated both as pretransplant preparation (in kidney and in liver transplantation) and for the treatment of steroid-resistant kidney rejection. Though some encouraging results have been observed, the efficacy of this form of intervention cannot yet be evaluated.

Plasmapheresis has been used preoperatively to deplete cytotoxic antibody titers and postoperatively when ABO-incompatible kidneys have

---

[12] *See the tenth edition of* Harrison's Principles of Internal Medicine, *chap. 294.*

been inadvertently implanted. In the latter situation, some surprising successes have occurred. Plasmapheresis has been used also to treat recurring glomerulonephritis in kidney transplants; this has included anti-GBM disease and mesangial IgM nephropathy.

Other renal conditions Renal failure in myeloma patients can be of many types, but "myeloma kidney" due to precipitation of large amounts of protein in the renal tubules is common. Plasmapheresis to deplete high circulating levels of paraproteins appears to benefit renal function in some cases. The specific nodular glomerulopathy of kappa light-chain disease may also be improved by intensive and prolonged plasmapheresis.

Among other nephrological diseases treated with plasmapheresis, there has been some enthusiasm for attempting to prevent renal damage in cases of rhabdomyolysis.

Metabolic diseases

Familial hypercholesterolemia Homozygotes for defective genes at the receptor locus for low-density lipoproteins (LDL) have severe hypercholesterolemia and usually succumb to atherosclerotic complications before reaching adulthood. Conventional therapies are inadequate, and prolonged lowering of LDL cholesterol has been achieved by weekly or biweekly plasmapheresis. This has been sufficient to decrease xanthomas, and it is hoped that the long-term prognosis will be significantly improved. If a permanent vascular access site can be constructed (e.g., arteriovenous fistula), this regimen over many years may interfere minimally with a normal childhood and is the treatment of choice for homozygotes.[13] In heterozygotes for familial hypercholesterolemia, other cholesterol-lowering measures are available, and plasmapheresis is effective only if pursued intensively and may be indicated only for unusually severe problems.

Other inborn metabolic defects Plasmapheresis is being explored as a means of removing

accumulated metabolites in various other genetically determined diseases. The best studied is Refsum's disease (heredopathia atactica polyneuritiformis), in which a defect in α oxidation of fatty acids causes a buildup of phytanic acid, which then can be neither metabolized nor excreted, and leads to retinitis pigmentosa, chronic polyneuropathy, and icthyosis. The phytanic acid is carried on lipoproteins and can be removed by plasmapheresis, which, with good dietary restriction, may be needed only every several months once control has been achieved. Removal of ceramide trihexoside by plasmapheresis in Fabry's disease (angiokeratoma corporis diffusum) appears less effective for the control or prevention of clinical problems.

Although massive infusion of normal plasma by plasma exchange in Hunter's syndrome (mucopolysaccharidosis II) has produced an increase in the missing enzyme activity (iduronate sulfatase), it has so far failed to produce clinically demonstrable benefit.

Liver failure Patients with primary biliary cirrhosis may develop xanthomas and neuropathy associated with hypercholesterolemia, and itching which may be ascribed to accumulation of bile acids. Regression of these symptoms with long-term plasmapheresis has been reported in several cases.

Both hepatic encephalopathy and Reye's syndrome have been treated with plasmapheresis for the removal of extreme concentrations of ammonia, bilirubin, and other toxic metabolites. In this setting, plasmapheresis may buy time for the liver to begin to regenerate.

Diabetes mellitus Diabetics may develop severe hypertriglyceridemia, which may be complicated by acute pancreatitis and other lesions ascribable to hyperviscosity. Plasmapheresis can correct the hypertriglyceridemia and may help control acute complications.

Plasmapheresis is also being studied for the purpose of removing anti-islet-cell antibodies in early type I diabetes, and anti-insulin-receptor antibodies in type II diabetes.

Thyrotoxicosis Removal of thyroid hormones by plasmapheresis has been described both in thyrotoxic crisis and with L-thyroxine overdose,

---

[13] *See the tenth edition of* Harrison's Principles of Internal Medicine, *chap. 103.*

and this treatment should be considered when all else fails. The exophthalmos of Graves' disease has responded inconsistently to plasmapheresis. The rationale is the removal of autoantibodies that may specifically cause this lesion and of thyroid-stimulating antibodies and other auto-antibodies demonstrated in Graves' disease.

Miscellaneous diseases

Pemphigus vulgaris Pemphigus vulgaris is caused by an autoantibody directed against intercellular glycoproteins in the skin. The pemphigus antibody (P Ab) is usually an IgG; it causes acantholysis and a blistering disease of skin and mucous membranes that is often severe and may be fatal. The pathogenicity of P Ab has been confirmed by lesions induced by transfer of pemphigus serum to tissue cultures and experimental animals. Prednisone doses as high as 300 mg per day are used together with azathioprine to reduce P Ab levels. When this fails, the addition of intensive plasmapheresis has produced stepwise reductions in P Ab levels that have generally correlated with clinical improvement (Fig. 4*B*). Marked benefit from plasmapheresis has been documented in several recent series of patients, though some patients resynthesize P Ab at alarming rates even with maximal immunosuppression.

Other skin conditions Many cases of uncontrollable psoriasis have been treated with plasmapheresis. Although some spectacular improvements have been ascribed to this intervention, a small double-blind trial using sham-plasmapheresis as a control has been unable to detect any significant clinical effect. Other skin diseases in which plasmapheresis has been used too infrequently to be judged include porphyria, bullous pemphigoid, herpes gestationis, dermatitis herpetiformis, pyoderma gangrenosum, and hyperglobulinemic purpura.

Malignant diseases Despite rationales involving removal of antibodies, CIC, or other blocking factors interfering with tumoricidal immunity, regression of tumors has not been achieved by plasma-removal techniques. Some interesting results attributable to passing plasma over protein A columns are described below under "Plasma Processing."

There are several recent claims that pruritus and night sweats in patients with hematological malignancies may be controlled by plasma exchange.

Immunological disorders Several patients with acquired immunodeficiency syndrome (AIDS) are currently undergoing experimental treatment with plasmapheresis in at least two centers. No results have been published, but depressed T-cell helper/suppressor ratios have apparently returned to normal in some cases. However, no clinically demonstrable benefit has been observed. Other immunological diseases in which plasmapheresis therapy has been reported include hyper-IgE syndrome, asthma, some hypereosinophilic syndromes, hereditary angioneurotic edema, familial erythrophagocytic lymphohistiocytosis, and allergen-related angioimmunoblastic lymphadenopathy. A number of these reports describing successes in these diseases may be overly enthusiastic.

Lepromatous leprosy Leprosy (Hansen's disease) in the lepromatous form may be complicated by damaging "reactions" that are characterized by the presence of CIC. One of these, Lucio's phenomenon, may represent an Arthus reaction arising when increased antibody production occurs in the presence of the massive antigenic load typical of lepromatous leprosy. Plasmapheresis in this situation has proved efficacious on several occasions when standard therapy (including steroids) has been insufficient.

Poisoning and drug overdose Protein-bound nondialyzable drugs and poisons may be removed efficiently. Among the many applications described, those in which clinically useful results are possible include *Amanita* mushroom poisoning, methyl parathion poisoning, renal failure due to low-molecular-weight dextrans, protein-bound aluminum intoxication, paraquat poisoning, and phenylbutazone overdose.

Other diseases A role for plasmapheresis therapy has been suggested in Crohn's disease, rheumatic fever, Weber-Christian disease, and many other diseases. A complete listing is impossible, as new applications are being explored all the time, and further experience and rigorous trials will gradually either validate or disprove some of the many speculations and hopes that remain untested.

THERAPEUTIC CYTAPHERESIS IN LEUKEMIA

Centrifugal call separators were initially conceived for the removal of leukemic cells. It was hoped that repeated leukapheresis would help control chronic myeloid leukemia (CML) and would improve the outcome. Unfortunately, granulocyte production is too rapid to allow adequate control of peripheral counts by this means over a long period; also leukapheresis appears not to alter the underlying biology of the disease, so that blast crisis is not prevented or postponed. Therefore, the main use of leukapheresis is the acute reduction of very high counts of leukemic cells, either to treat leukostasis syndromes or to avoid the adverse effects of massive cell lysis when chemotherapy is given.

Modern machines are capable of selective removal of various cell types; centrifugal separation of cells depends on their different densities, which are shown in Table 2. Techniques used in donors to increase white cell harvest, such as steroid pretreatment or hydroxyethyl starch infusion, are not appropriate for cytoreduction procedures, with the possible exception that hydroxyethyl starch, which is a sedimenting agent for red cells, may on rare occasions be used to

TABLE 2
Approximate specific gravities of different blood components

Specific gravity	Cell type
1.027	Plasma
1.04	Platelets
1.06	Monocytes
1.05—1.07	Lymphocytes
1.07	Myelocytes, promyelocytes
1.07—1.08	Blasts
1.08	Metamyelocytes
1.09	Mature granulocytes
1.095	Erythrocytes
1.8	Perfluorochemicals ("blood substitutes")

improve the separation when mature granulocytes are being removed. Citrate anticoagulation is preferable, because heparin may increase platelet aggregation. Volume replacement is often necessary with leukapheresis because the leukocrit may exceed 10% in some patients and the volume of white cell product may be substantial; red cell transfusion may be relatively safe once the white cell load has been reduced.

Uses of white cell reduction

Cerebral leukostasis Patients with acute (or chronic) myelogenous leukemia presenting with very high peripheral blast-cell counts are at high risk of developing leukostasis syndromes. Even when whole-blood viscosity is not noticeably increased, the usually very large size and relative nondeformability of myeloblasts may cause blockage of the microcirculation, with evidence of decreased perfusion of critical organs. This particularly affects the brain, causing neurologic deficits and impaired consciousness, and also affects the pulmonary circulation, causing hypoxemia. These effects may be dangerous or even fatal, and even the fastest-acting cytotoxic drugs require at least 2 or 3 days to be effective. Leukapheresis may greatly improve early management,[14] and one or two treatments may achieve a major reduction of peripheral cell counts (Fig. 5). Leukapheresis is indicated for counts in excess of about 70,000 myeloid blasts per microliter or when leukostasis is diagnosed. Sometimes only headache is present, and it clears rapidly during the leukapheresis procedure. Patients with more serious neurologic symptoms also improve rapidly. Because the effects of leukapheresis are short-lived, cytotoxic drugs should be instituted concurrently. Lymphoblasts and other cell types are smaller and less likely to cause leukostasis syndromes.

Hyperleukocytosis prior to chemotherapy Cytotoxic agents used for remission induction may cause side effects due to massive lysis of circulating cells. In addition to hyperuricemia and renal failure, which are usually preventable

---

[14] *See the tenth edition of* Harrison's Principles of Internal Medicine, *chap. 128.*

LEUKOCYTAPHERESIS FOR HYPERLEUKOCYTOSIS

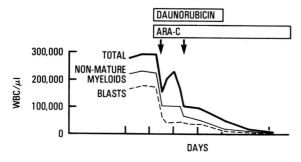

FIGURE 5

In a patient presenting with acute myeloid leukemia and severe hyperleukocytosis, two daily leukocytapheresis procedures (↓) averted early signs of cerebral leukostasis and reduced the peripheral blood white cell mass being subjected to cytolytic drug therapy. The procedures employed an IBM 2997 continuous-flow machine using a large-bore white blood cell extraction tube. The number of myeloblasts collected during each procedure exceeded the calculated number present in the circulation at the start of each run.

by allopurinol, disseminated intravascular coagulation (DIC) may be precipitated, particularly in acute promyelocytic leukemia. Moreover, acute lung dysfunction has been described as a consequence of cell lysis in myeloblastic leukemias, and other organs may be susceptible to similar postlysis syndromes. Therefore, leukapheresis may be beneficial for any severe hyperleukocytosis (> 200,000 leukocytes per microliter) prior to cytolytic therapy. In untreated chronic myelogenous leukemia, in addition to peripheral blood counts of several hundred thousand, relatively mature granulocytes may be present in vast numbers sequestered in many organs and tissues. In these patients, leukapheresis may induce these cells to return to the circulation, so that many procedures are needed before the peripheral cell count begins to fall.

Sézary syndrome This is a T-lymphocyte malignancy characterized by lymphocytic infiltration of the skin as well as raised peripheral blood counts. Reports are conflicting whether repeated lymphocytapheresis is useful in depleting lymphocytes from the skin and in overall management. Patients with Sézary syndrome and peripheral lymphocyte counts > 10,000 lympho-

cytes per microliter may be considered for this treatment.

Hairy-cell leukemia Leukapheresis for hairy-cell leukemia has been credited with marked resolution of several complications. There is some evidence to suggest that intensive cytoreduction by repeated procedures may have an overall beneficial effect on the course of the disease.

Other chronic treatment Although long-term treatment for CML appears unhelpful, there is controversy regarding possible benefit in chronic lymphocytic leukemia (CLL). Production of malignant cells occurs at a much slower rate in CLL than CML, and blast transformation is not a major problem in CLL. Chronic leukapheresis usually depletes malignant-cell counts in CLL and may improve anemia, thrombocytopenia, lymphoadenopathy, and constitutional symptoms. However, it is doubtful whether any alteration of the long-term outcome can be achieved.

Uses of platelet reduction

Therapeutic thrombocytapheresis has proved valuable in treating essential thrombocythemia, and other myeloproliferative disorders in which platelet counts > 1 million platelets per microliter occur with evidence of thrombosis or hemorrhage. Thrombocytapheresis may also be indicated for patients with high platelet counts who are about to undergo surgery, particularly if the bleeding time is prolonged.

THERAPEUTIC APPLICATIONS OF ERYTHROCYTAPHERESIS

Manual exchange transfusion used in the 1960s for sickle cell disease has been superseded by erythrocytapheresis. Red cells removed from blood-cell separators usually have about an 80% hematocrit, similar to the washed packed cells used to replace them. If the patient's hematocrit needs to be increased, the last part of the erythrocytapheresis is done in a "supertransfusion" mode, when, instead of exchanging the patient's packed cells for donor packed cells, a few units of donor packed cells are used to replace a similar volume of the patient's whole blood. Citrate anticoagulation is preferred, and transfusion reactions must be recognized and treated immediately because of the rapidity at which donor red cells are infused.

Sickle cell disease

Vascular occlusive crises in patients with sickle cell disease (homozygous SS) are frequent and are often debilitating. Standard management includes rehydration, analgesics, and oxygen therapy. Hypertransfusion therapy has been applied in numerous situations, and red cell exchange appears to be equally applicable and more practical. Most erythrocytapheresis procedures will utilize 6 to 10 units of washed packed cells for an adult, and a single procedure is sufficient to reduce the hemoglobin S (Hb S) from 100% to less than 40% in most instances. An exchange of this magnitude can be accomplished in as little as 2 h using a modern continuous-flow centrifuge machine. Clear indications include hepatic cholestasis, priapism, and crisis during pregnancy. Erythrocytapheresis is probably appropriate for painful vascular occlusive crises and for "acute chest syndrome" when these do not respond to conventional therapy. Chronic cutaneous ulcers are often unhealable in sickle cell patients, but some have improved rapidly after erythrocytapheresis. When surgery is proposed, preparative red cell exchange may be useful and is especially important before retinal surgery or when vascular occlusion is a necessary part of the procedure. Cerebral vascular occlusions occur in 10 percent of sickle cell patients, and survivors have a 60 percent risk of recurrent stroke. In this situation, in pregnant patients and in patients with frequent painful crises, the merits of regular prophylactic red cell exchanges are controversial. Because of the half-life of donor red cells, the effect of a single erythrocytapheresis procedure should be visible for several weeks. Treatments at monthly or bimonthly intervals appear to be unable to prevent crises indefinitely in patients with recurrent disease. This may reflect the fact that microcirculatory beds that have previously been damaged by sickling are more likely to be ischemic and thus to cause future recurrences.

Other red cell diseases

Thalassemics have been treated with erythrocytapheresis, but the efficacy is uncertain. Erythrocytapheresis (without red cell replacement) has also been used in patients with polycythemia, although the advantages compared to simple phlebotomy seem to be minor.

TECHNICAL INNOVATIONS AND FUTURE TRENDS

Plasma processing

As an alternative to plasma exchange, various techniques are under development to "purify" the patient's own plasma; this would circumvent the cost, potential infectivity, and possible scarcity of plasma replacement solutions and would limit the depletion of essential plasma constituents. Sometimes, plasma obtained at one plasmapheresis can be processed in the laboratory and used as replacement volume for the patient's next treatment. More recently, on-line methods have been explored so that plasma separated by an ordinary centrifugal or membrane-plasmapheresis machine can be passed through a purification device before being reinfused as the replacement solution. Some purification systems are designed to remove a particular antibody or plasma constituent known to be pathogenic in the disease under treatment, whereas others aim to be less specific and to produce essentially an albumin-based replacement solution. All of these techniques remain experimental, and the costs still exceed those of routine plasmapheresis. Moreover, the efficacy of these methods has to be proved or at least compared with the efficacy of ordinary plasma exchange.

Cascade filtration and cryogelation   Plasma obtained from whole blood (usually by a membrane separator) can be passed sequentially through another membrane filter of smaller pore size which in principle will hold back the larger plasma proteins and will allow passage of a solution mainly of albumin.. The Parker-Hannefin Corporation has marketed the Cryomax machine, which combines this principle with cooling of the separated plasma to 4°C, which, in the presence of heparin, causes cryoprecipitation of globulins within the second filter and thereby removes a major fraction of the plasma immunoglobulins and other large proteins. Removal of circulating immune complexes and macromolecules has been demonstrated, and in clinical trials of patients with rheumatoid arthritis, systemic vasculitis, and other immunological disease, this system seems as promising as conventional plasmapheresis.

Physical and chemical separation techniques Zinc diglycinate and other salts specifically able to precipitate immunoglobulins from whole plasma are under investigation with a view to on-line plasma processing. The general approach is to remove the precipitate by centrifugation or filtration and to remove residual salts by on-line dialysis. Convective electrophoresis and other systems are also being studied.

Plasmaperfusion Hemoperfusion, in which whole blood is passed over coated charcoal or resin columns, is already a standard therapy for selected drug poisonings. Platelet adherence and cell damage are features that limit the material that can be employed. Plasmaperfusion, in which cellular elements are already excluded by centrifugal separation or membrane filtration, can employ a variety of other chemical agents for specific adsorption of plasma constituents. These have included heparin-agarose columns for removal of LDL and activated charcoal columns for bile acid absorption.

Removal of specific antibodies by plasmaperfusion columns containing immobilized antigens is attractive but may be difficult because any release of antigen into the plasma may further stimulate immune reactivity. This has apparently occurred with deleterious effects when maternal plasma has been adsorbed on Rh-positive cells for the removal of anti-D and anti-C antibodies in pregnancy. However, anti-M removal by a similar method has allowed very successful therapy during at least one pregnancy. Experimental antigen columns that have been used successfully for on-line plasmaperfusion include DNA colloidion, for the removal of anti-DNA antibodies in the treatment of SLE, and synthetic blood group A and B substances, for the removal of anti-A and anti-B antibodies in patients about to receive ABO-incompatible bone marrow transplants.

Another approach, which has attracted considerable interest because of the expansion of monoclonal antibody technology, is the removal of specific plasma constituents using columns containing antibodies linked to sepharose beads or similar immobilized matrices. For instance, LDL has been successfully depleted by columns containing sepharose-linked anti-apoprotin antibody.

Protein A produced by some strains of *Staphylococcus aureus* has a strong affinity for the Fc region of IgG antibodies, and has been used in experimental plasmaperfusion protocols for removal of circulating immune complexes and putative blocking antigens. However, apparent beneficial effects in animals and patients with breast cancer have apparently occurred when even very small volumes of plasma have been reacted in vitro with protein A and then reinfused. The effect is not seen with simple plasma removal and appears to be a pharmacological rather than an apheresis effect. Nevertheless, large-volume protein A columns are capable of substantial immunoglobulin binding and may be useful for apheresis in immune-mediated diseases.

Selective cytapheresis

White cells Differential centrifugation techniques have been perfected in modern continuous-flow machines mainly to improve the purity and yield of cell products harvested from healthy donors. Similar refinements can also be employed for therapeutic purposes. For instance, the slight difference in density between T and B lymphocytes has been exploited to attempt selective depletion predominantly of T cells in some diseases. Further purification of T-cell subsets is conceivable, perhaps by subsequent processing using monoclonal antibodies against specific surface markers.

Red cells Similar to the separation of neocytes from donors for special transfusion purposes, there has been some success in separating sickle cells from Hb A cells by special centrifugal techniques in sickle cell disease patients. However, this has not yet been perfected to the point of having practical utility. Perfluorocarbons that are under development as red cell substitutes for life-threatening hemorrhage can be administered safely only in limited quantity; their high density (see Table 2) allows their subsequent removal by centrifugal apheresis, which may allow larger amounts to be given acutely and to be removed again when transfusion becomes available.

REGULATION OF THE UTILIZATION OF APHERESIS THERAPY

The high cost of therapeutic plasmapheresis and other apheresis procedures has attracted critical attention. Clinical investigation of the efficacy of these promising modalities has been unfettered and productive, but also it has been difficult to distinguish established indications from experimental ones. The temptation to offer hope, to do something and to believe that it is helping, has been difficult to resist when faced with devastating and often incurable illnesses. However, the argument that it cannot hurt to try plasmapheresis or lymphocytapheresis when all else has failed is dangerous, because like other dramatic interventions, these procedures clearly entail the risk of morbidity and mortality.

The problem of balancing uncertain benefit to an individual patient against the cost to society in general of providing extraordinarily expensive treatment is a difficult ethical dilemma which physicians face increasingly in many aspects of medical practice. Economic forces in all countries of the world in one way or another limit the supply of resources for plasmapheresis therapy, and the physician, though always required to provide the best care for the individual patient, must also use those resources wisely.

The greatest difficulty, however, in deciding whether to employ plasmapheresis or similar treatments results from the continuing inadequacy of knowledge regarding the medical efficacy of these interventions. Many immunological diseases are very difficult to study; for instance, even for commonly employed steroid and immunosuppressive therapies, it has been difficult to demonstrate the efficacy of these drug treatments in prospective controlled trials. Nevertheless, controlled studies of plasmapheresis need to be supported, and it is regrettable that several current multicenter trials cannot recruit adequate numbers of patients because the potential subjects are being advised to have plasmapheresis therapy anyway.

Patient selection for apheresis treatment within a hospital is best monitored by a committee of interested specialists representing expertise in the management of all diseases in question, together with physicians experienced in the practicalities and familiar with the risks of the procedure. Each patient must be fully evaluated before any commitment to provide treatment is made. The judgment must give due regard to data about the efficacy of apheresis versus other possible treatments for the patient's illness, whether these have been tried, have failed, or should not be tried, and the severity of the specific feature that is an indication for apheresis. Against this must be balanced the patient's overall health and ability to withstand the stress of apheresis treatment and the patient's ability to understand and consent when the application is experimental or unproved. In general, one of these three conditions must be met before apheresis is proposed: (1) it is established that the procedure is beneficial for the patient's disease and specific indications; (2) the patient consents to be a subject in a peer-reviewed prospective clinical trial; or (3) the patient has a bad prognosis and has no other viable choice of therapy available, and apheresis is of potential but unproven efficacy.

The problem of making appropriate choices when medical knowledge is not complete is, of course, not new. Burton, questioning the excessive and uncontrolled use of bloodletting in his *Anatomy of Melancholy* (1601) states, "In letting of blood three main cautions are to be considered, who, how much, when . . . ." The answers to the questions "how" and "why" are easier, though they have changed immeasurably with the introduction of sophisticated apheresis technology and with rationales based on complex modern understanding of immunology and biochemistry. However, the answers to the three questions that Burton asked, when applied to apheresis, are still only partially known and will require continued controlled observations during the next several years.

References

ABEL JJ et al: Plasma removal with return of corpuscles (plasmaphaeresis). J Pharmacol Exp Ther 5:625, 1914

AUFEUVRE JP et al: Clinical tolerance and hazards of plasma exchanges: A study of 6200 plasma exchanges in 1033 patients, in *Plasmapheresis in Immunology and Oncology,* JH Beyer et al (eds). Basel, Karger, 1982, pp 65–77

BERKMAN E: Issues in therapeutic apheresis. N Engl J Med 306:1418, 1982

BRECKENRIDGE RL et al: Treatment of thrombotic thrombocytopenic purpura with plasma exchange, antiplatelet agents, corticosteroid, and plasma infusion: Mayo Clinic experience. J Clin Apheresis 1:6, 1982

BROOKS BD et al: Therapeutic plasma exchange in the immune hemolytic anemias and immunologic thrombocytopenic purpura, in *Progress in Clinical and Biological Research.* 106: *Therapeutic Apheresis and Plasma Perfusion,* RSA Tindall (ed). New York, Alan B. Liss, 1982

CERCERE FA, SPIVA DA: Combination plasmapheresis/leukocytapheresis for the treatment of dermatomyositis/polymyositis. Plasma Ther Transfus Technol 3:401, 1982

GOLDFINGER D: Clinical applications of therapeutic cytapheresis, in *Therapeutic Hemapheresis,* EM Berkman and J Umlas (eds). Washington, DC, American Association of Blood Banks, 1980, pp 65–78

HAUSER SL et al: Intensive immunosuppression in progressive multiple sclerosis. N. Engl J Med 308:173, 1983

HAWKEY CJ et al: Plasma exchange and immunosuppressive drug treatment in myasthenia gravis: No evidence for synergy. J Neurol Neurosurg Psychiatry 44:469, 1981

HUESTIS DW: Mortality in therapeutic haemapheresis. Lancet 1:1043 1983

KEY TC et al: Automated erythrocytapheresis for sickle cell anemia during pregnancy. Am J Obstet Gynecol 138:731, 1980

LICHTMAN MA, ROWE JM: Hyperleukocytic leukemias: Rheological, clinical, and therapeutic considerations. Blood 60:279, 1982

LOCKWOOD CM, PETERS DK: Plasma exchange in glomerulonephritis and related vasculitides. Annu Rev Med 31:167, 1980

MCCULLOUGH J et al: What are the established clinical indications for therapeutic plasma exchange and how important is the choice of replacement fluid for efficacy of therapeutic plasma exchange in these situations? Vox Sang 43:270, 1982

POWLES R et al: Method of removing abnormal protein rapidly from patients with malignant paraproteinaemias. Br Med J 3:664, 1971

ROCK GA: Plasma exchange in the treatment of rhesus hemolytic disease: Review. Plasma Ther Transfus Technol 2:211, 1981

WALLACE D et al: A double-blind controlled study of lymphoplasmapheresis versus sham apheresis in rheumatoid arthiritis. N Engl J Med 306:1406, 1982

WEI N et al: Randomized trial of plasma exchange in mild systemic lupus erythematosus. Lancet 1:17, 1983

WENZ B, BARLAND P: Therapeutic intensive plasmapheresis. Semin Hematol 18:147, 1981

NON-A, NON-B HEPATITIS

LAWRENCE S. FRIEDMAN and JACK R. WANDS

Merely one decade ago viral hepatitis was thought to be caused primarily by two hepatotropic agents, hepatitis A virus (HAV) and hepatitis B virus (HBV), with occasional cases resulting from infection by the Epstein-Barr virus and cytomegalovirus. Since then, however, the application of specific serologic tests for the diagnosis of infections caused by HAV and HBV has led to the conclusion that significant numbers of cases of acute and chronic hepatitis in humans occur in the absence of infection with any known, serologically identifiable virus. These cases have been tentatively designated *non-A, non-B (NANB) hepatitis* to indicate that the diagnosis is based on exclusion of infection caused by HAV or HBV. Furthermore, the term non-A, non-B, rather than hepatitis C, was chosen to reflect the likelihood that more than one etiologic agent may ultimately be identified.

In the 10 years since the recognition of NANB hepatitis as an entity, the infectious nature of the causative agent(s) has been clearly established by transmission of the disease to chimpanzees. Progress has been made in defining the epidemiologic and clinical features of NANB hepatitis, including its important contribution to sporadic hepatitis and its principal role in post-transfusion hepatitis (PTH). NANB hepatitis has indeed been identified as the primary impediment to the delivery of safe blood. Despite intensive efforts to isolate and characterize the agents responsible for NANB hepatitis, however, no NANB hepatitis virus has been unequivocally demonstrated ultrastructurally or serologically.

In this article, the current state of knowledge about NANB hepatitis is reviewed. Epidemiologic, clinical, and preventive aspects of NANB hepatitis are discussed, and results of efforts to identify the etiologic agent(s) are summarized. In addition, results of preliminary investigations employing recombinant DNA technology and monoclonal antibodies to identify a NANB hepatitis agent related to HBV are described.

HISTORICAL OVERVIEW

Hepatitis-like illnesses have been recognized since antiquity, but not until the early twentieth century was the viral etiology of hepatitis proposed. The concept of two types of viral hepatitis derived from epidemiologic observations and volunteer studies of the 1940s. Infectious hepatitis, or type A, was defined by a short incubation period of 2 to 6 weeks and oral transmission. Serum hepatitis, or type B, was defined by a long incubation period of 6 weeks to 6 months (average 12 to 14 weeks) and percutaneous transmission. This theory of viral hepatitis predominated until the end of the 1960s, although earlier doubts were occasionally raised when the theory failed to account for the occurrence of multiple attacks of hepatitis in drug addicts and hemophiliacs and for an average incubation period of 7 weeks for hepatitis which followed blood transfusions.

The landmark discovery of Australia antigen by Blumberg and his colleagues in 1965 and its identification as hepatitis B surface antigen (HBsAg) led to the development of serologic tests to detect HBV antigens and antibodies. Testing of serum for HBV markers in turn led to the revelations that 50 to 75 percent of cases of PTH were not serologically related to HBV and that up to 50 percent of cases of sporadic hepatitis, heretofore assumed to be type A, were actually caused by type B. A further blow to the traditional two-virus concept of viral hepatitis came when mandatory exclusion of donor blood positive for HBsAg by increasingly sensitive assays resulted in a reduced frequency of posttransfusion HBV infection but failed to alter significantly the overall frequency of PTH. Moreover, the presence of anti-HBs in donor blood did not appear to protect the recipient from developing PTH.

Were cases of non-B PTH caused by percutaneously transmitted HAV infection? This question was answered with a resounding *no* following the identification of HAV in 1973, and the application of serologic tests to exclude HAV as the cause of PTH. In addition, protective anti-HAV could be demonstrated in the sera of many individuals prior to transfusion, and such individuals were not protected from PTH. Similarly, Epstein-Barr virus (EBV) and cytomegalovirus (CMV) could not be implicated as etiologic factors except in a minority of patients with PTH. In the case of EBV, protective antibodies were present in the sera of most blood recipients prior to transfusion. In the case of CMV, serologic evidence of recent CMV infection could be found as frequently in transfused patients in whom hepatitis developed as in those in whom it did not, and such fluctuations in antibody titer were felt to be insignificant.

The overwhelming implication of the preceding observations was that there was another virus, or group of viruses, that accounted for most cases of PTH. Additional evidence for an NANB agent came from the demonstration that the frequency of PTH could be reduced substantially by the substitution of commercially obtained blood from paid donors with blood obtained solely from volunteers. Because commercially available blood is obtained from individuals likely to be of a lower socioeconomic background than volunteer donors, it was argued that such paid donors might be more likely to have been exposed to a percutaneously transmitted blood-borne virus. The exclusion of commercial blood donors, in fact, resulted in a 70 percent reduction in the incidence of PTH. Such a reduction in the incidence of PTH as a result of eliminating commercial donors, but not as a result of HBsAg testing, supported the notion that

the NANB agent, not HBV, likely accounted for most cases of PTH all along.

Thus, by the mid-1970s there was compelling evidence for the existence of at least one more major hepatitis virus. The features of NANB hepatitis included (1) a variable but defined incubation period intermediate between that of HAV and HBV; (2) hepatic histology indistinguishable from hepatitis of other causes; and (3) a positive correlation between the development of NANB hepatitis and the source of donor blood (up to 10 times more frequent after transfusion of blood from commercial than from volunteer donors). Additional studies since then have helped define further the epidemiologic, clinical, and biological properties of this virus.

EPIDEMIOLOGY OF NANB HEPATITIS

Transfusion of blood and blood products was the first recognized and remains the most visible means of dissemination of NANB hepatitis. Table 1 lists the variety of blood products associated with transmission of NANB hepatitis. In general, the risk of transmission is greater for products pooled from multiple donors than for those derived from single donors. According to most studies of PTH since 1975, NANB hepatitis accounts for over 90 percent of PTH; the remaining 10 percent of cases are caused principally by HBV infection, despite universal HBsAg screening with sensitive "third-generation" radioimmunoassays. (Failure to detect HBsAg in donor blood subsequently found to cause acute HBV infection may result either from the presence of HBsAg in titers too low to be detected by conventional assays or from the absence of HBsAg and anti-HBs during the "window" period of acute hepatitis B, when anti-HBc is the only serologic expression of HBV infection.)

The attack rate of NANB hepatitis in individuals transfused with volunteer blood only is approximately 7 percent, with a range of 5 to 13 percent in various studies. Such an attack rate is considerably less than previous rates of 17 to 54 percent associated with transfusion of commercially obtained blood. Geographic differences in the incidence of PTH have been noted; for example, in one study of PTH the incidence was 10.2 percent in Los Angeles, but only 5.4

percent in St. Louis. Whether such variations in attack rate reflect different prevalences of asymptomatic carriers, different socioeconomic levels of donors, or the effect of an outbreak of NANB hepatitis in one city at the time of the survey is unknown.

Following the discovery that NANB hepatitis is associated with transfusion of blood products, other epidemiologic settings for the transmission of NANB hepatitis were identified (see Table 1). Like hepatitis B, but unlike hepatitis A, epidemiologic studies of NANB hepatitis suggested that percutaneous exposure, rather than fecal-oral transmission, was the principal means of dissemination. For example, NANB hepatitis was reported in patients undergoing hemodialysis and in renal transplant recipients. Subsequently, NANB hepatitis was observed in intravenous drug addicts, and in several surveys of drug addicts, NANB infection accounted for as many as 50 percent of the clinical cases of hepatitis. Moreover, the demonstration of two or three episodes of NANB hepatitis in the same individual provided circumstantial evidence for the existence of multiple NANB agents.

NANB hepatitis has also been responsible for institutional and nosocomial outbreaks of hepatitis and for cases of hepatitis among plasma donors participating in a plasmapheresis program. Health care workers and investigators have contracted NANB hepatitis not only following accidental needlesticks but also in the absence of overt parenteral exposure. Hospitalization per se has been shown to increase the risk of NANB hepatitis; in one study of hospitalized patients undergoing surgery but not requiring blood transfusion, the incidence of NANB hepatitis was 2.2 percent. This increased risk of hepatitis in hospitalized patients could not be related to the type of surgery, anesthesia, or medications used.

Transmission to heterosexual and homosexual contacts of individuals with NANB hepatitis has been documented. On the other hand, and consistent with the absence of fecal-oral transmission, intrafamilial and household transmission, while reported, is uncommon, and except for some rare exceptions (see below), common-source epidemics do not occur.

Vertical maternal-neonatal transmission has been described in six of nine infants born to women with acute NANB hepatitis during the third trimester of pregnancy. The diagnosis of

TABLE 1
Modes of transmission of non-A, non-B hepatitis

I Tranfusions
  A Lower risk products*
    1 Whole blood
    2 Packed red blood cells†
    3 Fresh frozen plasma
    4 Single-donor platelet concentrates
    5 Single-donor granulocyte concentrates
    6 Cryoprecipitate
    7 Fibrinogen
  B Higher risk products
    1 Factor IX complex
    2 Antihemophilic factor
    3 Multiple-donor platelet concentrates
II Hemodialysis
III Renal transplantation
IV Illicit self-injection
V Institutional (nosocomial outbreaks)
VI Plasmapheresis programs
VII Health care providers
VIII Intrafamilial
IX Homosexual and heterosexual contacts
X Vertical (maternal-neonatal)
XI Waterborne (India)
XII Sporadic

No risk generally associated with albumin, plasma protein fraction, immune serum globulin, hyperimmune globulin [if heat-treated for 10 h at 60°C or prepared by Cohn fractation (cold ethanol)].
† Risk may be decreased further by washing, freezing, and/or deglycerolization (see text).

hepatitis in the infants was made on the basis of abnormal liver function tests at 4 to 8 weeks of age and exclusion of infection due to other viruses, namely HAV and HBV.

A significant fraction of hepatitis cases that meet the exclusion criteria for NANB hepatitis occur in the absence of a well-defined outbreak or an epidemiologic setting. That such sporadic cases of NANB hepatitis must exist was first inferred from the observations that most blood donors who transmit NANB hepatitis have not themselves been transfused and they do not fall into any of the other epidemiologic categories described above. NANB hepatitis accounts for 15 to 25 percent of sporadic hepatitis, has a worldwide distribution, and is endemic in many areas, especially among lower socioeconomic groups. Because intrafamilial spread is infrequent, transmission is thought to result from inapparent parenteral exposure rather than from fecal-oral transmission. However, the understanding of precise transmission patterns awaits the development of serologic markers.

Although common-source outbreaks of hepatitis have always been attributed to HAV infection, recent studies from India implicate NANB hepatitis as a cause of some epidemics of viral hepatitis. In several common-source waterborne epidemics of viral hepatitis, an incubation period of 10 to 40 days, the frequent occurrence of secondary cases of hepatitis within households, and the absence of development of chronic hepatitis suggested a diagnosis of hepatitis A; however, serologic evidence of either hepatitis A or B was lacking. Moreover, distinctive pathologic features and a high incidence of fulminant hepatitis in pregnant women were inconsistent with a diagnosis of hepatitis A. An NANB agent related to HAV is presumed to be responsible for such epidemics.

Finally, the transmission of NANB hepatitis by asymptomatic blood donors has provided strong evidence for an asymptomatic carrier state. The potential size of this carrier reservoir is enormous. Based on an incidence of NANB hepatitis of 3 to 7 percent in the United States following single-unit blood transfusions, the carrier rate of NANB hepatitis could be 30 to 70 times greater than that of HBV!

CLINICAL FEATURES

Most clinical information about NANB hepatitis comes from studies of transfusion-transmitted disease. Among the different types of viral hepatitis there is considerable overlap of clinical features, so that etiologic distinctions (HAV, HBV, or NANB) cannot be predicted solely on clinical grounds. In general, NANB hepatitis resembles hepatitis B but has a shorter incubation period, less severe course, and greater propensity to become chronic with subsequent development of hepatic fibrosis and cirrhosis.

Acute NANB hepatitis

The mean incubation period from the time of exposure (transfusion) to the onset of symptoms or first abnormal liver function test [usually the serum alanine aminotransferase (ALT)] is 7 to 8 weeks, with a range of 2 to 26 weeks. For the majority of patients, the incubation period falls within 5 to 10 weeks. This incubation period is intermediate between those of hepatitis A (4 weeks) and hepatitis B (12 to 14 weeks). Varying incubation periods among individuals with NANB hepatitis are postulated to result from different infecting agents or different doses of infecting virus. The shortest incubation times are observed following infusions of factor VIII concentrates or cryoprecipitates (1 to 4 weeks) and in the waterborne epidemics in India (2 weeks).

Acute NANB hepatitis is generally a mild disease, on average less severe symptomatically and biochemically than hepatitis B and indistinguishable from hepatitis A. Jaundice is observed in only 25 percent of cases. The mean peak serum ALT level is below 800 IU in two-thirds of patients and above 2000 IU in fewer than 10 percent, although more severe biochemical abnormalities are common in immunocompromised hosts. Fatalities occur, but less commonly than in acute hepatitis B. Nevertheless, among 188 cases of fulminant hepatitis in one series, 34 percent were felt to be caused by NANB hepatitis; a lower survival rate (13 percent) was observed among patients with fulminant NANB hepatitis than among those with either fulminant hepatitis A or B (33 percent), although the possibility that some cases of apparent NANB hepatitis were actually caused by drugs or toxins cannot be excluded.

As in other types of hepatitis, symptoms include anorexia, malaise, nausea, and right upper quadrant pain and follow the onset of serum ALT elevation by 1 to 4 weeks. Many individuals with acute NANB hepatitis are probably asymptomatic. Unlike hepatitis A, fever, headache, and myalgias are uncommon. Lymphadenopathy and splenomegaly are rarely noted. Despite the presence of circulating immune complexes in up to 70 percent of individuals with NANB hepatitis, extrahepatic manifestations typical of hepatitis B (serum sickness, urticaria, purpura) are unusual. Marked elevations of serum IgM levels, typical of hepatitis A, are not observed in patients with NANB hepatitis. However, a recent study suggests that NANB hepatitis may account for many cases of hepatitis-related aplastic anemia.

The mean duration of disease in patients who recover from acute NANB hepatitis is 10 to 12 weeks. This is slightly longer than the mean duration of transfusion-transmitted hepatitis B (8 weeks) but shorter than the duration of sporadic

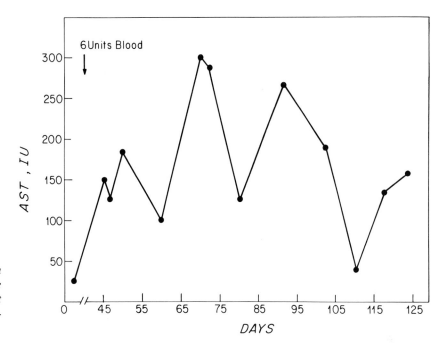

FIGURE 1

Fluctuating course of serum aspartate aminotransferase (AST) activity in a patient with posttransfusion hepatitis.

hepatitis B. In one study of epidemic waterborne NANB hepatitis, most patients recovered within 2 to 6 weeks.

In many individuals with NANB hepatitis, the course is marked by a distinctive pattern of waxing and waning serum aminotransferase activity not generally observed in other types of viral hepatitis. Episodic and multiphasic elevations in aminotransferase activity may alternate with periods of normal or nearly normal activity (see Fig. 1). In some patients episodic clinical deterioration parallels the biochemical flares, while in others biochemical exacerbations are unassociated with symptoms or signs of illness. Other patients experience a monophasic elevation of aminotransferase activity, which is characterized by a rapid elevation of the serum aminotransferase level to a peak that coincides with the intensity of the clinical illness and followed by a gradual resolution to normal. In still other patients the serum aminotransferase activity increases slowly to a plateau and remains abnormal at this level for weeks; the duration of illness is prolonged in these patients.

Chronic hepatitis

The most striking clinical feature of NANB hepatitis is its propensity to become chronic. De-

pending on the clinical setting, elevated aminotransferase levels may persist for longer than 1 year in 10 to 60 percent of patients. For individuals with posttransfusion and intravenous drug-transmitted NANB hepatitis, the incidence of chronic hepatitis is 40 to 60 percent, and if asymptomatic chronic NANB carriers with normal serum aminotransferases are considered, the incidence of chronic NANB viral infection 1 year after acute exposure may be as high as 75 percent. This incidence of chronic infection compares with values of 10 percent following acute hepatitis B and virtually zero percent following acute hepatitis A. Chronic infection is less likely to follow sporadic acute NANB hepatitis than transfusion-related disease, and the incidence ranges from zero to 20 percent in various series. Among immunosuppressed patients, however, chronic NANB hepatitis may develop in as many as 80 percent following acute NANB hepatitis. No instances of chronic hepatitis have been reported among patients with epidemic NANB hepatitis in India.

In the majority of patients (60 percent) with chronic posttransfusion NANB hepatitis, liver morphology is compatible with chronic active hepatitis on the basis of piecemeal necrosis (erosion of the limiting plate of hepatocytes surrounding the portal tracts). However, bridging and multilobular necroses are not usually observed, except in immunosuppressed patients, and the histologic lesion is considered to be mild. One-third of individuals with chronic NANB hepatitis demonstrate chronic persistent hepatitis or nonspecific hepatic changes on liver biopsy. In early studies of NANB hepatitis, cirrhosis was reported infrequently, but more recent studies suggest that the development of cirrhosis may not be uncommon. Long-term prospective studies are required to clarify the natural history of NANB hepatitis.

NANB hepatitis not associated with blood transfusion may have a different outcome from posttransfusion NANB hepatitis. Besides a lower predilection for chronicity than PTH, chronic sporadic NANB hepatitis is more likely to be associated with histologic changes of chronic persistent hepatitis. Whether these differences are related to differences in infecting viral dose, viral agents, or the severity of initial illness is unknown.

Regardless of the epidemiologic setting or histologic findings, most individuals with chronic NANB hepatitis have mild or no symptoms. Unlike autoimmune (or "lupoid") hepatitis, serum globulin levels are elevated minimally (if at all), autoantibodies are absent, and clinical evidence of autoimmune disease is lacking. Because of the paucity of symptoms and signs, most patients with chronic NANB hepatitis probably go undetected, unless studied prospectively. The course in most patients appears to be clinically indolent, often slowly resolving rather than chronically progressing, and cases of biochemical and histologic resolution after several years have been documented. Nevertheless, progression to cirrhosis has been found to occur in some patients. It is unclear whether hepatocellular carcinoma is likely to develop after prolonged chronic NANB infection, as in chronic hepatitis B.

Several investigators have attempted to predict the development of chronic NANB hepatitis based on the severity of the acute phase (Table 2). Factors shown in four major studies to predict the development of chronic hepatitis have included transfusion volume, the presence of

TABLE 2
Summary of studies on risk factors for development of chronic non-A, non-B hepatitis

Investigators	Number of patients with acute hepatitis	Number of patients in whom chronic hepatitis developed	Source of hepatitis	Risk factors for developing chronic hepatitis
Knodell et al. (1977)	44	10	Posttransfusion (military donors)	Large transfusion volume Presence of symptoms during acute illness (malaise, nausea, vomiting)
Rakela and Redeker (1979)	45	18	Posttransfusion (donor source not indicated) Illicit self-injection Sporadic	Absence of jaundice during acute illness
Berman et al. (1979)	26	12	Posttransfusion (volunteer donors)	Serum alanine aminotransferase > 300 IU/liter in anicteric patients only during acute illness
Koretz et al. (1980)	66	26	Posttransfusion (donor source not indicated)	No predictive factors identified

symptoms during the acute illness, the absence of jaundice, and a peak serum ALT level of greater than 300 IU. However, no two studies yielded identical results, and the inclusion criteria of the studies differed in terms of the source of hepatitis (posttransfusion, illicit self-injection, sporadic) and donor sources of blood (volunteer, commercial). When the results of the four studies are pooled, however, a striking increase in the incidence of chronic hepatitis is found to be associated with a peak serum ALT level greater than 300 IU during the acute phase (70 percent) compared with a peak ALT level less than 300 IU (22 percent). Caution is indicated in interpreting this result because the data may merely indicate that a higher serum ALT level is likely to reflect a true NANB infection rather than a nonviral hepatic abnormality.

Chronic carrier state

The prediction of an asymptomatic chronic viral carrier state for the NANB agent on the basis of transmission by asymptomatic blood donors was confirmed by chimpanzee transmission studies. In one well-described case, transmission of NANB hepatitis was achieved by inoculation of chimpanzees with serum from a patient 6 years after an acute episode of NANB hepatitis and at a time when the patient's serum aminotransferase activity was normal. Similarly, serial transmission of NANB hepatitis by inoculation of serum from one chimpanzee into another has occurred up to 16 months following acute infection in the donor chimpanzee and also at a time when the serum aminotransferase level was not elevated. These results imply that, like HBV, the NANB agent may circulate in the serum in the absence of clinical or biochemical disease.

DIAGNOSIS OF NANB HEPATITIS

In the absence of a virus-specific test for NANB hepatitis and of diagnostic clinical features, the diagnosis of NANB hepatitis is made by the exclusion of known viral and nonviral causes of liver disease in the proper clinical setting. In the research setting, inoculation of chimpanzees or marmosets with serum from persons suspected of having NANB hepatitis may be used to confirm the diagnosis, but this method is obviously impractical for general use. Pathologic exami-

nation of liver biopsy specimens from patients with suspected NANB hepatitis has a limited role in establishing the diagnosis.

Exclusion of other viral causes of hepatitis

In patients with suspected NANB hepatitis, exclusion of acute hepatitis A is demonstrated by the absence in serum of HAV IgM, the acute-phase antibody. Acute or chronic HBV infection may be excluded by demonstrating the absence in serum of HBsAg and anti-HBc. However, it is possible for an individual with chronic HBV infection (asymptomatic carrier or chronic hepatitis) to have acute NANB hepatitis as well. At present, there is no reliable means to differentiate acute hepatitis B from acute NANB hepatitis superimposed on chronic HBV infection, unless the chronic HBV infection is known to have preceded the acute hepatitis. The recent development of an IgM anti-HBc assay that may be specific for acute HBV infection may enable such a distinction to be made more easily in the future. In some individuals with chronic HBV infection, especially certain high risk groups like drug addicts, an exacerbation of liver disease may be caused by the recently identified delta agent. In such patients testing for anti-delta antibody in serum during flares of hepatitis is indicated.

In some instances it may be necessary to exclude EBV infection. This agent is capable of producing sporadic and posttransfusion hepatitis and has also been responsible for an outbreak of hepatitis in a hemodialysis unit. Features suggestive of infectious mononucleosis, including rash, pharyngitis, splenomegaly, lymphadenopathy, and atypical lymphocytosis, are occasionally absent in patients with EBV hepatitis. A negative heterophile antibody test excludes the diagnosis of EBV with up to 90 percent certainty, and absence of IgM antibodies to the viral capsid antigen by immunofluorescence testing excludes the diagnosis in all. The incidence of posttransfusion EBV infection is very low, however, because most transfusion recipients already have protective antibodies. In several studies of transfusion-associated hepatitis, a serologic association between EBV and PTH was not demonstrated.

TABLE 3
Clinical parameters: Posttransfusion hepatitis

Parameters	Hepatitis B virus	Non-A, non-B hepatitis	Cytomegalovirus
Number of cases	4	45	9
Mean incubation (weeks)	17.5	10.5	7.3
Percent icteric	75	24	0
Mean peak serum alanine aminotransferase (ALT), IU/liter	1050	655	177
Percent serum ALT > 300 IU/liter	100	73	0
Percent chronic hepatitis	25	58	0

SOURCE: *HJ Alter et al, in Viral Hepatitis, 1981 International Symposium, W Szmuness et al (eds), Philadelphia, Franklin Institute Press, 1982.*

The role of CMV in PTH has been difficult to evaluate because of the existence of multiple, partially related CMV serotypes and the typical pattern of fluctuating antibody levels in normal individuals. Moreover, CMV reactivation is known to occur under conditions of surgical stress and massive transfusion. In the past, serologic evidence of recent CMV infection was found to be as frequent in transfused patients in whom hepatitis developed as in those in whom it did not develop. Similarly, CMV seroconversion was seen to occur during some cases of typical posttransfusion hepatitis B. Except for immunosuppressed renal transplant patients, the role of CMV in posttransfusion liver disease was felt to be small.

Recent studies suggest that CMV infection may be playing a larger role in PTH than previously thought. Older studies determined serologic responses to CMV by a complement fixation method, which yielded inconsistent results and was often rendered unreliable by anticomplementary activity in the serum. More recent studies of CMV-antibody activity have made use of an indirect hemagglutination method, which is more sensitive, reproducible, and measurable in serum that is anticomplementary by complement fixation techniques. These studies have revealed that CMV infection may account for up to 15 percent of PTH. Preliminary analysis of such cases of PTH associated with CMV seroconversion suggests that they are clinically distinct from other forms of NANB hepatitis. In general, PTH associated with CMV is characterized by a short incubation period, very mild clinical and bio-

chemical abnormalities (ALT < 300 IU, no jaundice), and the absence of chronicity (Table 3).

The recognition that CMV plays a significant role in PTH has important implications. For example, it may now become easier to define cases of PTH which are caused by NANB agents other than CMV and which require monitoring for the development of chronic liver disease. On the other hand, the clinical relevance of CMV hepatitis appears to be minor in otherwise healthy transfusion recipients; efforts to prevent a mild, transient disease may not be warranted, except for defined populations in which CMV transmission by transfusion may be deleterious (e.g., immunodeficient patients). Prospective studies of transfusion recipients of blood screened for CMV may help clarify these issues.

Aside from HAV, HBV, EBV, and CMV, there appears to be little role for other viruses in causing hepatitis. Similarly, bacterial or parasitic infections rarely present a clinical picture which might be confused with NANB hepatitis. However, in any patient in whom NANB hepatitis is suspected, a careful search for toxic, drug, or allergic causes of hepatitis should be made, and congestive heart failure should be excluded.

Histologic features of NANB hepatitis

Because the liver is rarely biopsied in cases of acute hepatitis, the histologic features of acute NANB hepatitis, unlike chronic NANB hepatitis, are not well-characterized. In general, the histologic findings are typical of other types of viral hepatitis and include Kupffer cell reactivity, mild portal round-cell infiltration, and foci of intralobular mononuclear cells. Severe hepatocellular necrosis and marked cholestasis are generally absent. Recently, histologic features felt to be distinct for NANB hepatitis have been described. Eosinophilic alteration of the hepatocyte cytoplasm associated with many acidophilic bodies and microvesicular fat and unaccompanied by a significant inflammatory response was found in about 40 percent of cases of acute NANB hepatitis. Also noted in some cases of acute NANB hepatitis was a conspicuous sinusoidal cell proliferation. These changes were not observed in liver biopsy specimens from individuals with acute hepatitis A or B. However, they were also not present in many specimens from patients with acute NANB hepatitis, and the specificity of these findings has not yet been confirmed by others.

Unique histologic features have been observed in liver specimens from patients with epidemic NANB hepatitis in India. Some, but not all, specimens have revealed intracanalicular bile stasis and rosette, or "glandlike," formation of hepatocytes. These changes have not been observed in cases of NANB hepatitis outside India.

TRANSMISSION STUDIES

The best evidence for the existence of NANB agents derives from the successful experimental transmission of infection to human volunteers and certain animals. Transmission of the disease to animals has fostered the development of experimental assays designed to detect antigen-antibody systems present in serum.

Human volunteer studies, conducted in the early 1950s and reported after analysis of stored sera in 1977, included the inoculation of nine human volunteers with icterogenic HBsAg-negative serum from three donors. An incubation period of 18 to 89 days was observed, six of nine recipients became jaundiced, and two of six who were followed long enough showed evidence of chronic hepatitis. Infection caused by HBV, HAV, CMV, and EBV was excluded by serologic studies. Rechallenge experiments demonstrated the development of homologous immunity, and

the absence of an anamnestic anti-HBs response in patients convalescent from hepatitis B and inoculated with the NANB sera confirmed the specificity of the NANB agent. The existence of an infectious chronic carrier state for NANB hepatitis was implied by the transmission of hepatitis by serum from donors 6 months to 1 year after their initial blood donation had been implicated in transmitting hepatitis. Further studies demonstrated the serial passage in volunteers of an NANB agent and added support to its viral nature.

Animal studies

Transmission of NANB hepatitis from humans to chimpanzees and serial passage of the agent(s) in chimpanzees in 1978 provided the first assay for the infectious agent and an animal model for the disease. NANB hepatitis has been transmitted to chimpanzees by intravenous inoculation of acute- and chronic-phase sera from patients with NANB hepatitis, sera from blood donors implicated in cases of NANB hepatitis, and clotting-factor concentrates.

The hepatitis produced in such chimpanzees is generally mild and self-limited, and exclusion of infection by HBV, HAV, CMV, and EBV has been confirmed serologically. The severity of illness is unrelated to the volume of inoculum or the stage of disease (acute or chronic) at which the donor serum is obtained. Incubation periods are constant for a given inoculum but vary among the inocula from short (2 to 6 weeks) to long (10 to 20 weeks) intervals. As in cases of human NANB hepatitis, biphasic or episodic patterns of serum aminotransferase activity elevation are observed in infected chimpanzees, but there is no consistent relation between the pattern of ALT level changes in the chimpanzees and the pattern in the patients from whom the inocula were derived. Liver biopsies from chimpanzees with NANB hepatitis show a histologic picture typical of viral hepatitis with variation in size and staining quality of hepatocyte nuclei, irregularly clumped cytoplasm, focal necrosis of hepatocytes, acidophilic bodies, portal inflammation, and marked activation of sinusoidal lining cells.

A number of features of NANB hepatitis observed in human cases have been confirmed and further characterized in the chimpanzee model. A long period of viremia, preceding the onset of clinical illness by as many as 12 days and following the onset of clinical illness by as long as 9 weeks, has been demonstrated in chimpanzees with acute NANB hepatitis. Moreover, viremia may persist for months following resolution of acute illness and return of serum ALT activity to normal. Serial passage of NANB hepatitis in chimpanzees has also revealed a marked propensity for the development of chronic hepatitis. In one study, 6 of 11 chimpanzees had persistent serum ALT elevations 1 year after acute infection, and in ongoing studies serum ALT elevations have been shown to persist for up to 4 years. Histologically chronic NANB hepatitis in chimpanzees is characterized by a lesion similar to chronic persistent hepatitis in humans; the development of cirrhosis is rare. Histologic evidence of chronic persistent hepatitis may be observed even after serum ALT activity has returned to normal.

Transmission of hepatitis to chimpanzees by inoculation of sera from asymptomatic human donors with normal serum ALT levels has confirmed the existence of healthy human carriers. In addition, the persistence of the agent in the blood of one patient was documented over a 6-year period following acute hepatitis even when serum ALT activity was normal. The specificity of NANB inocula have been established by the demonstration of homologous immunity, the inability to alter susceptibility to infection by HBV after convalescence from NANB infection, and the induction of NANB disease in animals already immune to both type A and type B hepatitis. That a single agent may be responsible for many cases of PTH in the United States has been suggested by the observation that homologous immunity could be induced in chimpanzees to three inocula obtained from chronically infected humans residing in different geographic areas.

Recently NANB hepatitis has been transmitted successfully to the marmoset, a small monkey that is more readily available, less expensive, and more convenient to handle than chimpanzee. However, marmosets cannot be infected as regularly as chimpanzees, and the incubation period is long (13 to 24 weeks). At this time the use of either chimpanzees or marmosets to evaluate individual cases of human hepatitis is impractical, but these animals remain important research tools.

ATTEMPTS TO IDENTIFY AND CHARACTERIZE NANB AGENTS

The successful transmission of the NANB agent(s) to animals has spurred intensive efforts to identify the causative agent or other diagnostically useful markers of the agent. To date no NANB agent has been identified with certainty, but a number of candidate virus particles have been observed, ultrastructural hepatocyte abnormalities specific for NANB hepatitis have been described, and potential serologic assays for the NANB agent have been developed. These studies have provided further insight into the biology of the NANB agent. More recently, monoclonal antibodies and DNA hybridization techniques have been applied to the study of the NANB agent.

Particles associated with NANB hepatitis

The use of electron microscopy and immune electron microscopy to examine infected sera and liver tissue has revealed a variety of viruslike particles associated with NANB infection. In different studies these particles have ranged in size from 15 to 25 nm to 60 to 80 nm. It is not known whether the size differences are the result of multiple infecting agents, differences in methodology, differences in the source of particles, or the unrelatedness of the particles to actual NANB agents. Particles have been observed in infectious blood products and healthy donor serum with elevated ALT levels, as well as sera and liver specimens from individuals and animals with acute NANB hepatitis. On the basis of only limited observations, these particles may be specific for NANB hepatitis.

Several viruslike particles have been proposed as candidates for the actual NANB virus. One example is the finding of Bradley and colleagues of 27-nm spherical particles in the serum and hepatocyte cytoplasm of chimpanzees and in human sera infected with an NANB hepatitis agent in factor IX concentrates. These particles are similar in appearance, buoyant density, and cytoplasmic location to small RNA viruses (picornaviruses) like HAV. Another example is the finding of Trepo and others of particles with the appearance of HBV forms in the sera of patients with NANB hepatitis. They have observed small (15- to 25-nm) spherical and long filamentous particles as well as larger (35- to 45-nm) spherical double-shelled (Dane-like) particles, analogous to particles found in sera of HBV-infected patients. In addition, particulate DNA polymerase activity has been detected in some sera and in homogenates of liver tissue containing these HBV-like particles, and intranuclear particles with the appearance of HBV cores (22 to 27 nm) have been identified in the liver sections. On the basis of these findings there is speculation (but no proof) that the HBV-like particles represent infection with an HBV-like virus, similar to other "hepadna" (or HBV-related) viruses found in woodchucks, ground squirrels, and Pekin ducks. If there is such an HBV-related NANB virus, its surface antigen does not cross react with HBsAg by conventional radioimmunoassays. Further characterization of these particles is needed to establish their identity with the infectious agent of NANB hepatitis or their relation to other hepatitis viruses.

Although little is known about its physical and chemical properties, the NANB agent has been shown to be inactivated by formalin, suggesting that the formalin used in the preparation of the HBV vaccine may eliminate the risk of transmitting NANB agents by vaccination. Moreover, the development of a formalin-inactivated NANB vaccine may be possible. The NANB agent is also inactivated by heat, which may provide a way of reducing the high risk of hepatitis transmission by pooled plasma products, such as clotting-factor concentrates.

Ultrastructural studies

A number of ultrastructural alterations, initially thought to be specific for NANB hepatitis, were observed in liver cells of chimpanzees inoculated with NANB-containing sera or plasma products. In chimpanzees infected with an NANB hepatitis inoculum derived from acute-phase sera of patients with PTH and designated strain H, hepatocyte nuclei were condensed and irregular and were found to contain viruslike spherical particles (20 to 27 nm). In chimpanzees infected with a different NANB inoculum designated strain F, hepatocyte cytoplasm were found to contain tubular, double-membraned structures, which appeared to be part of the endoplasmic reticulum.

Initially, the intranuclear particles and the intracytoplasmic tubular structures were not seen in the same chimpanzees, and the possibility of two distinct NANB agents was suggested. Cross-challenge experiments at first further supported the existence of at least two immunologically distinct NANB agents. Infectious preparations of a factor VIII concentrate induced a short-incubation illness in chimpanzees and were associated with only hepatocyte nuclear changes typical of strain H. On the other hand, contaminated factor IX preparations induced a long-incubation illness and were associated with tubular cytoplasmic alterations typical of strain F. Infection with one agent prevented a second infection by the same agent (homologous immunity) but did not protect against challenge by the other infectious agent. Furthermore, each strain could be serially passaged in chimpanzees and marmosets, and the ultrastructural pattern for a given strain (nuclear or cytoplasmic) remained the same.

Subsequent studies questioned the strain-specificity of the ultrastructural findings. Both nuclear and cytoplasmic changes were observed in the same liver biopsy specimen from infected chimpanzees, and one inoculum was found to provoke either nuclear or cytoplasmic changes in different infected chimpanzees. In addition, some animals infected with an inoculum specific for one type of change failed to show evidence of infection when challenged with material known to produce the other type of change. More recently, even the virus-specificity of the ultrastructural changes has been challenged, and nuclear particles have been observed in liver specimens from chimpanzees with acute and chronic hepatitis B.

Electron-microscopic examination of liver specimens from humans with NANB hepatitis has also revealed ultrastructural alterations in hepatocytes. In individuals with acute NANB hepatitis intranuclear particles only have been observed, while in individuals with chronic NANB hepatitis both intranuclear particles and intracytoplasmic fused, circular membranes have been observed, often in the same specimen. However, the nuclear particles have also been identified recently in liver specimens from individuals with acute hepatitis A and B, CMV hepatitis, and even nonviral liver disease, including alcoholic cirrhosis, alpha$_1$ antitrypsin deficiency, and Reye's syndrome.

In sum, the specificity of the ultrastructural changes for NANB hepatitis has not been confirmed, and it is possible that they represent host cellular responses to a variety of stimuli rather than disease-specific markers.

Serologic assays

There have been a number of attempts to develop serologic tests for presumed NANB hepatitis virus antigen and antibody in serum and liver of humans and chimpanzees. The methods employed have included agar gel immunodiffusion, counterelectrophoresis, radioimmunoassay, enzyme-linked immunosorbent assay (ELISA), and immunofluorescence staining of liver tissue. Human convalescent sera or sera from multitransfused patients have been used as sources of antibody in these experimental assays. In general, the NANB antigen assays have been reported to share the following features: (1) antigen is not found in pretransfusion specimens or before clinical or laboratory evidence of infection; (2) antigen is absent in patients with serologic evidence of HAV and HBV infection; (3) antigenic material identified in patients with acute NANB hepatitis disappears with resolution of hepatitis or persists if infection becomes chronic; and (4) antibody appears on resolution of the acute disease.

Unfortunately problems exist with each of the assays developed thus far. They lack specificity, reproducibility, and confirmability by independent laboratories. None of the tests has successfully identified sera known to contain NANB agents from a panel of coded sera, although the radioimmunoassay shows the most promise. It is probable that some of the "antigen" and "antibody" detected by these assays represents immune complexes or other non-virus-specific reactions, such as complement-breakdown products. Evaluation of the assays has been further complicated by the unavailability of sufficient quantities of reagent antigens and antibodies.

The relationship of putative antigens and antibodies to the infectious agents of NANB hepatitis and the diagnostic usefulness of conventional assays remains unclear. The inability to detect virus-specific antigen in sera known to contain NANB agents implies that the antigen concentration must be significantly lower than that of HBsAg in individuals with HBV infection. The antigens may in fact be masked within immune complexes. The failure to detect a specific NANB antibody in convalescent sera may be due to an inadequate humoral response to the antigen, which may account for the high incidence of chronic hepatitis following acute NANB infection.

DNA hybridization and monoclonal antibody studies

The application of recombinant DNA technology to the study of hepatitis viruses has provided a better understanding of HBV and compelling evidence for the existence of an NANB agent(s) virologically related to HBV. The entire nucleic acid sequence of HBV has been determined and the HBV genome has been cloned in both prokaryotic and eukaryotic cells. Chronic carriers have been found to contain both free viral DNA in infected hepatocytes and, in some instances, viral DNA integrated into host hepatocyte DNA. Moreover, chronic HBV carriers in whom primary hepatocellular carcinoma (HCC) develops almost always have HBV DNA integrated into the HCC cellular genome. Integration of viral DNA into the host genome is thought to initiate the process which results in malignant transformation of normal hepatocytes.

Further observations are relevant to individuals with NANB hepatitis. Persons with acute and chronic viral hepatitis not attributable by conventional tests to infection by HAV or HBV (negative serum HAV IgM, HBsAg, anti-HBc, and anti-HBs) have been evaluated by molecular hybridization techniques for the presence of HBV DNA in the liver and serum. In preliminary studies, liver specimens and serum samples from some of these individuals have been found to contain DNA sequences which hybridize to the HBV DNA probe. This finding suggests that some instances of presumed acute or chronic NANB hepatitis may in fact be caused by HBV, without serologic expression of viral markers, or by an HBV-related agent(s), which presumably shares some DNA sequences with the HBV genome. Further studies of patients with NANB hepatitis to determine the extent of viral DNA homology with HBV DNA may help distinguish infection caused by HBV from infection caused by a distinct HBV-related–NANB agent.

The use of monoclonal antibodies has also provided information about viral antigenic structure. For example, subtle but important antigenic differences among closely related strains have now been identified for rabies, influenza, herpes, and adenoviruses. High-affinity monoclonal antibodies have been produced as well to antigenic determinants on the HBsAg. Such antibodies have been used to develop sensitive and specific radioimmunoassays (RIAs) for the measurement of HBsAg-associated determinants in serum. In preliminary studies, serum samples from some individuals with acute and chronic NANB hepatitis (on the basis of negative commercial RIAs employing polyvalent antibodies to HBsAg) have been found to contain HBsAg-associated determinants when tested with the monoclonal antibody RIAs. Serum specimens from some of these individuals have also been found to contain HBV DNA sequences by hybridization with recombinant-cloned HBV DNA. These results cannot be explained solely by the greater sensitivity of monoclonal antibody RIAs for HBsAg determinants, because in many such individuals with NANB hepatitis, other monoclonal RIAs have detected additional peptides distinct from those detected in individuals with hepatitis B. It has also been observed that the monoclonal antibody RIAs, unlike conventional RIAs for

HBsAg, may detect HBsAg-related determinants in immune complexes formed in anti-HBs excess, even in the absence of conventional serologic evidence for HBV infection. Thus, use of monoclonal antibody RIAs to HBsAg-associated determinants suggests that some cases of NANB hepatitis are caused by an HBV-related agent not detected by conventional serologic assays.

The molecular hybridization and monoclonal antibody techniques described above have been used to study chimpanzees inoculated with a clotting-factor concentrate previously shown to transmit NANB hepatitis. In these studies an incubation period of approximately 60 days from inoculation to first appearance in serum of HBsAg-determinant-reactive material was observed. Serum ALT elevations were found to precede by several weeks the appearance of HBsAg-determinant-reactive material (Fig. 2). The presence of antigen in serum, as measured by the monoclonal antibody RIA, coincided with the appearance in serum of HBV DNA-like sequences, as determined by molecular hybridization analysis. The period of presumed antigenemia persisted for weeks to months and disappeared with recovery from clinical and biochemical illness, although antigenemia was still detectable for a short time after return of ALT levels to normal. Most important, the above sequence of events following inoculation of the NANB agent-containing concentrate has been shown to occur in chimpanzees presumably immune to HBV infection on the basis of preexisting serum anti-HBs. In such inoculated animals, the conventional HBsAg RIA remains negative despite the demonstration of HBsAg-associated determinants by monoclonal antibody RIA.

Thus, DNA hybridization and monoclonal antibody techniques have provided evidence that at least one NANB agent shares nucleic acid sequences and antigenic determinants with HBV, but the exact relation of such an NANB agent to HBV remains to be elucidated. Furthermore, the biologic significance in the chimpanzee model of the appearance of HBsAg-related antigenic material after evidence of hepatic injury (serum ALT rise) is unclear. Further studies employing DNA hybridization and monoclonal antibody techniques should provide additional insights into the nature of NANB hepatitis.

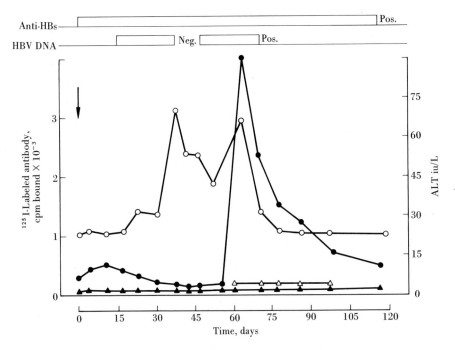

FIGURE 2
Clinical and virologic course of non-A, non-B hepatitis in chimpanzee. Note that elevations in alanine aminotransferase (AlaATase) values (o) precede the appearance of antigen and HBV-related DNA sequences in the blood. Radioimmunoassays: ●, monoclonal IgM; △ Ausria II; ▲ monoclonal IgG1 and IgG2a; ↓, point of inoculation. (From JR Wands et al, Proc Natl Acad Sci USA 79:7552, 1982.)

EVIDENCE FOR MORE THAN ONE NANB AGENT

Several lines of evidence suggest that there must be more than one NANB agent. First, incubation periods for NANB hepatitis in transfused patients have been observed to vary with the type of donor blood product; the incubation period for posttransfusion hepatitis following red blood cell infusions averages 7 to 8 weeks, while the incubation period following infusions of factor VIII concentrates is 1 to 4 weeks. Second, the high frequency of chronicity and minimal secondary spread in posttransfusion NANB hepatitis contrasts with the rapid dissemination and absence of chronicity in the waterborne epidemic NANB hepatitis in India. Third, multiple distinct bouts of biopsy-proven acute NANB hepatitis have been documented in intravenous drug abusers, hemophiliacs given multiple doses of factor VIII, and renal transplant recipients; individual bouts of hepatitis have been separated by intervals of good health and normal liver function tests, and during the episodes of acute hepatitis infections by HAV, HBV, EBV, and CMV have been serologically excluded. Fourth, the two types of ultrastructural hepatocyte changes in chimpanzees inoculated with infectious material from different patients and the ability to induce second episodes of hepatitis on cross-challenge with inocula from different sources suggest the existence of more than one NANB agent. Finally, molecular hybridization techniques using a cloned HBV DNA probe and monoclonal antibodies directed against HBsAg determinants have suggested that some, but not all, cases of NANB hepatitis may be caused by an agent related to HBV.

PREVENTION OF NANB HEPATITIS

Posttransfusion NANB hepatitis represents an important public health problem in the United States. An estimated 3.3 million blood recipients receive an average of 3 units of blood products resulting in 230,000 new cases of PTH each year. Efforts to prevent PTH have been hindered by the inability to document serologically the sources of infection, the susceptibility of contacts, or the existence of antibodies to NANB agents in globulin preparations. Nevertheless, a number of general measures can be undertaken to limit the transmission of NANB hepatitis, and several specific methods have been proposed as interval measures to decrease the incidence of PTH until a virus-specific test is widely available.

General measures

General hygienic precautions used for HBV infection have been applied to NANB infection because of the similarity in transmission patterns of both agents. Recommended guidelines include proper handling of contaminated needles and syringes, sterilization of reusable medical and dental instruments, and avoidance of shared needles in drug addicts. Renal dialysis machines used for patients with NANB hepatitis should be isolated. In epidemics of NANB hepatitis, such as those in India, public health measures to prevent fecal contamination of water supplies are suggested.

For the prevention of transfusion-transmitted NANB hepatitis, the optimal use of blood and blood products is crucial. It is important to transfuse only when necessary, using low-hepatitis-risk products whenever possible and avoiding pooled blood products and concentrates. The most effective measure by far to date has been the use of blood solely from volunteer donors and the exclusion of commercial, paid donors. Also encouraged are the indentification and exclusion of donors whose blood is the only unit transfused to a patient in whom hepatitis develops, or of donors whose blood is implicated in more than one case of hepatitis in multitransfused patients.

Specific measures

In the absence of a specific NANB marker, a number of nonspecific tests have been proposed to identify blood-donor carriers of the NANB agent. The most promising of these is the ALT level. Two recent studies have shown the incidence of PTH in transfusion recipients to be proportional to the ALT level in donor blood. In a study by the Transfusion-Transmitted Viruses Study Group, the attack rate among individuals receiving at least 1 unit of blood with an elevated ALT level (>45 IU) was 39 percent, compared to an attack rate of only 3.4 percent for those receiving blood with normal ALT levels (Fig. 3). Despite this impressive difference, the nonspecificity of ALT as a marker of NANB hepatitis is shown by the finding that in 60 percent of patients who received blood with an ALT level above 45 IU, hepatitis did not develop. Moreover, a normal donor ALT level did not preclude the development of PTH in the recipient; in fact, because 95 percent of all donors had normal serum ALT activity, the majority of cases of PTH in recipients followed transfusion of blood with normal serum ALT levels.

Taking into account that discarded blood units with elevated ALT levels would be replaced by units with normal ALT levels which still carry a risk of hepatitis, a second study showed that an ALT exclusion level of 2.25 standard deviations greater than the mean log level of ALT for normal subjects would exclude 29 percent of donors who transmitted PTH and only 1.6 percent of all donors. Further cost-benefit analysis discloses that a 30 percent reduction in hepatitis cases per year in the United States would result in 70,000 to 95,000 fewer cases of PTH and 3500 to 4500 fewer cases of cirrhosis. On the other hand, ALT testing and exclusion of 1.6 percent of all donor units would add an additional $20 billion to the cost of health care delivery, would decrease the number of blood donors (many of whom are not NANB carriers), and would raise ethical concerns about informing blood donors of elevated serum ALT levels when the significance may not be clear.

Thus, ALT screening of donor blood eliminates a significant fraction of noninfectious donors, does not appear to prevent most cases of NANB hepatitis, and is at best an interim measure. However, until a specific NANB test is widely available, ALT testing of donor blood may be warranted. Some blood-transfusion centers have in fact begun to withhold blood with elevated ALT activity, and prospective studies of the incidence of PTH following exclusion of donor blood with elevated ALT activity are in progress.

A variety of other serum markers have been evaluated as potential indirect indicators of NANB infection. Limited studies have shown

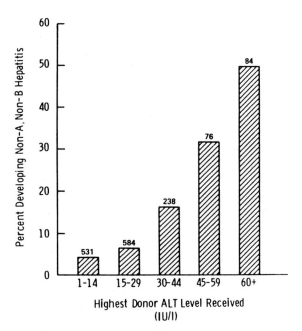

FIGURE 3

Incidence of non-A, non-B posttransfusion hepatitis in relation to donor alanine aminotransferase (ALT) level. (From FB Hollinger et al, in W Szmuness et al (eds), Viral Hepatitis: 1981 International Symposium, Philadelphia, Franklin Institute Press, 1982.)

that serum cholylglycine and plasma carcinoembryonic antigen levels correlate with the risk of transmitting NANB hepatitis, but the routine use of these markers to screen donor blood would involve considerable expense and is unlikely to be introduced. Interest has been expressed in the measurement in serum of anti-HBs and anti-HBc as indicators of NANB infection. The presence of anti-HBc in serum in the absence of HBsAg and anti-HBs may be associated with transmission of HBV infection, but this accounts for a small precentage of cases of PTH and routine testing of donor serum for anti-HBc is generally not undertaken. Reports that both anti-HBc and anti-HBs in donor serum are associated with transmission of NANB hepatitis have prompted speculation that an increased risk of NANB infection in individuals with serologic evidence of HBV exposure relates to the predilection of both agents for lower socioeconomic groups. To date in one prospective study in the United States anti-HBc-containing blood resulted in a higher

recipient incidence of NANB hepatitis than blood without anti-HBc, regardless of the presence or absence of anti-HBs. However, these results were not confirmed in a second study from the Netherlands, possibly because of the much lower incidence of NANB hepatitis there. In general, anti-HBc screening of donor blood has not been adopted because combining ALT and anti-HBc testing would probably not prevent as much NANB hepatitis as predicted by the sum of the two alone; blood donors with elevated ALT activity are more likely to have anti-HBc in their serum than are donors with normal ALT levels, and ALT screening appears to result in greater prevention of PTH than anti-HBc testing.

Other techniques to reduce the risk of hepatitis infection from blood products have been tested. The use of frozen, deglycerolized, and washed blood has resulted in a trend in favor of a decreased incidence of hepatitis, but these methods clearly do not prevent PTH. In chimpanzees, ultraviolet irradiation combined with β-propiolactone treatment of transfused blood known to be infectious caused a reduction, but not elimination, of infectivity for type B and NANB viruses.

Early studies of the efficacy of immune serum globulin in the prevention of PTH were complicated by the inability to distinguish hepatitis B from NANB hepatitis, and conflicting results were obtained. Since the advent of sensitive serologic tests to exclude infections caused by HAV and HBV, three large-scale prospective controlled trials comparing immune serum globulin with placebo in the prevention of PTH have been undertaken. The results of these three studies are summarized in Table 4. In the study by Kuhns et al., immune serum globulin prepared from individuals convalescing from NANB hepatitis and given after exposure had no effect on the prevention of transfusion-associated hepatitis. Knodell et al. found that immune serum globulin and hyperimmune gamma globulin administered before transfusion were equally effective and significantly better than placebo in reducing the frequency of total and icteric, but not anicteric, hepatitis. They also found that the frequency of chronic hepatitis was lower in patients with PTH who had received one of the gamma globulin preparations than in those who had re-

TABLE 4
Summary of controlled studies on immune globulin prophylaxis of postransfusion hepatitis

	Kuhns et al. (1976)	*Knodell et al. (1976)*	*Seeff et al. (1977)*
Source of immune globulin (IG)	Convalescent NANB hepatitis serum	Standard IG and hyperimmune globulin (HIG)	Standard IG
Timing of dose	Two doses, 7 and 30 days after transfusion	One dose, before transfusion	Two doses, up to 4 days and 1 month after transfusion
Source of donor blood	Volunteer and commercial donors	Volunteer and military donors	Volunteer and commercial donors
Incidence of total hepatitis in recipients (incidence of icteric hepatitis)			
Placebo	16.7% (7.8%)	13.8% (8.5%)	9.5% (2.5%)
IG	18.3% (6.4%)	6.4%* (1.1%)*	7.7% (1.3%)†
HIG		5.4%* (1.1%)*	

* *Statistically significantly less than corresponding incidence for placebo group.*
† *Incidence of hepatitis less for IG group than placebo group only for recipients of commercial blood.*

ceived placebo. Finally, Seeff et al. observed that immune serum globulin given after transfusion reduced the frequency of icteric, but not anicteric and total, cases of PTH compared to placebo. However, further analysis of the data showed that the beneficial effect of immune globulin was limited to recipients of commercial donor blood; there was no beneficial effect on recipients of volunteer blood, for whom the incidence of hepatitis was much lower than commercial blood recipients regardless of immune globulin administration. Taken together, these three studies suggest that immune serum globulin may ameliorate icteric hepatitis or result in anicteric hepatitis rather than prevent NANB PTH, but that the use of all volunteer blood has a much greater impact on preventing PTH. On the basis of these studies no specific guidelines can be made for the use of immune serum globulin after needlestick exposure, sexual contact, or neonatal exposure, but because of its safety and lack of expense, some authorities recommend the administration of immune serum globulin 0.06 ml/kg in these situations.

Clearly, adequate prevention of PTH awaits the development of a practical, commercially available NANB detection system. In the meantime, measures such as ALT screening of donor blood may serve as means of preventing some cases of PTH. Figure 4 summarizes the potential impact of the various techniques discussed above to decrease the incidence of PTH.

TREATMENT OF NANB HEPATITIS

In the absence of specific, effective therapy for viral hepatitis, treatment of individuals with NANB hepatitis is supportive and symptomatic until spontaneous resolution occurs. Bed rest and mild restriction of activities may be all that is necessary for most symptomatic patients, while hospitalization may be required for those who cannot maintain adequate hydration and nutrition at home. Rarely, complications of fulminant hepatitis, such as coagulopathy, bleeding, and encephalopathy, must be treated.

Close surveillance of individuals with chronic hepatitis is recommended, but in the absence of serologic markers, the natural history is unknown. Despite some evidence that chronic NANB hepatitis may be unresponsive to corticosteroid therapy, a trial of corticosteroid therapy may be attempted in individuals with symptomatic chronic active NANB hepatitis associated with marked aminotransferase elevations. Controlled studies of immunosuppressive or antiviral therapy for chronic NANB hepatitis are needed.

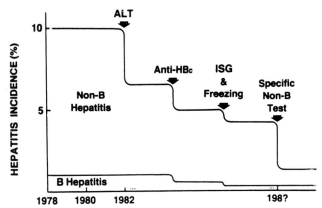

FIGURE 4

Estimation of the cumulative effects of alanine aminotransferase (ALT) testing, anti-HBc testing, use of immune serum globulin (ISG), and use of frozen-deglycerolized red blood cells (freezing) on the incidence of posttransfusion hepatitis. A specific non-A, non-B hepatitis virus(es) test would likely be the most effective preventive measure. (From PV Holland, in W Szmuness et al (eds), Viral Hepatitis: 1981 International Symposium, Philadelphia, Franklin Institute Press, 1982.)

Acknowledgment

The authors are grateful to Ms. Mimi Kindelmann and Mrs. Hilda Gardner for their excellent assistance in the preparation of this article.

References

AACH RD, KAHN RA: Post-transfusion hepatitis: Current perspectives. Ann Intern Med 92:539, 1980

—— et al: Serum alanine aminotransferase of donors in relation to the risk of non-A, non-B hepatitis in recipients: The transfusion-transmitted viruses study. N Engl J Med 304:989, 1981

ALTER HJ et al: Transmissible agent in non-A, non-B hepatitis. Lancet 1:459, 1978

—— et al: Donor transaminase and recipient hepatitis: Impact on blood transfusion services. JAMA 246:630, 1981

BERMAN M et al: The chronic sequelae of non-A, non-B hepatitis. Ann Intern Med 91:1, 1979

DIENSTAG JL et al: Etiology of sporadic hepatitis B surface antigen-negative hepatitis. Ann Intern Med 87:1, 1977

——: Non-A, non-B hepatitis. Gastroenterology 85:439, 1983

——: Diagnosis and prevention of viral hepatitis, in *Update IV: Harrison's Principles of Internal Medicine,* KJ Isselbacher et al (eds). New York, McGraw-Hill, 1983, 165–196.

FEINSTONE SM et al: Transfusion-associated hepatitis not due to viral hepatitis type A or B. N Engl J Med 292:767, 1975

GERETY RJ (ed): *Non-A, Non-B Hepatitis.* New York, Academic, 1981

HOLLAND PV, ALTER HJ: Non-A, non-B viral hepatitis. Hum Pathol 12:1114, 1981

HOLLINGER FB et al: Transfusion-transmitted viruses study: Experimental evidence for two non-A, non-B hepatitis agents. J Infect Dis 142:400, 1980

KNODELL RG et al: Etiologic spectrum of post-transfusion hepatitis. Gastroenterology 69:1278, 1975

—— et al: Efficacy of prophylactic gamma-globulin in preventing non-A, non-B post-transfusion hepatitis. Lancet 1:557, 1976

KORETZ RL et al: The long-term course of non-A, non-B post-transfusion hepatitis. Gastroenterology 79:893, 1980

KUHNS WJ et al: A clinical and laboratory evaluation of immune serum globulin from donors with a history of hepatitis: Attempted prevention of post-transfusion hepatitis. Am J Med Sci 272:255, 1976

PRINCE AM et al: Long-incubation post-transfusion hepatitis without serological evidence of exposure to hepatitis-B virus. Lancet 2:241, 1974

RAKELA J, REDEKER AG: Chronic liver disease after acute non-A, non-B viral hepatitis. Gastroenterology 77:1200, 1979

ROBINSON WS: The enigma of non-A, non-B hepatitis. J Infect Dis 145:387, 1982

SEEFF LB ET AL: A randomized, double blind controlled trial of the efficacy of immune serum globulin for the prevention of post-transfusion hepatitis: A Veterans Administration cooperative study. Gastroenterology 72:111, 1977

SHAFRITZ DA et al: Monoclonal radioimmunoassays for hepatitis B surface antigen: Demonstration of hepatitis B virus DNA or related sequences in serum and viral epitopes in immune complexes. Proc Natl Acad Sci USA 79:5675, 1982

SZMUNESS W et al (eds): *Viral Hepatitis: 1981 International Symposium.* Philadelphia: Franklin Institute Press, 1982

TABOR E et al:Transmission of non-A, non-B hepatitis from man to chimpanzee. Lancet 1:463, 1978

——— et al: Chronic non-A, non-B hepatitis carrier state: Transmissible agent documented in one patient over a six-year period. N Engl J Med 303:140, 1980

WANDS JR et al: Detection and transmission in chimpanzees of hepatitis B virus-related agents formerly designated ''non-A, non-B'' hepatitis. Proc Natl Acad Sci USA 79:7552, 1982

HEPATITIS B VIRUS AND HEPATOCELLULAR CARCINOMA

DAVID A. SHAFRITZ and MORRIS SHERMAN

Although hepatocellular carcinoma (HCC) is not a common tumor in Europe and North America (it accounts for less than 1 percent of all malignancies in the United States), it is the most common neoplasm in China, in much of the rest of Asia, and in parts of sub-Saharan Africa. Some estimates have put the worldwide incidence of HCC at 250,000 new cases per year, making it one of the most common, if not the commonest, lethal tumor in the world.

The pathogenesis of HCC is at present uncertain, but the surprising differences in incidence in different geographic areas and among different cultural groups have implicated environmental factors in the etiology of this tumor. Epidemiological studies have provided evidence for an association of HCC with two environmental agents: hepatitis B virus (HBV) and aflatoxin B_1, a potent chemical carcinogen found in certain molds growing on grain and nut food products.

The association between aflatoxin and HCC rests upon the epidemiologic finding of high levels of food contamination and intake of aflatoxin in some countries where HCC is common (e.g., Maputo, formerly Mozambique). Aflatoxin is one of the most potent known hepatic carcinogens in several species of experimental animals. Initial evidence for an association of persistent HBV infection with HCC was also largely epidemiologic, but recent application of molecular biology techniques has resulted in elucidation of the organization and expression of the HBV genome and of the state of HBV DNA in malignant and nonmalignant human liver tissue. In this chapter, we review the biology of HBV and the epidemiological evidence for an association between HBV and HCC, and we discuss recent findings on the basis of recombinant DNA and molecular hybridization technology which suggest mechanisms whereby HBV might cause neoplastic changes in human hepatocytes.

BIOLOGY OF HEPATITIS VIRUS

Humans are the only known natural host for HBV, although chimpanzees can be infected experimentally. This limited host specificity, coupled with the inability to propagate HBV in tissue culture, has hampered elucidation of the biology of the virus and its replication cycle.

One of the most important discoveries concerning this virus was the detection in human serum in 1964 of an antigen, first known as Australia antigen, which was later shown to be associated with acute HBV infection. It was subsequently renamed hepatitis-associated antigen (HAA) and is currently designated *hepatitis B surface antigen (HBsAg)*. Soon thereafter, it was recognized that HBsAg could be detected in the serum of some patients who had recovered from acute hepatitis, and who may or may not have chronic liver disease, and even in some individuals with no history of previous acute hepatitis infection. Obviously such patients still retain the virus (i.e., are carriers of HBV) and may still be infectious to their immediate contacts. It also soon became apparent that in these patients chronic liver disease was related to persistence of HBV infection. Currently, a hepatitis B carrier is defined as an individual showing HBsAg in the serum for a minimum of 6 months using sensitive third-generation immunoassay testing. The carrier state may persist for life but remits spontaneously in approximately 10 percent of patients per year.

117

HBV gene products

Several viral gene products have been identified; these include HBsAg, hepatitis B core antigen (HBcAg), and hepatitis B e antigen (HBeAg). HBsAg is found in the serum in a variety of particulate structural forms. Most commonly found are small (16- to 25-nm) spherical particles and filamentous structures of 22-nm diameter and length ranging up to 1000 nm (Fig. 1*A*). These particles do not contain nucleic acid but are aggregates of viral envelope protein. Less frequently found in serum are 42-nm particles orig-

inally described by Dane (the so-called Dane particle). These compromise an outer envelope and an inner 27-nm core structure or viral nucleocapsid (Fig. 1*B*). The outer envelope of the Dane particle contains membrane lipids and proteins, some of which are glycosylated. The exact protein composition of the envelopes is not well defined, except for two major HBsAg-containing polypeptides (PI and PII), considered in more detail below. The inner nucleocapsid contains a major polypeptide, HBcAg, HBeAg, nucleic acid, and other components (also to be described below). Nucleocapsid particles distinct from

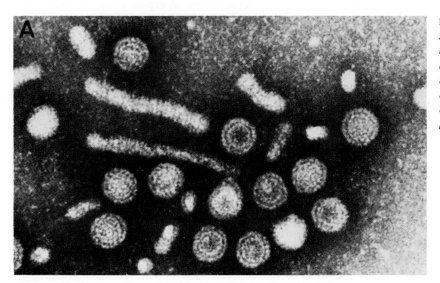

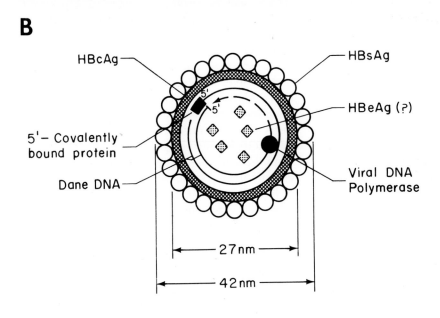

FIGURE 1
A. Electron micrograph showing the particulate forms of hepatitis B virion found in serum. B. Schematic representation of the hepatitis B virion showing the constituent proteins and nucleic acid.

Dane particles have been observed by electron microscopy in the nucleus of infected hepatocytes but are not found in serum.

HBsAg HBsAg antigenic activity has been found in two major polypeptides, PI (~23,000 daltons) and PII (~27,000 daltons). Both are constituents of the viral surface envelope and are present in about equal quantity. Similarity in amino acid composition and identity of NH_2-terminal and COOH-terminal sequences suggests that PI and PII are identical, except that PII is glycosylated. This relation was confirmed by identification in cloned HBV DNA of a single nucleotide sequence which codes for a 25,400-dalton polypeptide consisting of 226 amino acids with NH_2-terminal and COOH-terminal amino acids identical to those known for HBsAg. A third envelope polypeptide of 70,000 daltons is present in HBsAg preparations, but this protein cross reacts with antialbumin antibodies and its origin is uncertain. Other envelope polypeptides of higher molecular weight have been described but are thought to be aggregates of PI and PII.

Several antigenic determinants on the HBsAg polypeptide have been described, leading to a classification of virus subtypes. There is one well-characterized group-specific determinant called *a* and two sets of mutually exclusive subtype determinants *d* or *y* and *w* or *r*. Thus, four major subtypes of HBsAg (i.e., adw, ayw, adr, and ayr) denote the phenotypes of the virion. Further subdivision of the a-determinant subspecificity into a_1, a_2, a_3, and other intermediate specificities has led to serologic classification of HBsAg into 10 known categories. Determination of subtypes is of limited clinical value and is used primarily in epidemiological or transmission studies.

HBcAg *Hepatitis B core antigen (HBcAg)* is a single polypeptide of 19,000 daltons. Although the amino acid sequence has not been determined directly, it has been deduced from the nucleotide sequence of the HBcAg gene and consists of 183 to 185 amino acids. HBcAg is found in the blood only as an internal component of Dane particles and is not found free in the serum. Particles with the electron-microscopic appearance of Dane particle cores (viral nucleocapsids) and containing HBcAg by immunohistochemical analysis have been isolated from homogenates of

HBV-infected liver. Such methods (electron microscopy and immunohistochemical staining for viral antigens), however, are relatively insensitive, require specialized technical skills, and are not used routinely in clinical practice. Nucleocapsid particles have also been shown to contain DNA polymerase activity similar to that of Dane particles (see below). There is an early and brisk antibody response to HBcAg during infection (anti-HBc), and both IgM and IgG isotypes of anti-HBc have been observed. The presence of anti-HBc IgM denotes active infection, whereas anti-HBc IgG signifies previous infection.

HBeAg The *hepatitis B e antigen (HBeAg)* was first described in 1972. It is antigenically distinct from HBsAg, although it occurs exclusively in HBsAg-positive sera. An antibody response to HBeAg is often observed following HBV infection, suggesting that HBeAg is also a virus-coded antigen. HBeAg is present transiently in the serum of most patients with acute HBV infection, and it frequently persists in the serum of chronic HBV carriers who have high concentrations of Dane particles. The presence of HBeAg in the serum has been shown to correlate with infectivity. Before hyperimmune γ-globulin was used to prevent vertical transmission of HBV, approximately 95 percent of infants born to HBeAg-positive mothers in Taiwan showed evidence of HBV infection within the first year of life. However, a small proportion of anti-HBe–positive patients have also been reported to transmit HBV infection via blood transfusion, and approximately 20 percent of anti-HBe–positive mothers transmit infection to their infants. The persistence of HBeAg in serum also correlates with active liver disease, although chronic persistent and chronic active hepatitis have also been described in some anti-HBe–positive patients. Because of these exceptions, measurement of HBeAg is of limited use as an indicator of chronic liver disease in individual patients.

HBeAg can be generated in vitro by proteolytic digestion of HBcAg, although at present it is not clear whether HBcAg and HBeAg represent different antigenic determinants of a single polypeptide or are separate proteins. The question of the exact physical relationship of HBeAg to Dane particles also remains unsettled, because

HBeAg can sometimes be detected free in the plasma. The association of HBeAg with various plasma proteins and the antigenic heterogeneity or subdivision of HBeAg into distinct subgroups e_1, e_2, and e_3 has also been reported.

Other potential viral polypeptides Associated with the Dane particle is an endogenous DNA polymerase activity. This DNA polymerase is located in the nucleocapsid core and can fill in nucleotides missing in one strand of HBV virion DNA (Fig. 1*B*). Polymerase activity is measured in Dane particles by first removing the viral coat with a detergent (Triton X-100) and then incubating the remaining nucleocapsids with radioactively labeled deoxyribonucleotides. In addition to DNA polymerase, there has recently been a report of a protein kinase activity associated with the core of Dane particles and of a protein covalently bound to the 5′ terminus

of the complete Dane DNA strand. Although the latter two proteins have been found associated with the Dane particle, their viral origin and function remains uncertain.

Organization of the HBV genome

The Dane particle contains a small, circular DNA molecule. The complete genome is about 3200 to 3300 base pairs but has an unusual structure (Fig. 2). One strand, the *long (L) strand*, is of fixed length and is complete, except for a nick of one or a few nucleotides. The nick is located at a fixed position in the nucleotide chain. The second strand, referred to as the *short (S) strand*, is incomplete and lacks 15 to 50 percent of its nucleotide complement. The 5′ end of the S strand is also at a fixed position within the HBV genome. The double-stranded molecule is held in circular configuration by base pairing of the 5′

FIGURE 2
Schematic diagram of the hepatitis B virus genome showing the known viral genes and open translational reading frames coding for potential viral polypeptides. (From P Tiollais. Copyright 1981 American Association for the Advancement of Science.)

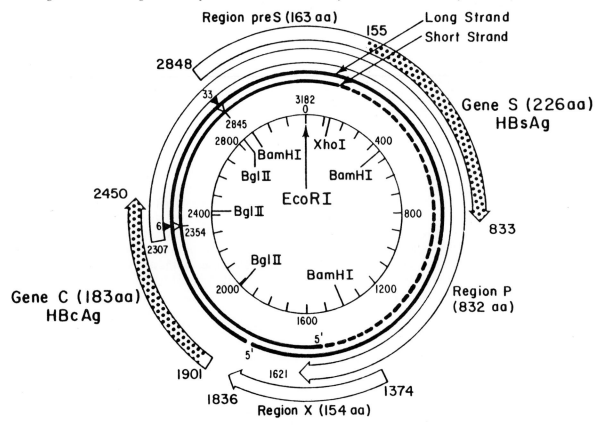

extremities of the L and S strands which overlap for a length of 250 to 300 nucleotides, the so-called cohesive-end region (Fig. 2). The DNA polymerase of the nucleocapsid can fill in the gap of missing nucleotides in the S strand and presumably can repair the nick in the L strand but cannot join the 5' to the 3' end of either strand to form a covalently closed, circular, double-stranded molecule.

Studies of cloned HBV DNA have revealed significant heterogeneity in the HBV DNA nucleotide sequence. Although particles isolated from a single patient are generally homogenous with respect to DNA sequence, immunological subtypes with different restriction endonuclease maps have been reported. Heterogeneity has also been demonstrated even within a single subtype in isolates from different patients.

The L strand has four open-reading frames (sequences of nucleotides containing a start and stop codon signal for polypeptide synthesis) called the *S, C, P,* and *X regions* (Fig. 2). The S region codes for HBsAg, and a pre-S sequence, for which no polypeptide has yet been identified. The C region codes for HBcAg. The HBcAg-coding sequence is located on the same strand (L strand) and in the same orientation and translational (trinucleotide codon) reading frame as the HBsAg-coding sequence. The P region covers 75 percent of the genome, and because of its large size, could possibly code for the DNA polymerase. The P region overlaps the other three regions and completely covers the S region. The X region has no known polypeptide product. The S strand has only short open-reading frames, which could code for polypeptides shorter in length than 10,000 daltons.

HBV-related viruses in animals

Recently, three additional viruses which are phylogenetically related to human hepatitis B virus have been discovered: woodchuck (*Marmota monax*) hepatitis virus (WHV), ground squirrel (*Spermophilus beecheyi*) hepatitis virus (GSHV), and duck hepatitis B virus (DHBV). Features which all four species (including human) have in common include (1) virus morphology, (2) size and structure of the viral DNA, (3) a virion DNA polymerase which repairs the single-stranded region in the incomplete double-stranded circular genome, (4) cross-reacting viral surface antigens, (5) an antigen-antibody system similar to hepatitis B core antigen, and (6) persistent infection with continuous expression of viral antigen(s). This evolutionarily related class of DNA viruses has been termed *hepadna* (*hep*atitis *a*ssociated *DNA*) *viruses*. Each of these viruses has a unique host specificity, and only the human virus (HBV) has been found to infect an alternate species, the chimpanzee. Since only limited studies can be performed in chimpanzees, these related animal viruses may provide valuable models for the study of viral replication and/or pathogenesis of HBV infection.

Although these HBV-like viruses have many similar properties, there are important differences. It has been shown that the two major polypeptides of GSHV surface antigen are smaller than their HBV counterparts. Only one-third of the tryptic peptides of the GSHV and HBV surface antigens are identical, and the viral DNAs show only limited cross hybridization or DNA sequence homology. There are also differences in the degree and activity of liver disease. Although persistent infection of liver has been observed in ground squirrels, woodchucks, and ducks, histological evidence of chronic persistent or chronic active hepatitis has been reported in the woodchuck and possibly also in the duck. Both human and woodchuck hepatitis B viruses have been associated with primary liver cancer in their respective hosts, whereas ground squirrel and duck hepatitis viruses have not so far been shown to be associated with hepatic malignancy. Duck hepatitis virus has been shown to replicate in the pancreas as well as in the liver. DHBV infection can be acquired by either horizontal or vertical transmission (the virus has been found in unhatched duck eggs, as well as in newborn ducklings), and finally, DHBV has been shown to replicate via an RNA intermediate, which may have significant implications (see below).

Replication cycle of HBV and related viruses

Lack of suitable tissue-culture systems has prevented complete study of replication of these viruses, and consequently little is known about this aspect of HBV infection. It has been suggested that replication of HBV within the hepatocyte requires that at least one copy of the genome be integrated into host DNA. Integrated HBV DNA has been reported in acute hepatitis and has been conclusively demonstrated in both chronic hepatitis and asymptomatic HBV carriers. In all of these situations, virus replication occurs.

More recently, a full-length RNA transcript of DHBV has been identified in duck liver. By convention, the primary mRNA transcript is called the *plus strand,* and the DNA from which it is copied (i.e., the DNA strand containing the actual gene-coding sequence for the mRNA) is called the *minus strand.* The complementary DNA strand is also designated as a plus strand. The DHBV RNA transcript is polyadenylated, and there is evidence that viral DNA is synthesized from this RNA transcript by a reverse transcriptase-like enzyme. This DNA, the minus strand, forms the L strand of the DHBV genome. The DNA plus strand (the S strand) is then synthesized from the DNA minus strand (the L strand). Therefore, the duck system has certain properties similar to RNA tumor viruses, which integrate into host DNA as part of their normal replication mechanism.

THE EPIDEMIOLOGICAL ASSOCIATION BETWEEN HBV INFECTION AND HCC

An association between HCC and preexisting hepatitis, with or without cirrhosis, was described more than 30 years ago. More recently, the presence of HBsAg in serum has also been strongly associated with HCC. Based on the incidence determined by sensitive immunoassays, it has been estimated that there are more than 2.25 million carriers of HBV worldwide. Three lines of epidemiological evidence have linked HBV infection to HCC. There is a strong geographic concordance between the prevalence of HBV infection and the incidence of HCC, there is a high prevalence of HBV markers in the serum of patients with HCC compared to control populations, and recent prospective studies have demonstrated an increased risk of developing HCC among patients who are HBV carriers.

Geographic concordance

In North America and western Europe, the prevalence of HBV infection in the general population is low (0.1 to 1.0 percent of blood donors are HBV carriers). In central and eastern Europe, the Mediterranean basin, and the middle east, the prevalence of the carrier state is somewhat higher, ranging up to 5 percent of the total population. However, in sub-Saharan Africa, the carrier rate of HBV infection in the general population varies from 6 to 13 percent. In Asia, the prevalence of chronic HBV infection is 2 to 6 percent in Japan, 14 to 20 percent in Taiwan, and up to 25 percent in Vietnam. Thus, there is a marked variation in the prevalence (or carrier rate) of HBV infection in various parts of the world as determined by radioimmunoassay or counterimmunoelectrophoresis assay for HBsAg.

The incidence of HCC in different regions is difficult to estimate with accuracy because existing data are on the basis of either autopsy studies or mortality figures. Autopsy studies have an inherent bias since patients who do not die in hospitals are less likely to have autopsies and thus would not be included in estimations of HCC incidence. Mortality figures may be overestimated because they often include patients with metastatic liver disease and are culled from registries of death or from cancer registries, which usually cover only selected population groups. Furthermore, in many areas where HCC is common, these statistics are poorly kept, if kept at all.

Despite these objections, certain general observations can be made. In North America and western Europe (i.e., areas of low HBV prevalence), the proportion of HCC in autopsies ranges from 0.22 to 1.65 percent. However, in Africa and east Asia, where HBV is common, HCC is found in from 2 to 8 percent of autopsies, a difference of up to tenfold compared to western countries. Whereas HCC makes up 2 to 2.5 percent of total cancers in the United States and western Europe, in areas of Africa and southeast Asia it accounts for 20 to 40 percent. In many underdeveloped countries where HBV infections are common, HCC is the commonest lethal cancer of males. In females it may be exceeded in incidence only by cancers of the breast and re-productive organs.

Mortality data indicate that the mortality rate from HCC varies from 3 to 7 deaths per 100,000 population per year in most western countries. In certain high HCC prevalence areas, notably southern Africa and southeast Asia, the mortality rate from HCC is between 20 to 100 deaths per 100,000 population per year. The highest death rates from HCC in the world (130 per 100,000) have been recorded in Maputo. The in-creased death rate in high-incidence countries is even more marked in younger age groups (e.g., in the 15- to 25-year age group in Maputo, the HCC mortality is 150 per 100,000 per year and is the leading cause of death in this age group). HCC is also the leading cause of death for adult males in Taiwan, where the HBsAg carrier rate is approximately 15 percent. The general con-cordance between the HBsAg carrier rate in dif-ferent areas of the world and the death rate from HCC is depicted in Fig. 3.

FIGURE 3
A. Worldwide distribution of hepatitis B virus (HBV).
B. Worldwide distribution of the incidence of primary-hepatocellular carcinoma (PHC). (From P Maupas and JL Melnick, Prog Med Virol 27:1, 1981.)

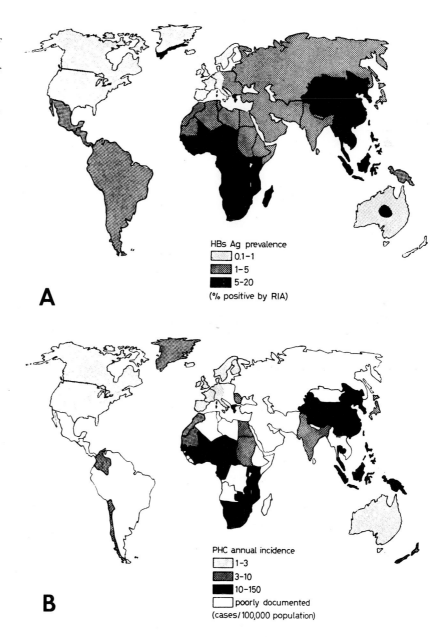

TABLE 1
Hepatitis B virus markers in patients with hepatocellular carcinoma (HCC) in different countries

	Percent of patients with HCC	*Percent of control populations*
HBsAG		
Greece	55	4.7
Spain	19.3	2.0
United States	14.7	1
Senegal	51.9	12.0
Mozambique	62.1	14.3
Uganda	47.0	6.0
Zambia	63.0	7.5
South Africa	59.5	9.0
Taiwan	54.8	12.2
Singapore	35.8	4.1
Japan	37.3	2.6
Vietnam	80.3	24.5
ANTI HBc		
Greece	70.0	31.9
Spain	87.0	14.8
United States	48.5	1
Senegal	87.3	26.0
South Africa	86.0	31.7
Hong Kong	70.3	36.2

SOURCE: *After B Bloomberg and WT London, Curr Probl Cancer 6:1–23, 1982.*

However, not all geographic evidence confirms the relationship between high HBV-carrier rates in the general population and HCC. It is possible that some countries may be too large a geographical area to be considered as a single unit. Indeed, in those countries which have been studied (Maputo, Kenya, and China), although the prevalence of HBV infection may be uniform throughout the country, the incidence of HCC shows remarkable internal geographic variation. In Maputo, the eastern coastal lowlands have an incidence of HCC considerably higher than the national average, but in the inland mountainous areas, the incidence is lower than the national average. In China, areas of high HCC prevalence are very localized; for example, the highest rates are found in Kee Dong and the coastal and southern provinces. However, if whole provinces in China are considered as units, the correlation between HBV and HCC is poor. Furthermore, Egypt and Greenland are countries with high HBV prevalence, yet they do not have an unusually high reported incidence of HCC.

Other evidence from South Africa suggests that factors apart from HBV must be involved.

Although the prevalence of infection is similar in rural and urban black African populations, the incidence of HCC is much higher in the rural as compared to the urban black population and HCC occurs at an earlier age in rural blacks.

Serum HBV markers in patients with HCC

The increased frequency of HBV markers, in particular HBsAg, in serum of patients with HCC is remarkable, particularly in those areas of the world where HCC is common (Table 1). Between 40 and 80 percent of African patients with HCC are positive for HBsAg. Excluding Japan, in the far east between 66 and 90 percent of patients with HCC are positive for HBsAg. In the same areas, the prevalence of HBsAg in individuals without HCC ranges from 6 to 14 percent (Africa) and 7 to 25 percent (far east). However, if a high titer of anti-HBc is taken as evidence of active infection, then even more HCCs are associated with intercurrent HBV infection. If alcoholics with cirrhosis are excluded, even in the United States and Europe 31 to 71 percent of patients with HCC have HBsAg in the serum compared to less than 2 percent in control populations.

Anti-HBs is more frequently found in control populations than in patients with HCC. When accompanied by HBsAg, the presence of anti-HBc is more commonly observed in patients with HCC than in controls, although a correlation with HCC does not hold true if anti-HBc is the only marker of HBV infection or if anti-HBc is accompanied by anti-HBs.

It is noteworthy in patients with HCC that, when present, the amount of circulating HBsAg is relatively low compared to titers found in carriers without HCC. This is probably because HCC develops only after prolonged HBsAg carriage, by which time HBsAg titers have usually decreased.

It is also remarkable that in all populations which have been studied, the bulk of patients with HCC have at least one HBV marker. HBsAg has been detected in the cytoplasm of nontumorous hepatocytes in up to 94 percent of HBV carriers with HCC but only occasionally has been found in the tumor itself. HBcAg is found frequently in the nucleus of nonmalignant hepatocytes but is not found in tumor tissue.

Prospective studies

Epidemiological evidence presented thus far indicates an association between HBV and HCC but says nothing about a causal relationship. Before such a relationship can even be considered, HBV infection must be shown to be present before the onset of HCC and a close association must be maintained between these two entities during evolution of the malignant process (unless HBV were to trigger neoplastic transformation which was then self-sustaining). Relevant information on these matters has been obtained by prospective studies. The most convincing evidence for a causal association has come from a study performed in Taiwan, which involved 22,707 male government employees, all of whom were tested for HBV markers at the time of entry into the study. A remarkable 95 percent follow-up was achieved. Of the 22,707 men, 3454 (15.2 percent) were HBsAg-positive on admission to

the study. According to the most recent update of this study (a follow-up period ranging from 4 to 7 years), 95 cases of HCC have occurred, 92 in patients who were HBsAg-positive. Of the three patients with HCC who were HBsAg-negative, one had anti-HBc in the serum and the other two were anti-HBc– and anti-HBs–positive.

From an epidemiological viewpoint, the best evidence for a causal association between a disease and a putative etiological factor is the relative risk, which in this case is the ratio of the risk of HCC among those individuals with active HBV infection. In the Taiwan study, the estimated relative risk of HCC in patients with active HBV infection was 223. A separate prospective study in Japan estimated the relative risk of HCC in HBV carriers to be about 350. Others have derived more conservative estimates from case control studies, but even so, the least estimate of relative risk is 10 to 30, making HBV second only to cigarette smoke as the most common known agent associated with carcinogenesis in humans.

HBV and age of onset of HCC   In those areas of the world where HCC and HBV infection are common, HCC occurs in considerably younger individuals than in low-incidence areas. In Maputo, for example, the peak onset of HCC is between ages 25 and 35. In Taiwan, the average age of onset is 41 years. However, in western countries the incidence of HCC rises with age, so that the peak age of onset is above 60 years.

The development of HCC in patients with HBsAg is related to the duration of virus carriage. On the average, 10 to 30 years of persistent infection seem to be required, although the earliest reported case of HCC in an HBsAg carrier is in a 6-year-old child in Japan. Six adolescents with HCC between ages 10 to 16 have recently been described from South Africa. All of these patients were HBsAg carriers.

In Taiwan, HBV transmission from mother to infant occurs predominantly in the perinatal period. In rural southern Africa, the bulk of transmission appears to occur not in the perinatal period, but in early childhood. By the age of 5 years, the majority of rural southern African children have been exposed to HBV, have become carriers, or have developed antibodies. Mothers of HCC patients are HBsAg-positive more frequently than the fathers of these patients (71 vs. 18.5 percent) and more frequently than mothers of matched controls (71 vs. 14.3 percent), suggesting that maternal transmission of HBV is important in the pathogenesis of HCC. If neonatal infection or early childhood infection truly enhances either the likelihood of HBV persistence or the progression of the HBV carrier state to HCC, then these data may explain the difference in age of onset of HCC in different parts of the world. In western countries, where HBV infection is acquired much later in life, after 20 to 30 years of persistent infection, competing causes of death will reduce the incidence of HCC.

HCC and cirrhosis   That persistent HBV infection results in cirrhosis in a significant proportion of carriers seems beyond doubt. That the majority of HCCs, whether related to HBV or not, arise in cirrhotic livers is also well established, although in Africa about 40 percent of HCCs arise in noncirrhotic livers, compared to less than 20 percent in western countries. Clearly, cirrhosis is not a necessary stage in the evolution of HCC, but the question arises as to whether cirrhosis is a premalignant condition under certain circumstances (e.g., in HBV carriers). If alcoholics are excluded, the majority of cirrhotic livers bearing HCCs are of macronodular or postnecrotic type, and many of these patients show evidence of intercurrent or previous HBV infection. Indeed, one study has shown that the incidence of HCC in cirrhotics who are HBV carriers is higher than the incidence of HCC in non-HBV-infected cirrhotics (23 vs. 6 percent). In patients with postnecrotic cirrhosis without HCC, the prevalence of HBV markers is approximately the same as in patients with HCC. Also, the geographic distribution of the incidence of macronodular cirrhosis is similar to that described for HCC and HBV. Other conditions associated with cirrhosis (e.g., lupoid chronic active hepatitis and Wilson's disease) are not associated with an increased incidence of HCC. The above evidence suggests that postnecrotic cirrhosis and HCC are distinct end results from a variety of etiological agents, and that although cirrhosis may often precede development of HCC, it is not an obligatory stage in the pathogenesis of HCC.

MOLECULAR STUDIES WITH RECOMBINANT HBV DNA PROBES

When, at the end of 1978, National Institutes of Health guidelines for recombinant DNA research were revised to permit cloning of DNA from pathogenic human viruses, HBV DNA was soon cloned and the complete nucleotide sequence determined. ^{32}P-labeled HBV DNA was then used as a highly sensitive and specific hybridization probe to detect HBV DNA sequences in human hepatoma cell lines, in human liver, and in human hepatocellular carcinoma tissue. The procedure, known as *molecular hybridization* or the *Southern blot,* is illustrated schematically in Fig. 4. Total cellular DNA is extracted from the tissue of interest and is electrophoresed in an agarose gel before or after digestion with restriction endonucleases. Restriction endonucleases are enzymes which recognize specific nucleotide sequences, usually a hexanucleotide segment, in double-stranded DNA. These enzymes cleave each strand of the DNA at a unique position in the hexanucleotide segment and produce a series of smaller molecules containing a staggered or overlapping sequence at each end. For example, one of the first-described restriction enzymes, EcoRI (restriction enzyme RI isolated from *Escherichia coli*), recognizes the sequence

$$5'G\!AATTC3'$$
$$3'CTTAA\!G5'$$

On digestion of high-molecular-weight DNA with this enzyme, a series of double-stranded DNA molecules with an average length of 5000 to 10,000 nucleotide base pairs is produced. More than 200 restriction endonucleases have been described, each with unique specificity. By using a series of restriction enzymes and a hybridization probe specific for the DNA of interest, the properties and basic organization of DNA molecules containing this sequence can be defined (a so-called restriction map).

Figure 4 shows how these methods have been used to identify and characterize HBV DNA sequences in liver or hepatocellular carcinoma tissue. A critical question in analyzing for HBV DNA sequences was whether this DNA is integrated into the host cellular DNA. This is because it had been shown previously in animal

STRATEGY FOR RESTRICTION ENZYME ANALYSIS OF HEPATITIS B VIRUS DNA

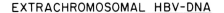

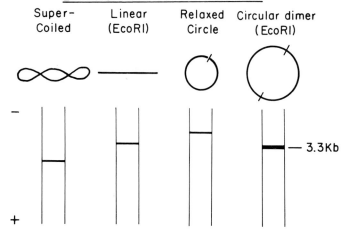

FIGURE 4

Technique of restriction-enzyme digestion, Southern transfer, and molecular hybridization to show the state of hepatitis B virus DNA in extracts from human liver. (From DA Shafritz and MC Kew, Hepatology 1:1, 1981. Copyright 1981 American Association for the Study of Liver Diseases.)

DNA tumor virus systems, such as simian virus 40 (SV40), that integration of viral sequences into host DNA occurred during oncogenic transformation of virally infected cells. To distinguish between nonintegrated (free virion) and integrated HBV DNA, restriction enzyme Hind III is utilized. Hind III does not recognize any site within the HBV genome, which as stated previously is 3200 to 3300 base pairs. Ignoring subtle differences in the migration of linear versus circular versus supercoiled genomes (Fig. 4), the size of molecules containing HBV sequences can be analyzed before or after Hind III and EcoRI digestion and compared to DNA standards of known length. If HBV DNA is not integrated, it will migrate in the gel as a unique band at 3200 to 3300 base pairs and the migration position will not be influenced by Hind III digestion. However, digestion with EcoRI, which recognizes

one site in the HBV genome, will linearize all nonintegrated HBV DNA molecules and cause them to migrate as a single band at 3200 to 3300 base pairs (Fig. 4, upper portion). In contrast, if HBV DNA sequences are integrated into host cellular DNA, entirely different results will be obtained. Since cellular DNA is of very high molecular weight, undigested material will show HBV DNA sequences in a very diffuse pattern near the top of the gel (Fig. 4, lower portion). Digestion with Hind III will cleave these molecules, so that HBV DNA sequences will be spread randomly throughout the gel and may or may not be detectable by hybridization. If, however, the HBV DNA sequences are located within specific locations in the cellular genome, then Hind III digestion will produce discrete hybridization bands representing these unique integration sites. Since HBV DNA is not cleaved by Hind III, all integrated HBV DNA sequences should remain in molecules larger than the viral genome (except for small fragments of HBV DNA which may become integrated and still migrate in molecules smaller than 3200 to 3300 base pairs).

The particular use of EcoRI is to distinguish truly integrated HBV genomes from a variety of HBV concatomers (fully replicated genomes which have remained linked together), oligomers (tandem repeats), and other high-molecular-weight circular or linear forms which may be produced during persistent infection and may be difficult to distinguish from integrated molecules. EcoRI digestion will break all of these high-molecular-weight forms producing linear molecules that are 3200 to 3300 base pairs long, so that after EcoRI digestion all molecules longer than 3300 base pairs and containing HBV DNA sequences must be covalently linked to host

chromosomal DNA (Fig. 4, lower portion). The only possible exception would be oligomers which have lost their EcoRI restriction site, and such molecules have not to date been identified for HBV in native hosts (human or chimpanzee).

Integration of HBV DNA in human HCC

Initial studies showing integration of HBV DNA into human tissue were performed in a hepatocellular carcinoma cell line, PLC/PRF/5, derived from a 24-year-old Mozambican black male who was an HBsAg carrier. The PLC/PRF/5 cell line also produces HBsAg, but no other HBV marker, and does not secrete live virus. When DNA was extracted from these cells and subjected to the above analysis, undigested DNA showed hybridization in the high-molecular-weight region (Fig. 5). No free genome band was

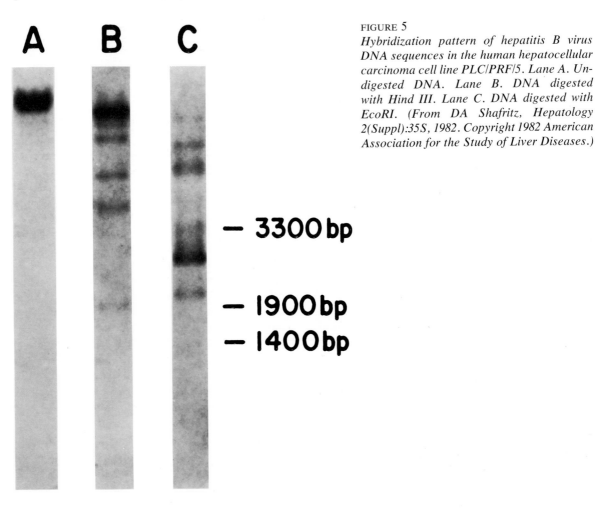

FIGURE 5

Hybridization pattern of hepatitis B virus DNA sequences in the human hepatocellular carcinoma cell line PLC/PRF/5. Lane A. Undigested DNA. Lane B. DNA digested with Hind III. Lane C. DNA digested with EcoRI. (From DA Shafritz, Hepatology 2(Suppl):35S, 1982. Copyright 1982 American Association for the Study of Liver Diseases.)

seen in undigested material (Fig. 5, lane A). After Hind III digestion, five or six clearly defined bands larger than 3300 base pairs were seen (Fig. 5, lane B), each representing all or part of the HBV genome covalently linked to varying amounts of host DNA. Another cell line, Hep3B, also secretes HBsAg and has one or two uniquely integrated HBV DNA bands.

Since HBV DNA integration could have occurred during the process of establishing these cell lines or the actual cell line established may not have been representative of the major malignant cell type in the original tumor, conclusions which can be reached from these studies are limited. However, a large number of human HCCs from patients persistently infected with hepatitis B virus have been studied directly and have shown similar results. Each tumor studied so far has a unique HBV-DNA-banding pattern, although bands of similar size have been found in different tumors (Fig. 6). In most HCCs associated with HBsAg-positive serum, HBV DNA has been found in the tumor, and in most instances in which HBV DNA has been found in

tumors, integrated viral sequences have been identified. Free HBV DNA has also been found in some tumors, but this may be due to cross contamination with nontumorous liver tissue.

When tumor and liver specimens from the same patient have been examined, the pattern of integration in the tumor has been either identical to or different than that seen in the liver (Fig. 6). Some specimens of liver and tumor have one or a few bands in common, but the patterns are otherwise largely different. Irrespective of whether the same or different integration patterns are present in liver and tumor, the presence of unique banding patterns, indicating that many cells in the specimen had identical HBV DNA integration sites, suggests that cells (either tumor or liver) are clonal in origin (i.e., derived from single cells which have been stimulated to divide). Free viral DNA has also been found in the nontumorous liver of HBsAg-positive patients with HCC.

Some HBsAg-negative and anti-HBs–positive patients with HCC may also contain integrated HBV DNA in their tumor cells. Most anti-HBs

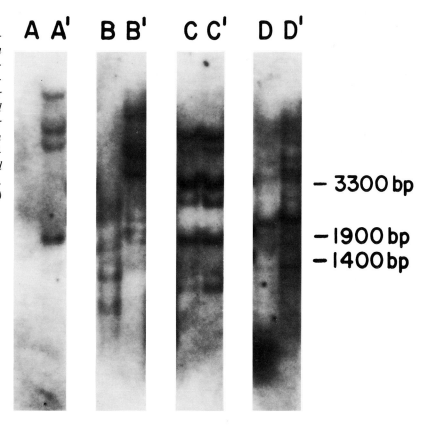

FIGURE 6
Hybridization pattern of hepatitis B virus DNA sequences in liver and tumor tissue from patients with hepatocellular carcinoma. In each pair of cellular DNA extracts, the left-hand track is from nontumorous liver and the right-hand track is from adjacent tumor. (From DA Shafritz and MC Kew, N Engl J Med 305:1067, 1981. Copyright 1981, Massachusetts Medical Society.)

A A'   B B'   C C'   D D'

– 3300 bp

– 1900 bp
– 1400 bp

patients, however, do not have evidence of either chronic liver disease or HCC, and it is possible that those who are anti-HBs–positive at the time of tumor development may have been HBsAg-positive for many years with seroconversion occurring as a relatively late event. In one series of alcoholic patients with HCC from France, many patients had no serum HBV markers, yet each tumor was reported to contain integrated HBV DNA. This finding, which has major implications, has not yet been confirmed in other studies.

HBV DNA in the liver of HBsAg carriers

Hepatitis B virus carriers are defined clinically as individuals showing the presence of HBsAg in their serum for a period of longer than 6 months. Such patients have persistent infection and may or may not show evidence of liver disease. In short-term HBsAg carriers (i.e., positive for HBsAg for more than 6 months but less than 2 years), HBV DNA is usually not integrated into the host genome, irrespective of the presence or absence of liver disease. These patients are generally HBeAg-positive and DNA-polymerase–positive, and free viral DNA is invariably present in the liver at this stage. In these HBV carriers it is possible that integration of HBV DNA has occurred at low frequency into multiple, nonspecific, or random sites in the host genome or into a unique site in such a small number of hepatocytes that it cannot be detected. However, in patients positive for HBsAg for several years, integrated HBV DNA has been found in a significant number of individuals. In some cases, HBV DNA is diffusely integrated into high-molecular-weight cellular DNA, whereas in others discrete integration bands are found (Fig. 7). Integration of HBV DNA can occur in the absence of clinical or histological evidence of liver disease, and it would be from this group of patients that HCC could develop in the absence of cirrhosis.

In most long-term HBV carriers (HBsAg-positive for more than 2 years) the cytoplasm of hepatocytes exhibits the so-called ground-glass histological appearance which correlates with the presence of cytoplasmic HBsAg. Many of

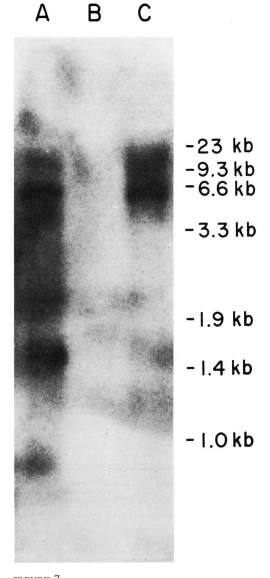

FIGURE 7

Lanes A and C. Hybridization pattern of hepatitis B virus (HBV) DNA from the liver of long-term HBV carriers. Lane B. Control. Integration of HBV DNA into unique hybridization bands is present. (From DA Shafritz, J Cell Biochem 20:303, 1982.)

these patients are anti-HBe–positive, only integrated viral DNA can be demonstrated in the liver, and Dane particles are absent from the serum. This implies that HBsAg in these patients may be produced from an integrated HBV DNA template; therefore, the presence of serum

HBsAg does not necessarily indicate active viral replication or virion production.

Chimpanzees infected with HBV may become chronic carriers and may develop liver disease including chronic active hepatitis. They do not develop HCC. It is interesting that, to date, integrated HBV DNA has not been found in the liver of chimpanzee carriers, although the duration of the carrier state in those animals examined (4 to 13 years) was still relatively short compared to humans and studies performed were not exhaustive.

HCC in woodchucks

As mentioned previously, woodchuck hepatitis virus, like HBV, is associated with HCC in its natural host, and these tumors also contain integrated viral DNA sequences in almost every instance in which viral sequences have been found.

Approximately 16 percent of woodchucks trapped in eastern Pennsylvania and about 25 percent of a colony maintained at the Philadelphia zoo are chronically infected with WHV. The bulk of these animals develop HCC by the time they reach 3 to 4 years of age. In contrast to humans, the livers of woodchuck hepatitis carriers show histological features of acute inflammation as well as chronic hepatitis at the time at which the primary neoplasm is observed. As in humans, the HCC often appears multifocal in origin, although this has not been studied in detail.

As a first step to determine how the integrated WHV sequences contribute to tumor formation, cellular DNA containing integrated WHV DNA sequences from two different tumors has been cloned. The structures of these cloned, integrated WHV DNA molecules have been determined by restriction-endonuclease mapping and electron-microscopic techniques. The integration patterns seen in these two woodchuck clones resemble the integration patterns found with DNA tumor viruses (e.g., SV40, polyoma, and others). Integrated WHV sequences do not occur at fixed sites in either the cellular or the viral genome and contain inversions, deletions, and translocations of viral sequences, as well as alterations in cellular flanking sequences.

HBV DNA in Serum

Using molecular hybridization techniques, HBV DNA can be detected in the serum of many HBsAg-positive carriers. Although serum HBV DNA has not been extensively characterized, it is thought that this DNA is derived from virus particles and its presence is thought to indicate active viral replication, as well as potential infectivity. In immunosuppressed patients, such as renal dialysis or transplant recipients in whom viral replication is expected to be increased, HBV DNA is often found in serum in high concentration. During acute hepatitis B infection when HBsAg and HBeAg are present, HBV DNA is always detectable in serum, although in varying amounts. From the available data it is presumed that all chronic HBsAg carriers, who are also HBeAg-positive, are infectious. Most have some form of chronic liver disease, either chronic persistent or chronic active hepatitis (with or without cirrhosis), and virtually all of these patients have HBV DNA in serum and nuclear HBcAg in liver biopsy specimens, indicating continued viral replication. Patients who are HBsAg-positive and anti-HBe–positive are generally thought to have passed the stage of active viral replication and were previously considered to be noninfectious, although exceptions have been found. Indeed, patients who are HBsAg-positive and anti-HBe–positive with normal histology on liver biopsy do not have detectable HBV DNA in serum. However, some patients who are anti-HBe–positive do have HBV DNA in serum. These individuals frequently have chronic liver disease and continued virus replication as evidenced by the presence of both nuclear HBcAg on liver biopsy and HBV DNA in the serum. The implications of these findings are (1) that viral replication is suppressed or inactive in long-term HBsAg carriers with anti-HBe and normal liver histology, and (2) that viral replication persists and may be associated with development of chronic liver disease in HBsAg-positive and anti-HBe-positive patients who continue to release particles containing HBV DNA into the serum. These patients may also be potentially infectious in spite of being anti-HBe-positive. A determination of the level of HBV DNA in serum of individual

HBeAg-positive and anti-HBe–positive patients versus infectivity (maternal-infant or chimpanzee transmission) could shed further light on this question. Serum HBV DNA is less frequently detected in the serum of patients with HCC and, when present, is generally at very low levels suggesting that viral replication is suppressed or inactive. It is becoming increasingly obvious that the use of immunological markers of HBV has certain limitations (especially when both viral antigens and their specific antibodies are present in serum at the same time). With advances in molecular hybridization technology, it is likely that HBV DNA determinations will be used clinically as an adjunct to, or a replacement for, some of these immunological measurements.

RELATION OF HBV DNA INTEGRATION TO POTENTIAL ONCOGENICITY

All published studies are consistent with the interpretation that integration of HBV DNA into the hepatocyte genome precedes the development of HCC by months or years. The exact time at which integration occurs, the relationship between integration and HBV serum markers (as well as their progression), and the frequency with which integration leads to development of HCC require further study. From epidemiological evidence, it would appear that 10 years of the HBV carrier state (and more often 20 to 30 years) are usually required for HCC to develop. Therefore, individuals contracting the carrier state in the first years of life may be at greatest risk to develop HCC.

Although the published studies do not prove that HBV is oncogenic, the finding of integrated HBV DNA in many hepatocellular carcinomas and in nearly all hepatocellular carcinomas in which viral sequences are present is highly suggestive that HBV is directly or indirectly oncogenic. An hypothesis based on current information is as follows. During the progression of the carrier state, it is possible that hepatocytes expressing all, or at least some, of the specific viral proteins are continuously being removed by host defenses, possibly mediated by HBcAg–anti-HBc complexes or by the recognition of viral polypeptides by cytotoxic lymphocytes. Integration of HBV DNA may be a random event, but

hepatocytes which contain integrated HBV DNA may not express the full virion or specific recognition factor(s) required for immunologic or other host responses. Therefore, cells containing integrated HBV DNA might be preferentially retained within the hepatic parenchyma, and with cell division this might eventually lead to an increased proportion of such hepatocytes in long-term HBsAg carriers. At this stage in persistent infection, HBV DNA would be integrated into multiple or nonspecific sites within the cellular genome (Fig. 8, stage I). These patients may be HBeAg- or anti-HBe–positive. The presence of liver disease is not essential at this stage.

Subsequently, a clone or several clones of hepatocytes might become selected for preferential survival and/or multiplication by factors which are at present unknown. Since they contain integrated viral DNA, these cells are by definition virally transformed but are not yet neoplastic. The DNA from these cells would show discrete integrated HBV DNA bands on restriction-enzyme analysis (Fig. 8, stage II). Under the influence of other factors, (e.g., host immune surveillance mechanisms, nutritional state, environmental toxins, chemical carcinogens, hormones, and so on), one or more of these clones will give rise to the eventual malignant clone(s). Chromosomal alterations during the evolution of malignancy could account for changes in the integration pattern as the tumor emerges, distinguishing it from that found in the hepatocyte of origin. Alternatively, different integration patterns in liver and tumor could be due to sampling from an area of liver distinct from that which gave rise to the malignant clone. In any event this hypothesis implies that factors other than HBV contribute to the development of malignancy.

HBV as a "DNA tumor virus"

The genome of DNA tumor viruses, such as polyoma and SV40, consists of covalently closed double-stranded circular molecules. These circles have extra twists conferred upon them by structural features of the genome and exist in superhelical form. In the HBV genome, superhelical forms have also been recently reported. DNA tumor viruses do not cause cancer in their natural hosts but are highly oncogenic in labo-

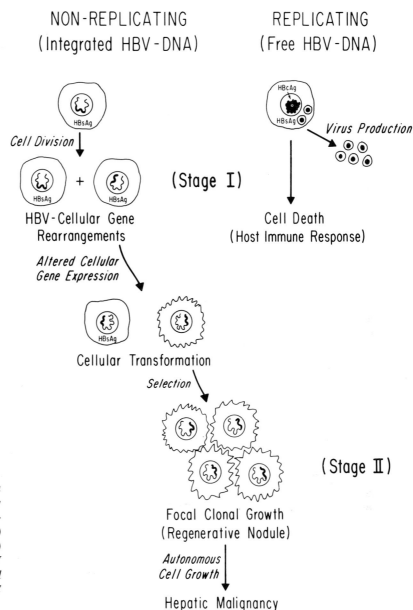

NON-REPLICATING
(Integrated HBV-DNA)

REPLICATING
(Free HBV-DNA)

FIGURE 8
Schematic model representing a hypothetical pathway which may explain the pathogenesis of hepatocellular carcinoma (HCC) related to hepatitis B virus (HBV) on the basis of patterns of HBV integration found in short- and long-term carriers and in HCC tissue.

ratory animals and may cause neoplastic transformation of cells in culture. Cells which permit viral replication (permissive) in general do not undergo malignant transformation. Only those cells which do not permit replication under a given set of conditions (nonpermissive) can be transformed. Defective (mutated) viruses and specific fragments of SV40 DNA are also capable of inducing neoplastic transformation. Transformation by DNA tumor viruses depends on the formation of certain virus-coded antigens, the

"transformation" on "T" antigens, although the precise mechanism of transformation is not known. A T antigen has not been described for HBV, but a nuclear antigen similar to that described in Epstein-Barr virus transformation has been recently described.

Integration of SV40 DNA appears to be a random event, occurring at no fixed sites in either the cellular or the viral genome. Similarly, HBV and WHV do not appear to have a fixed integration site in the host genome. SV40 viral DNA is integrated into host DNA in a complex fashion, with inversions, deletions, duplications, and translocations of viral DNA and rearrangement of cellular sequences at the site of integration. With viruses, such as SV40, it is clear that integration of viral DNA into the host genome occurs prior to, or at the time of, oncogenic transformation. As described previously, WHV DNA is integrated into woodchuck HCC DNA in a complex fashion with multiple inversions, deletions, and translocations, suggesting a series of events during evolution of malignancy which are similar to those observed for SV40.

HBV as an "RNA tumor virus"

The RNA tumor viruses (retroviruses) cause either sarcomas, lymphomas, or leukemias in susceptible experimental animals. These viruses are also able to transform fibroblasts in vitro. The retrovirus genome consists of a single-stranded RNA molecule. Following infection, a single-stranded complementary DNA (the *minus strand*) is produced from the RNA template (the *plus strand*) using reverse transcriptase. A viral DNA plus strand is then synthesized on the minus strand, using cellular DNA polymerase, to form a provirus. Proviral DNA has to be integrated into the host cell DNA before replication can occur. Full-length RNA plus strands are then transcribed from integrated proviral DNA and packaged into mature virus particles. All retrovirus proviral genomes are bound at both ends by repeat sequences, the long terminal repeats. These are important in the process of proviral DNA integration and also contain promotor sequences (i.e., sequences important in regulating expression of the viral genes).

Retroviruses may cause oncogenic transformation by several mechanisms, which have been described during the last few years. Many retroviruses contain sequences known as *onc genes,* which have no known replicative or structural function for the virus but which are associated with a transformed phenotype in cultured cells. These onc genes are viral homologues of cellular sequences from normal vertebrate cells (protooncogenes). Protooncogenes in some cells have been shown to code for a protein which functions as a tyrosine phosphorylase and may act upon proteins of the cytoskeleton (e.g., vin-

culin). Oncogenic change may thus result from an increased dose of the transforming gene, which accompanies retroviral infection. A second mechanism of retroviral oncogenicity was first described in avian leukosis virus, which lacks a transforming oncogene. These viruses induce transformation by integration of a viral promotor sequence adjacent to a cellular protooncogene. Transcription initiated at the viral promotor sequence causes enhanced expression of the protooncogene, leading to neoplastic transformation.

Some aspects of hepadna virus replication resemble those observed in retroviruses. In both cases, a DNA copy of an RNA molecule is made, and the second DNA strand is copied from the first. In HBV, the complete L strand corresponds to the minus strand and the S strand corresponds to the plus strand. Although integration does not appear to be necessary for hepadna virus replication, integration does occur, at least in HBV and WHV. The overlapping sequences of the HBV genome responsible for maintaining the circular configuration could, if the genome were linearized, serve a function analogous to a retroviral long terminal repeat.

Retrovirus oncogenes may be inserted into cells in culture (transfection) and cause neoplastic transformation. In eukaryotic cells, HBV DNA transfection has not yet been shown to cause neoplastic transformation. Therefore, HBV DNA may not contain an oncogene as such. However, two strong viral promotors have been identified in HBV DNA, one in the pre-S gene region and one in the cohesive-end region. In two woodchuck HCCs with integrated WHV DNA which have been studied, both tumors have sequences in common from the cohesive-end region. Therefore, it is possible that HBV becomes oncogenic when this region is integrated at or near a cellular oncogene, resulting in enhanced expression of that gene.

Alternatively, during persistent infection, cellular oncogenes may become integrated into replicating HBV mutant genomes, similar to those seen in SV40. These mutant HBV genomes could then be transferred to other hepatocytes, resulting in enrichment of oncogenic sequences in recipient cells and in increased expression of transforming properties. Finally, integration of HBV sequences could stimulate rearrangement of cellular sequences by acting as a fluid or transposable genetic element.

Possible role of chemical carcinogens

It is clear that HBV is not the sole cause of HCC, since many tumors arise in non-HBsAg carriers and do not contain HBV DNA. Although other putative hepatitis viruses (non-A, non-B) could potentially be involved, there is strong evidence for participation by other factors, notably alcohol consumption and dietary aflatoxin intake. Diseases such as hemochromatosis, tyrosinemia, and α_1-antitrypsin deficiency are also associated with HCC.

Interactions between viruses and chemical carcinogens in producing neoplastic transformation have been studied. Animals treated with a combination of chemical carcinogens and oncogenic viruses develop tumors more frequently than animals treated with virus or chemicals alone. For example, infection of newborn mice with polyoma virus, followed by cutaneous treatment with benzo[a]pyrene, increases the incidence and rate of appearance of malignant skin tumors over that seen with benzo[a]pyrene alone. When skin lesions in rabbits caused by intravenous administration of Shope papilloma virus are painted repeatedly with chemical carcinogens, malignancies develop, whereas administration of virus alone causes only benign tumors. Similarly, in cell cultures, treatment with chemical carcinogens increases the susceptibility of surviving cells to viral-induced cellular transformation. In addition, several polycyclic aromatic hydrocarbons which are oncogenic for hamster and mouse cells in vitro act synergistically with retroviruses to transform rat, hamster, and mouse cells. Similar findings have been reported in hamster ovary cells, using a DNA virus, simian adenovirus (SA7), and a number of different chemical carcinogens. A postulated mechanism for this synergistic interaction is that carcinogens induce breaks in cellular DNA which then serve as potential integration sites for viral DNA. Alternatively, genetic recombination following chromosome breaks secondary to exposure to chemical carcinogens may lead to reorganization of the cellular genome such that a repressed cellular oncogene is relocated next to a viral promotor, resulting in enhanced and/or altered expression of the cellular oncogene.

Chinese hamster ovary cells infected with SV40 and subsequently exposed to carcinogens show amplification of integrated SV40 DNA sequences as well as host DNA sequences. The patterns of molecular hybridization suggest that some viral sequences have been preferentially amplified. It is possible that similar mechanisms are involved in HBV-mediated oncogenicity. Aflatoxin B_1, a highly potent chemical carcinogen produced by the fungus *Aspergillus flavus*, is a common food contaminant in some areas of the world where HBV infection and HCC are common (e.g., Maputo, Kenya, and Thailand). In these areas, dietary aflatoxin intake may exceed 0.1 to 0.2 μg per day. It is possible that a low level of recurrent chromosome damage occurs, which in the presence of chronic HBV infection might increase the likelihood of HBV DNA integration.

Alcohol is thought to be a cocarcinogen. Many drug-metabolizing enzymes are induced by alcohol. This may result in enhanced activation of carcinogens and increased frequency of chromosome breaks. Alcoholics who are chronically infected with HBV might thus be more likely to develop integrated viral DNA. Alternatively, in patients who already have integrated HBV DNA, the increased exposure to carcinogens may result in amplification of HBV sequences (similar to SV40) and increased expression of a putative transforming protein.

A conclusion from the Taiwan study mentioned earlier is that HBV alone would seem to be sufficient to cause HCC. However, a cocarcinogen or tumor promotor could be acting within a given population but lead to HCC only in combination with HBV infection. Such a cocarcinogen or promotor would not be detected by this type of epidemiological study.

IMMUNOTHERAPY OF HCC

Current therapy of persistent HBV infection includes the use of interferon and adenine arabinoside. These agents are most effective when virus replication occurs at high frequency. In some patients, however, complete virions are no longer secreted, although HBsAg is still produced. In these patients, either HBV persists but does not replicate or HBsAg is produced from an integrated HBV DNA template. Eradication of virus DNA from cells in which HBV DNA is integrated but still expressed could be achieved by immunotherapy using monoclonal antibodies to proteins expressed on the cell surface. For example, when injected into athymic nude mice (BALB/c, nu/nu), the PLC/PRF/5 cell line produces well-vascularized, encapsulated tumors in nearly 100 percent of animals. In culture, it has been shown that monoclonal antibodies to HBsAg bind to viral determinants on PLC/PRF/5 cells and precipitate HBsAg in the culture medium. In the presence of complement, IgG2a or IgM monoclonal anti-HBs antibodies cause specific lysis of PLC/PRF/5 cells in culture but have no effect on other human hepatoma cells (Mahlavu or SK-Hep 1) which do not express HBsAg. When PLC/PRF/5 cells were injected into nude mice, the monoclonal antibodies caused suppression of tumor growth or prevention of tumor development in many animals. Although monoclonal antibodies have not been used for the treatment of human HCC or other HBV-related conditions, this remains an avenue for exploration. "Breakthrough" tumor growth (i.e., escape of the tumor from the inhibition caused by the monoclonal anti-HBs antibodies) was seen in some animals. This phenomenon has been found in other systems and may limit clinical application of monoclonal antibody immunotherapy. However, since HBV-infected hepatocytes and HBsAg-producing tumor cells have been shown to have HBsAg on their surface, the possibility exists that multiple monoclonal antibodies or monoclonal antibodies perhaps linked to cellular toxins could be therapeutically effective in killing tumor cells.

CONTROL OF HBV INFECTIONS BY VACCINATION

Based on the fact that antibodies to HBsAg confer immunity to the disease, several vaccines against hepatitis B are now available. The first generation of vaccines has been prepared by purifying HBsAg from the serum of HBV carriers. A variety of physical, chemical, and/or biologic methods were used to inactivate and remove potential pathogens from the vaccine, while retaining effective immunological activity.

These vaccines have been shown to be safe and highly effective, achieving an antibody response in up to 96 percent of normal recipients, although in immunologically compromised patients, such as renal dialysis patients, the vaccine is less effective. To date, only minor complications have been linked to the vaccine; nevertheless, since the vaccine is derived from human serum, there is a constant fear that some pathogen, at present poorly defined, may not be inactivated. Of particular concern are non-A, non-B hepatitis agents and the putative acquired immune-deficiency syndrome (AIDS) pathogen, both of which are likely to be present with some frequency in the serum of HBsAg carriers. To date, none of these diseases has been reported to be specifically transmitted by the vaccine.

Despite the efficacy of the vaccine, efforts are underway to produce second- and third-generation vaccines. The current vaccines are too expensive for large-scale use, particularly in underdeveloped nations. Several possible strategies may yield cheaper, yet effective, vaccines. The PLC/PRF/5 cell line secretes HBsAg but not intact virus. Other neoplastic and nonneoplastic cell lines can be induced to secrete HBsAg by introducing HBV DNA into the cell. Alternatively, the HBsAg gene can be isolated and introduced into prokaryotes, such as *E. coli,* or into eukaryotes, such as yeasts with expression of HBsAg. Recently, the HBsAg gene has been introduced into the vaccinia genome. Inoculation of rabbits with this vaccinia variant resulted in production of anti-HBs (in addition to antivaccinia) antibodies. Animals previously inoculated with the normal vaccinia strain did not produce anti-HBs. Although this vaccine might not be useful in an adult population and safety trials will need to be performed, this approach may have application in large-scale vaccination of children and in the prevention of vertical transmission of HBV. Short lengths of the hydrophilic portion of HBsAg are also mildly antigenic. These peptides are sufficiently small to be synthesized chemically but may need to be conjugated to adjuvants to be sufficiently antigenic to confer protection against infection. Whatever form of vaccine eventually becomes widely available, if HBV is truly oncogenic, widespread immunization should be followed 10 to 30 years later by a declining incidence of HCC.

SUMMARY

Until recently, human carcinogens have been identified largely as a result of epidemiological studies. In the absence of direct demonstration of the molecular mechanisms of oncogenicity, some doubt remains concerning whether many of these agents are truly oncogenic in humans. Available epidemiological data, although highly suggestive, do not prove a causal relationship between HBV and HCC, but the additional evidence provided by molecular studies supports and greatly strengthens the association. However, direct in vitro or in vivo experimental evidence for oncogenicity by HBV is still lacking. It is also not clear whether HBV may of itself induce tumors or whether some other factor(s), environmental or genetic, may also be necessary.

Whereas numerous potential chemical carcinogens affecting humans have been described, only a handful of the many viruses which infect humans has been linked to cancer. These include the Epstein-Barr virus, herpes simplex virus type 2, cytomegalic inclusion virus, and the recently described human T-cell leukemia-lymphoma virus. Because virus-induced alterations in cellular DNA may be more specific and therefore more easily measured than those caused by carcinogens, it is possible that elucidation of the pathogenesis of virus-induced cancer may provide information which may be applicable to the mechanisms of neoplastic transformation due to other causes. The relationship between oncogenes and retrovirus-induced transformation is a case in point. If a direct link can be established between some portion of the HBV genome or its expression and development of hepatic neoplasia, this may provide an important model of carcinogenesis, because the malignant cells often express a variety of viral and other protein markers associated with neoplastic change. Determining what controls expression of these various genes may lead to a better understanding of basic events in the origin of the malignant process.

References

BEASLEY RP et al: Hepatocellular carcinoma and hepatitis B virus: A prospective study of 22,707 men in Taiwan. Lancet 2:1129, 1981

BISHOP JM: Enemies within: The genesis of retrovirus oncogenes. Cell 23:5, 1981

BLUMBERG BS: Australia antigen and the biology of hepatitis B. Science 197:17, 1977

BONINO F et al: Hepatitis B virus DNA in the sera of HBsAg carriers: A marker of active hepatitis B replication in the liver. Hepatology 1:386, 1981

BRECHOT C et al: Detection of hepatitis B virus DNA in the liver and serum: A direct appraisal of the chronic carrier state. Lancet 2:765, 1981

KEW MC: The hepatitis B virus and hepatocellular carcinoma. Semin Liver Dis 1:59, 1981

MAGNIUS LO, ESPMARK JA: New specificities in Australia antigen positive sera distinct from the Le Bouvier determinants. J Immunol 109:1017, 1972

ROBINSON WS: The genome of hepatitis B virus. Annu Rev Microbiol 31:357, 1977

SHAFRITZ DA: Hepatitis B virus DNA molecules in the liver of HBsAg carriers: Mechanistic considerations in the pathogenesis of hepatocellular carcinoma. Hepatology 2(Suppl):35S, 1982

—et al: Integration of hepatitis B virus DNA into the genome of liver cells in chronic liver disease and hepatocellular carcinoma. N Engl J Med 305:1067, 1981

SHOUVAL D et al: Protection against experimental hepatoma formation in nude mice by monoclonal antibodies to hepatitis B virus surface antigen. Hepatology 2(Suppl):128S, 1982

SUMMERS J, MASON WS: Replication of the genome of a hepatitis B-like virus by reverse transcription of an RNA intermediate. Cell 29:403, 1982

SUMMERS J: Three recently described animal virus models for human hepatitis H virus. Hepatology 1:179, 1981

SZMUNESS W: Hepatocellular carcinoma and the hepatitis B virus: Evidence for a causal association. Prog Med Virol 24:40, 1978

TIOLLAIS P et al: Biology of hepatitis B virus. Science 213:406, 1981

TOOZE J (ed): *Molecular Biology of Tumour Viruses: DNA Tumour Viruses*, 2d ed. Cold Spring Harbor, NY, Cold Spring Harbor Lab, 1980, part 2

VARMUS HE: Form and function of retroviral proviruses. Science 216:812, 1982

GALLSTONE DISEASE: CURRENT CONCEPTS ON THE EPIDEMIOLOGY, PATHOGENESIS, AND MANAGEMENT

MARTIN C. CAREY and MICHAEL A. O'DONOVAN

Gallstones are the leading worldwide cause of gallbladder and biliary tract disease. In western societies, where gallstones represent a major health problem, their origins and natural history are incompletely understood; concepts regarding their treatment are in transition. Within the past few decades, major advances have occurred in defining the etiology and pathogenesis of cholesterol gallstones; in contrast, basic information on the pathobiology of pigment gallstone formation does not seem to have progressed substantially. During this period, dramatic new technological advances have enhanced the precision of radiological, ultrasonographic, and endoscopic diagnosis of stones and their associated diseases and have made the surgical treatment of gallstones safer and more effective. In the early 1970s, the introduction of specific bile acids for dissolving gallstones represented a benchmark pharmacological breakthrough for possible medical therapy of gallstones. This innovation not only added a new and evolving dimension to the management of gallstones, but further advances may eventually lead both to the prevention of gallstones in individuals at high risk of developing stones and to the rapid obliteration of gallstones in individuals who are at high risk of dying from the complications of surgery.

Despite these advances, the diagnosis and management of calculous biliary tract disease still represent a formidable challenge to the clinician. Irrespective of the diagnostic modality employed, the diagnosis of uncomplicated gallstones is still associated with a 5 percent margin of false-negative errors; and the diagnosis of complicated gallstone disease continues to rely chiefly on clinical judgment. Which patients with gallstones should be treated, when they should be treated, and how, are matters of heated controversy. Fueling this debate is the epidemiological evidence that surgery for gallstones is probably overutilized: cholecystectomy rates in the United States are threefold higher than in the United Kingdom or Scandinavia, despite the fact that gallstone prevalence rates are much higher in western Europe. Since the latter part of the last century, the management of gallstone patients has traditionally been the undisputed province of the surgeon and the literature, largely anecdotal, pointed to the hazards of harboring gallstones in one's gallbladder. A 1928 humorist in *Collier's Magazine* wrote:

An' now it's the gall bladder. Doctors are mad over it. The appendix, tonsils, teeth, auto-intoxication, acidosis—are all forgotten; an' that gall bladder is now the undisputed belle of the body. For a medical man it has all the lure an' emotional appeal of a Swinburne poem, a Ziegfeld chorus or a moonlight party in Hollywood.

During the past several years, prospective epidemiological evidence suggests that the "innocent gallstone is not a myth" and the gallstones may be much more benign than supposed.

Initial optimism for medical therapy of gallstones waned dramatically with publication of the results of the National Cooperative Gallstone Study (Schoenfield et al.). The efficacy of chenodeoxycholic acid in dissolving gallstones in highly selected patients was disappointingly small, and even though the dosage was suboptimal, the incidence of side effects was high and potentially serious. Nevertheless, medical therapy, especially with the safer ursodeoxycholic acid, has a place in the management of patients with gallstones, although the ideal patient for such therapy is the patient with asymptomatic ("silent") stones who probably requires no intervention whatsoever. Further, once stones are obliterated and therapy is discontinued, the rate of recurrence of stones is disconcertingly high. It has been suggested that stone dissolution may not radically change the natural history of gallstone disease. One of the greatest benefits of medical therapy may be the postponement of the biliary complication of gallstones, especially in the older gallstone patient.

To the epidemiologist, the gallstone problem is a major public health challenge. For example, there is strong evidence that the disease itself is in transition. Compared with the last century, the prevalence of gallstones is on the increase; not only is this the case in the west, but also in countries that are becoming westernized. In the orient, where gallstones were once infrequent and predominantly pigment in type, there is a progressive transition to the cholesterol variety and total stone prevalence has escalated. Moreover, the true age- and sex-related prevalence rates of gallstones in typical western countries still rely predominantly on autopsy studies, which by definition are biased and usually unrepresentative of the living population. More importantly, the age- and sex-related natural history of both microscopic stones ("sludge" or "gallsand") and macroscopic stones is still extremely sketchy. Nonetheless, rational decision making in clinical practice must be based on an accurate assessment of such data, incomplete as they are.

The dilemmas faced by the investigator are intertwined with all aspects of gallstones and their associated diseases. Our knowledge of the staging and evolution of cholesterol and pigment gallstone disease, from the initiation of the metabolic defect and the development of chemically abnormal bile to the formation of macroscopic stones, is still woefully inadequate. Risk factors for both categories of stones have been defined, but at least 80 percent of the gallstone population have, as far as is known, no identifiable risk factor. The role of diet in the etiology of stones is presumed but not proved, and its possible etiologic and pathogenetic mechanisms are totally obscure. Knowledge of what causes biliary tract pain from either sludge or stones is extremely vague, and the reasons why many (perhaps most) patients can silently carry gallstones to their graves are still not understood.

Finally, medical therapy for a relatively benign disease that necessitates 1 to 3 years of bile acid ingestion and physician monitoring with its attendant high failure and recurrence rates is unacceptable to many. New breakthroughs are needed to induce safe, noninvasive disintegration and/or dissolution of stones over a much-reduced time period. Further, the development of simple laboratory tests and interventions is needed to detect individuals and populations at risk and to prevent de novo stone formation and recurrence.

In this chapter, we will focus principally on current concepts in management of patients with gallstones. We will define the current status of therapy for gallstones in terms of the roles of expectant versus medical or surgical managements. We will base our recommendations concerning the role of each therapeutic modality on an analysis of the relevant pathophysiological, historical, clinical, and epidemiological evidence. We will weigh management decisions based on the natural history of stones against the risks and efficacy of surgery and chronic therapy with bile acids, and we will indicate what factors should influence these decisions. Finally, we will indicate what strategies for intervention are on the horizon for the rapid noninvasive disintegration and/or dissolution of stones and will speculate on possible modalities for preventing stone formation and recurrence.

PATHOPHYSIOLOGY
Classification of gallstones

Human beings are affected by two types of gallstones: (1) cholesterol stones, composed predominantly of crystalline cholesterol monohydrate, and (2) pigment stones, composed mainly of either noncrystalline calcium bilirubinates and/or a covalently linked polymer derived from bilirubin. In the west, the minority (5 to 10 percent) of stones are pure cholesterol monohydrate, often containing a pigmented center. Depending upon the population studied, about 5 to 25 percent of stones are pigment stones and contain less than 5 percent cholesterol monohydrate. Most gallstones are of mixed composition, containing cholesterol monohydrate, bilirubin salts and polymers, proteins, calcium salts of phosphate, carbonate, fatty acids, and traces of lecithin and bile acids. In classifying gallstones, the term "mixed" is now obsolete, since cholesterol monohydrate is the major component (>50 percent by weight) of these stones; stones which contain between 10 to 50 percent cholesterol are rare. Both pigment and so-called mixed cholesterol stones, in contrast to "pure" cholesterol stones, occur in multiples, with the pigment stones being generally smaller, spiculated, and darker.

Anatomic and radiologic considerations

In most patients, gallstones are usually of only one chemical type and a single distribution in size and are found at only one anatomical site. Most gallstones form primarily in an intact gallbladder and the surrounding bile is sterile. Ductal stones, including those which are retained following cholecystectomy, are usually stones which have migrated from the gallbladder. Most of these are cholesterol stones and, less commonly, pigment stones of the polymer variety ("black pigment" stones). Since cholesterol stones contain only small concentrations of calcium salts, they are usually radiolucent (80 percent). Radiopaque cholesterol stones contain calcium salts which are either aggregated in the nidus of the stones or distributed as shells surrounding a radiolucent core. Bilirubin polymer or black pigment stones form only in the gallbladder; since they often contain quantities of calcium bilirubinate, phosphate, and carbonate, most (75 percent) are radiopaque.

Primary or de novo biliary duct stones form either in the intrahepatic ducts (hepatolithiasis) or in the extrahepatic ducts. They are commonly associated with biliary tree infection or infestation, coupled with congenital or acquired bile duct obstruction. Hepatolithiasis without gallbladder involvement is common in the orient but

extremely rare in the west. Such stones are composed of mixtures of calcium bilirubinate and palmitate, contain little protein or other calcium salts, and contain virtually no cholesterol; they are usually radiolucent. In the west, the usual setting for primary duct stone formation is in patients who have undergone cholecystectomy several years previously. These stones are composed of mucin glycoproteins, calcium bilirubinate, and palmitate and contain more cholesterol than the intrahepatic variety. Primary duct stones are usually associated with bacterial infection and impaired ductal drainage and are radiolucent.

Migration of small gallbladder stones via the biliary tree into the duodenum is extremely common. Ductal migration of a large solitary stone is relatively rare: such stones usually enter the intestine via a spontaneous cholecystoenteric or choledochoenteric fistula. Thus, gallstones can be found at any anatomic site of the gastrointestinal tract including the stomach, small intestine, and colon and are commonly detected by ultrasound or sieving of the feces. Obstruction of the ampulla of Vater by a migrating ductal stone can lead to gallstone pancreatitis. Such migrant gallstones are the second-leading cause of acute pancreatitis in industrialized societies; a large stone, having passed through a cholecystoduodenal fistula, can become impacted in the ileocecal sphincter and result in small bowel obstruction (gallstone ileus). In the absence of a previous surgical history, gallstone ileus is one of the most common causes of small bowel obstruction unrelated to hernia in patients older than 65 years.

Cholesterol gallstone formation

The evolution of cholesterol gallstones follows five sequential stages: stage 1—a constitutional or acquired defect in the metabolism and secretion of biliary lipids; stage 2—cholesterol supersaturation of bile; stage 3—nucleation in the gallbladder; stage 4—agglomeration of cholesterol monohydrate crystals, possibly in gallbladder mucin gels; and stage 5—growth of the cholesterol microcrystals from gallsand into mature gallstones. Recent research has elucidated the etiologies and pathogenetic mechanisms which underlie stages 1 and 2, but much less is known concerning stages 3 through 5.

TABLE 1
Pathophysiologic abnormalities, etiologic mechanisms, and causes of cholesterol gallstones

Type	Abnormality	Mechanism	Causes
1	Reduced bile salt secretion	Defective bile salt synthesis	Congenital 12α-hydroxylase deficiency, cerebrotendinous xanthomatosis, estrogens, possibly type 2b hyperlipoproteinemia, chronic cholestatic liver disease, and primary biliary cirrhosis
2	Reduced bile salt secretion	Excessive alimentary bile salt loss	Ileectomy, ileal bypass, regional ileitis, cystic fibrosis with pancreatic insufficiency, primary bile salt malabsorption, possibly bile salt sequestering agents
3	Reduced bile salt secretion	Oversensitive bile salt feedback	Constitutional, genetic or acquired from unknown causes in otherwise normal patients with gallstones
4	Excessive cholesterol secretion	Excessive cholesterol synthesis or intake	Obesity, type 4 hyperlipoproteinemia, clofibrate therapy, high caloric intake, massive cholesterol intake, estrogens
5	Reduced bile salt secretion *and* excessive cholesterol secretion	Not known	Constitutional, genetic, or acquired from unknown causes plus obesity in American Indians (severe form) and many Caucasians with modest obesity and gallstones (mild form)
6	Bile salt and lecithin absorption and possibly cholesterol secretion in the gallbladder	Abnormal gallbladder function from stasis and infection	Cholecystitis (acalculous and bacterial), salmonellosis, somatostatinoma syndrome, post-truncal vagotomy, pheochromocytoma, other stasis syndromes, total parenteral nutrition

Cholesterol is insoluble in water; hence, special mechanisms are available to maintain biliary cholesterol in aqueous solution in bile. This is achieved by the combined physicochemical action of bile salts and membrane-derived phospholipids, principally lecithins. Bile salts and phospholipid molecules combine to solubilize cholesterol molecules in small water-soluble particles, named mixed micelles and liquid crystalline vesicles. Because cholesterol secretion is coupled to lecithin secretion which, in turn, is tightly coupled to bile salt secretion, the fluctuant rhythm of the enterohepatic circulation of bile salts principally controls the secretion rate of cholesterol into bile. Cholesterol secretion also varies with the predominant species of bile salt, the rate of hepatic and extrahepatic cholesterol synthesis, the rate of hepatic uptake of cholesterol-rich lipoproteins, and perhaps other intracellular and hormonal factors. Bile salt (and lecithin) secretion is controlled by the recycling frequency and size of the bile salt pool. Because the ratio of cholesterol to bile salt (and lecithin) in bile is controlled by the delicate balance of these factors, the resulting output of cholesterol often exceeds the solubilizing capacity of bile. Thus, any metabolic derangement which increases cholesterol secretion rates or reduces bile salt secretion rates, or produces a combination of both abnormalities, can give rise to supersaturated and potentially lithogenic bile. On this basis, bile lipid secretory abnormalities can be divided into five categories (types 1 through 5) as shown in Table 1. The etiologic factors corresponding to each pathophysiologic abnormality are several. In the sixth category (type 6) the pathogenetic mechanism does not relate to altered hepatic secretion of lipids but is entirely extrahepatic in origin, being due to altered gallbladder secretory, hormonal, or mechanical function. While cholesterol supersaturation of bile is a necessary prerequisite for the formation of cholesterol gallstones, it is not a sufficient condition in and of itself. The second abnormality in lithogenic gallbladder biles is that nucleation of the excess cholesterol takes place about five times faster than in nonlithogenic control biles for the *same degree* of cholesterol supersaturation. Possible gallbladder factors in lithogenesis are the addition of a nucleating agent, the removal of an antinucleating agent, or simply a change in physical state of bile by lipid concentration per se. As inferred from animal studies, mucin hypersecretion and poor contractility (hypotony) of the gallbladder may also play important roles.

Pigment gallstone formation

Much less is known concerning the etiology and pathogenesis of pigment stones. While the etiologic factors are most certainly different, the pathogenetic mechanisms may have many similarities to those giving rise to cholesterol stones. Technological advances, particularly high-performance liquid chromatography, have only recently allowed precise separation and quantitative measurement of bilirubin and its conjugates in bile. Phase equilibria and electrochemical studies to define the solubility of bilirubin and its conjugates in model bile systems are being pursued, but the results are not yet available. It is likely that the solubilities of bilirubin and its conjugates will vary as functions of pH, calcium concentration, lipid concentration, relative lipid composition, and mucin glycoprotein content of bile. Bilirubin, calcium, and bile salt secretory studies analogous to those carried out with the major biliary lipids in cholesterol stone patients have not yet been attempted in pigment stone patients. Hence, it is not known whether the biliary secretory rates of bilirubin, calcium, bile salts, and bicarbonate ions differ between pigment stone and control populations.

Bilirubin is soluble in bile because it is bound in ester linkage to one or two molecules of glucuronic acid to form bilirubin monoglucuronide or bilirubin diglucuronide, respectively; human bile also contains small amounts of mixed diconjugates of xylose, glucose, and glucuronic acid. In healthy human beings the diconjugate/monoconjugate ratio is about 4:1, and less than 2 percent of bile pigments is composed of the otherwise insoluble unconjugated (free) bilirubin. At physiologic pH this small amount of free bilirubin should be solubilized in bile by the detergent properties of bile salts; as a result, bile should become lithogenic with bilirubin only when there is increased secretion of unconjugated bilirubin, increased conversion of normal or elevated levels of conjugated bilirubin to the unconjugated

form, and/or a decreased secretion of bile salts. There are suggestions that noninfected biles of pigment stone patients in the west may contain increased concentrations of both unconjugated bilirubin and bilirubin monoconjugates, which are less soluble and chemically more labile than bilirubin diconjugates. Patients with chronic hemolysis apparently have a bile pigment composition similar to that of normal controls but excrete excess conjugated bilirubin in their bile. Studies in animal models of pigment stone formation have suggested that the concentrations of unconjugated bilirubin are higher than in control animals and exceed the solubilizing capacity of bile. As occurs in animal models of cholesterol stones, the gallbladder responds to the lithogenic stimulus with an increased synthesis and secretion of mucin glycoproteins. The predominant pigment stone in occidental patients, irrespective of whether they suffer from a chronic hemolytic state or not, appears to be the bilirubin polymer, or black pigment stone. The physicochemical basis for the formation of bilirubin polymer stones is not known.

The pathogenesis of pigment stones in patients with infected or infestated bile is clearer; these stones are invariably calcium bilirubinate in composition (often called brown or earthy pigment stones). The levels of monoconjugated pigments and unconjugated bilirubin in the bile of these patients are greatly increased. This has been shown to be the result of deconjugation of bilirubin conjugates by bacterial β-glucuronidases in the biliary tract. Glucaric acid, an inhibitor of this enzyme, is normally present in bile but its inhibitory capacity appears to be overwhelmed in the setting of rapid bacterial hydrolysis. The concentration of unconjugated bilirubin then exceeds the solubilizing capacity of bile salt-lecithin-cholesterol micelles and probably precipitates as the calcium salt. In the oriental pigment stone syndrome, the pigment composition of bile is apparently completely normal when secreted and becomes abnormal only within the biliary tree and gallbladder.

Biliary sludge and its relevance

Biliary sludge is a frequent finding on abdominal ultrasonography. The term refers to a sonographic feature of a crescent of low-amplitude intraluminal echoes arising from the dependent portion of a gallbladder. The echogenic crescent flows with a change in the position of the patient and is usually not associated with acoustic shadowing. Less often, gallbladder bile is diffusely echogenic. Despite the frequency of biliary sludge, its chemistry, etiology, pathogenesis, and natural history are not well-defined.

Physicochemical considerations Normal bile is a nonechogenic liquid admixed in the gallbladder with a dilute mucin glycoprotein solution to form a polymer solution. The normal gallbladder mucosa secretes mucin continuously, and since bile contains no enzymes for mucin degradation, the normal physical state of bile is dependent on gallbladder contraction for elimination of mucin glycoproteins into the upper small intestine. If the gallbladder does not empty normally, or if mucin glycoproteins are secreted in excessive amounts (e.g., in the setting of a lithogenic stimulus), then the concentrations of mucin glycoproteins can reach critical levels where the glycoproteins polymerize to form a gel. With this "phase transition," bile becomes a gel phase in addition to a liquid phase, and a gel-fluid level forms. Being much more viscous than liquid bile, the rate at which the gel-fluid level is reestablished after the position of the patient is changed is often very slow. In the gallbladder, this gel matrix is the major component of sludge. The mucin gel can apparently bind otherwise soluble conjugated bile pigments and can act as a nucleating matrix for calcium bilirubinate precipitation in pigment lithogenic bile or liquid crystalline vesicle and solid crystalline precipitation in cholesterol lithogenic biles. Studies in animals and in humans have shown that biliary sludge is a mucin gel dispersed with a variety of "microprecipitates," which are usually calcium bilirubinate and, less commonly, cholesterol monohydrate crystals. In vitro filtration studies of biliary sludge suggest that the particulate matter, and not the viscous mucin gel itself, is the source of sonographic echoes. The size of the dispersed microprecipitates can be as small as 5 to 10 μm.

Clinical associations Echogenic bile is most often seen in patients with extrahepatic biliary obstruction, patients with acute and resolving cholecystitis, and patients undergoing prolonged fasting after surgery or during severe intercurrent illness. The most dramatic causation of biliary sludge is prolonged parenteral hyperalimentation. Serial ultrasonographic studies of patients initially free of hepatobiliary disease and undergoing total parenteral nutrition (TPN) have shown that the percent of sludge-positive patients increases from 6 percent during the first 3 weeks to 50 percent between the fourth and sixth weeks, and reaches 100 percent in patients on TPN therapy for longer than 6 weeks. Gallstone formation occurs in 50 percent of sludge-forming patients but is not observed in patients who have negative ultrasonographic evidence for sludge.

All studies suggest that at least 50 percent of patients with stones resulting from prolonged TPN have a high complication rate that necessitates cholecystectomy; those at greater risk for complications of sludge and stone formation are those that have cholesterol lithogenic bile in the first place. Such patients are those with "small-bowel failure," usually from massive small-bowel resection ("short-bowel syndrome"), severe Crohn's disease, and refractory celiac sprue. Analysis of the biles and stones obtained at surgery has revealed thick mucin gels, cholesterol crystals, pigment precipitates, and blackish-brown, irregularly shaped, soft, friable stones that contain mainly bilirubin salts and some cholesterol. However, biliary sludge is not necessarily pathognomonic of an irreversible organic lesion. After prolonged fasting, sludge usually disappears when a normal diet is resumed. With the use of ultrasonographic evaluation, sludge is found to decrease from 88 percent during the first 3 weeks of oral refeeding to zero by the end of the fourth week in patients following TPN. It appears that in both adults and children intestinal "rest" and gallbladder stasis during TPN can lead to the production of biliary sludge which can result in eventual gallstone formation; in individuals not at risk for cholesterol gallstones, the microprecipitates appear to be mainly calcium bilirubinate. In patients at risk for cholesterol gallstones, the microprecipitates are mixed, presumably containing some cholesterol but still predominantly calcium bilirubinate. The etiologic roles of cholestasis, increased biliary levels of lithocholic acid, and hypersomatostatinemia in the formation of biliary sludge and stones during TPN are not established.

Role of sludge in stone formation   Since sludge is a physicochemical dispersion of solids and liquid crystals trapped in a three-dimensional gel network, it may well be the "primordial soup" in which all pigment and cholesterol stones are formed. Although never studied as such, mucin gels may change not only the equilibrium solubility of cholesterol and bilirubin in bile but may drastically alter the metastability of bile by inducing nucleation at lower degrees of supersaturation. For example, it is known that calcium bilirubinate, a bilirubin polymer, and sometimes mucin can be found at the central nidus of essentially all-human cholesterol gallstones but not all gallstones induced by diet in animal models. This suggests that the precipitation of calcium bilirubinate, or a bilirubin polymer, may be the initial event in human biliary lithogenesis. The development of cholesterol or pigment stones may then depend on the physicochemistry of the bile in which the initial nucleation has taken place. Even at this embryonic stage in the formation of stones, biliary sludge can give rise to severe biliary pain and, in some cases, acute cholecystitis.

EPIDEMIOLOGY

Reliable epidemiological data provide important clues as to the etiology of stone disease, the risk factors for the formation of stones, and the natural history of symptoms and complications. Other diseases which have similar high or low prevalences can be identified and, in certain situations, a common etiologic basis can be inferred. In the case of gallstones, solid epidemiological data, especially natural history data, are critical for decision making in practice. This information may also demonstrate that special populations exist, so that inferences concerning clinical outcome based on evaluation of unusual gallstone populations may not necessarily be extrapolated to all others.

Worldwide autopsy prevalence

Figure 1 displays the sex-related world distribution of gallstones based on age-adjusted autopsy prevalence rates since 1940. Chileans have an extremely high prevalence rate, and anecdotal

FIGURE 1
Age-adjusted autopsy prevalence of gallstones. (After AB Lowenfels, Gut 21:1090, 1980; M Brett, DJP Barker, Int J Epidemiol 5:335, 1976.)

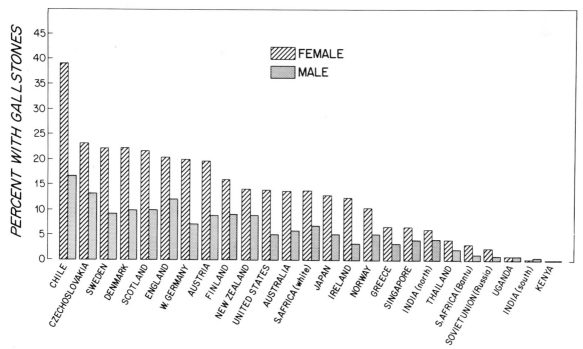

evidence suggests that similar prevalence rates might be found in other populations of Central and South America. Gallstones are very common in most of the industrial nations of western Europe, with Czechoslovakia, Poland (not shown), and Scandinavia (with the exceptions of Finland and Norway) having the highest prevalence rates. Curiously, New Zealand, the United States, and Australia have considerably lower prevalence rates compared with most countries of western Europe. Although accurate information is lacking, the middle east, eastern Europe, the Soviet Union, and the Baltic countries appear to have low prevalence rates. Prevalence rates in countries that are less developed are very low; gallstones are extremely rare throughout most of Africa, with the sole exception being the white population of South Africa, which has a prevalence rate similar to that of Australia. No recent epidemiologic information is available for most of Soviet Asia, the People's Republic of China, or Oceania, although studies from the older autopsy literature suggest that gallstones were rare. Prevalence rates of gallstones can vary considerably in different parts of the same country; for example, stones are moderately common in northern India, but are extremely rare in southern India.

Figure 1 also shows that throughout the world, prevalence rates of gallstones in females are about twice those in males. In countries with high prevalence rates, the majority of stones are cholesterol stones, whereas in countries with lower prevalence rates, the majority are pigment stones. There is good evidence for a change in frequency and type of gallstones in certain countries. In western Europe, autopsy prevalence rates before and after 1940 suggest that there has been a marked increase (in some instances greater than 80 percent) in occurrence of gallstones. Similar chronological changes have been documented in studies from Japan: between 1941 and 1948 the overall prevalence of stones was 5 percent, and 45 percent of stones were composed of calcium bilirubinate. Since 1974, only 10 percent of stones among Japanese are pigment stones, and cholesterol stones have shown both a relative and an absolute increase to reach the prevalence rates shown in Fig. 1. With rare exceptions, stones discovered at autopsy have not been typed on the basis of chemical analysis.

Nevertheless, it is safe to infer that the prevalence rates of pigment stones may be similar throughout the world at 2 to 5 percent on the scale displayed in Fig. 1 and that excess prevalence rates represent cholesterol stones.

True prevalence versus clinical prevalence

Apart from being unrepresentative of the living population, most autopsy studies cannot provide information as to what percentage of patients with stones had symptoms or complications during life. Despite the great medical interest in gallstones and their associated diseases, no scientific sample of a typical Caucasian, Asian, or Black population has been studied to determine both *true* prevalence *and* clinical prevalence rates of gallstone disease. However, epidemiological studies to determine true versus clinical prevalence rates have been carried out on two unique populations. We will show below that the results of these investigations are most instructive.

Cholesterol stones Certain tribes of North American Indians (Pima, Chippewa, Micmac) are known to have the highest prevalence rates of gallstones in the world; virtually all Indian gallstones are cholesterol stones. In the late 1960s, 600 male and female Pima Indians of all ages were surveyed by clinical evaluation, oral cholecystography, and surgical records. Rigorous epidemiological and evaluation criteria were employed and the true age- and sex-specific prevalence rates plus clinical prevalence rates of gallstones were derived (Fig. 2). This important study showed a dramatic increase in gallstone prevalence in females from ~12 percent in the 15 to 24 year age group to 73 percent in the 25 to 34 year age group; females in the higher age groups showed similar prevalence rates which increased to 90 percent beyond 65 years of age. Gallstones were first detected in Pima males at a slightly later age than in females, and a more gradual increase in prevalence rates was found with advancing age. Prevalence rates in Pima males increased from <1 percent in the 15 to 24 year age group to 66 percent in the 55 to 64+ year age group. The percentage of females with clinical evidence of disease (biliary pain and/or biliary complications) constituted ~2 percent in

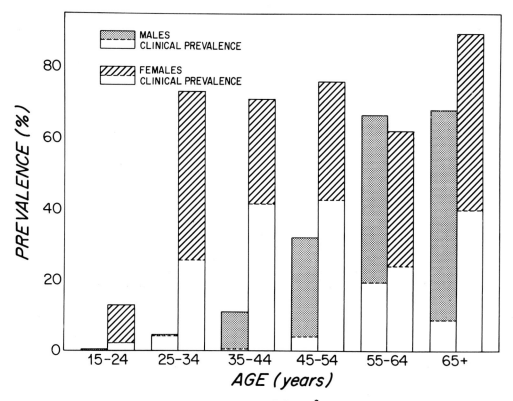

FIGURE 2

Age- and sex-related prevalence rates of gallstones in Pima Indians. Open sections of each histogram indicate prevalence of symptomatic disease. (After RE Sampliner et al, N Engl J Med 283:1358, 1970.)

the 15 to 24 year age group, 26 percent in the 25 to 34 year age group, and ~40 to 50 percent after the age of 35 years. The clinical prevalence rate in males was much lower in all age groups; symptoms or complications, when they arose, generally did so beyond the age of 45. The etiology of such epidemic proportions of gallstones in Pima (and other North American) Indians is unexplained; nevertheless, much insight into the pathogenesis of Indian gallstones has been acquired. Bile salt secretion rates are low, biliary cholesterol secretion rates are high; both combine to produce extreme degrees of biliary cholesterol supersaturation. The hyposecretion of bile salts has been associated with contraction of the bile salt pool, especially that of chenodeoxycholic acid, and may be related to constitutional and/or dietary factors. Biliary hypersecretion of cholesterol may, in part, be due to the very high prevalence rates of obesity in this population as compared with those for the average U.S. population (Fig. 3). It is interesting to note that, while obesity in the Pima Indians has been recorded for over 100 years, hospital records and missionary accounts do not suggest that gallbladder disease

was common at the turn of the century or in the early part of this century. Pima Indians are also characterized by high fertility rates and a high prevalence rate of diabetes mellitus, 10 times higher than in the general U.S. population (Fig. 3). While there has been no documented statistical correlation between fertility, diabetes, and gallstone prevalence in this population, it is possible that fertility and diabetes may be contributory factors to the very high prevalence rates of clinical symptoms in female Pima Indians (Fig. 2). Gallbladder hypotonicity is a frequent complication of diabetes mellitus and pregnancy.

Pigment stones As is well known, pigment gallstones are a common finding in patients with chronic hemolytic disease of any etiology, but apart from autopsy and cholecystectomy data, the true age- and sex-related prevalence of pigment gallstones in a homogeneous population

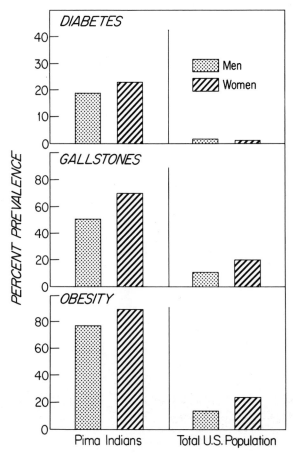

FIGURE 3

The American Indian's burden: age- and sex-adjusted prevalence of diabetes mellitus, gallstones, and obesity in Pima Indians vs. typical U.S. communities. (After GO Friedman et al: J Chronic Dis 19:273, 1966; JF Brody, The New York Times, Feb 5, 1980, pp C1 and C5.)

was not known until recently. At the Children's Hospital in Detroit, Mich., investigators surveyed their entire sickle cell population under the age of 18 years by ultrasonography. This population consisted of 226 individuals evenly divided between males and females with proven hemoglobin sickle cell disease. A diagnosis was considered positive when either gallstones (63) or biliary sludge (14) were found; the population was also evaluated for symptoms (history of right upper quadrant pain) and complications (documented right upper quadrant pain and tenderness, accompanied by an increase in blood levels of conjugated bilirubin). The results (Fig. 4) show a much higher than expected prevalence of gallstones even in the youngest (2 to 4 year) age

group. The prevalence of stones increases sharply with advancing age, reaching 45 percent in the case of 10- to 14-year-old males and 50 percent in the case of 15- to 18-year-old females. Stones were significantly more prevalent in prepubertal males than females, but this trend was reversed in the adolescent years. It is relevant that adult mice with congenital hemolytic anemias show a similar female preponderance. Of 14 patients (6.2 percent) who had biliary sludge at their initial examination, 4 developed definite stones at subsequent follow-up, whereas 4 others cleared their sludge and in 6 patients the amount of sludge remained unchanged. Despite the high prevalence of gallstones in these young patients, a history of right upper quadrant pain and/or cholestatic episodes was surprisingly infrequent. Only 14 patients (6 percent) were symptomatic for gallstone disease; 10 of these had definite stones, giving a 16 percent prevalence of clinical disease in patients with stones. In the patients with sludge, the clinical prevalence was 21 percent. Since this study demonstrated an unexpectedly high prevalence rate of cholelithiasis below the age of 10 years and a low incidence of clear-cut symptoms at all ages, the investigators raised doubts regarding the justification of early surgical intervention.

Comparable epidemiological information is not available for patients with hereditary spherocytosis and thalassemia major; however, cholecystectomy, oral cholecystography, and autopsy data suggest that stone prevalence rates in hereditary spherocytosis may be even higher than in thalassemia major and sickle cell disease, reaching 60 to 70 percent in the fifth to sixth decades.

Symptomatic gallstones at cholecystectomy

It is instructive to examine the age distribution of chemically analyzed stones obtained at consecutive cholecystectomies for symptomatic gallstones in a western urban population. Investigators at the Hospital of the University of Pennsylvania analyzed gallstones from 94 symptomatic patients, 38 percent of whom were black, admitted during a 6-month period. The age-related distribution of cholesterol and pigment stones is shown in Fig. 5. While these frequencies do not allow any conclusions concerning the

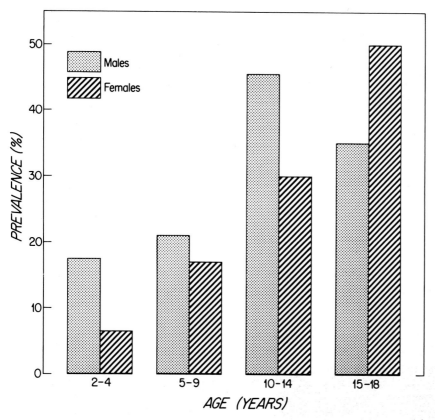

FIGURE 4
Prevalence of pigment gallstones detected by ultra-sonography in 224 patients with homozygous sickle cell disease. (After S Sarnaik et al, J Pediatr 96:1005, 1980.)

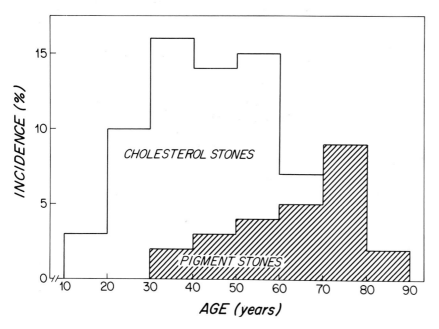

FIGURE 5
Incidence of chemically ana-lyzed cholesterol and pigment gallstones in 94 consecutive cholecystectomies for symp-tomatic gallstones over a 6-month period in Philadelphia. (From BW Trotman, RD So-loway, Am J Dig Dis 20:735, 1975.)

age-related prevalence of each stone type, the distribution suggests that symptomatic stones are generally cholesterol in type in the 20 to 60 year age group and are generally pigment in type in older age groups. Since autopsy prevalence rates of stones in western urban populations increase with advancing age, these data are consistent with the possibility that cholesterol stone formation has an abrupt onset in the general population in the third to fourth decades (as in the Pima Indians) and that nonhemolytic pigment stone formation may be delayed by several decades.

Risk factors for gallstones

The previous sections have dealt with a number of major determinants of gallstone prevalence such as geographic location, race, and hemolytic status. However, it is now appreciated that the risk factors in individual patients need to be extended substantially, as shown in Table 2. Most

TABLE 2
Risk factors for gallstones

1 Pigment stones
  a Demography: orient more than occident, rural more than urban
  b Chronic hemolysis
  c Alcoholic cirrhosis
  d Biliary infection
  e Congenital anomalies
  f Advancing age
  g Erythropoietic protoporphyria
2 Cholesterol stones
  a Demography: northern Europe; North and South America more than orient or Africa, North and South American Indians, familial predisposition
  b Obesity, especially during weight reduction
  c High-calorie diet
  d Hyperlipidemia, types 2b and 4
  e Clofibrate therapy
  f Gastrointestinal disorders involving major malabsorption of bile salts: ileal disease, resection, or bypass; cystic fibrosis with pancreatic insufficiency, primary bile salt malabsorption
  g Gallbladder stasis syndromes, somatostatinoma, post-tuncal vagotomy
  h Female sex hormones: females more than males after puberty, oral contraceptives and other estrogenic medications
  i Advancing age, especially among males
  j Probable, but not well established: pregnancy, hyperparathyroidism, diabetes mellitus, polyunsaturated fat diets, primary biliary cirrhosis

of these factors are associated with a higher than average prevalence rate of gallstones and are supported by strong epidemiological and, in some cases, pathophysiologic evidence. In the pigment stone category, the risks are associated with biliary infection and/or infestation, congenital anomalies, alcoholic cirrhosis, and erythropoietic protoporphyria, in addition to chronic hemolysis from any cause. In the cholesterol stone category, the risks are associated with (1) obesity, certain familial hyperlipidemia syndromes, hypocholesterolemic drugs, and estrogen medication, all of which lead to hypersecretion of biliary cholesterol; (2) constitutional and acquired hepatic defects leading to defective bile salt synthesis, and gastrointestinal syndromes associated with major malabsorption of bile salts, all of which lead to hepatic hyposecretion of bile salts; and (3) a host of syndromes associated with gallbladder stasis or hypotony. As in the pigment stone category, at least 80 percent of cholesterol stone patients have no identifiable risk factor.

Gallstones and cancer

Gallstone prevalence and the occurrence of specific cancers may be related in two ways: (1) the risk factor(s) implicated in the prevalence of certain cancers may also be involved in inducing an excess prevalence of gallstones; and (2) lithogenic bile or gallstones per se may be risk factors for cancers of the organs in which they are sequestered (e.g., the biliary tree) or where they are passively absorbed (e.g., stomach and colon). On the basis of reliable worldwide prevalence rates, evidence for a strong relationship of the first type is displayed in Fig. 6. The age-adjusted mortality rates from uterine cancer correlate strongly with the age-adjusted autopsy prevalence rates of gallstones in females. This correlation is not unexpected since both endogenous and exogenous estrogens are known to be risk factors for both diseases. It has been suggested that the prevalence of breast cancer and gallstones can be interrelated in a similar fashion.

A strong relationship of the second type is shown for females in Fig. 7. The worldwide age-adjusted incidence of gallbladder cancer correlates closely with the age-adjusted autopsy prevalence rate of gallstones. In countries with low

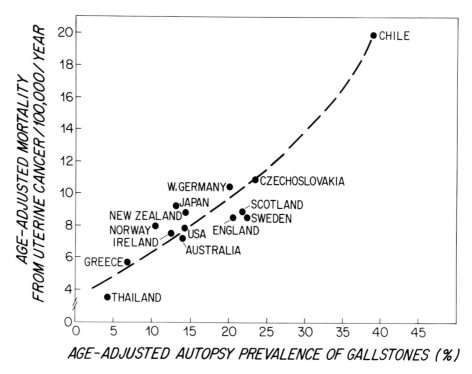

FIGURE 6
*Geographic relation-
ship betwween mortal-
ity rates from uterine
cancer and the autopsy
prevalence of gallstones
in females. (From AB
Lowenfels, Gut 21:1090,
1980.)*

FIGURE 7
*Geographic relationship be-
tween incidence of gallbladder cancer and autopsy prevalence of gallstones in
females. (From AB Lowen-
fels, personal communica-
tion, with additions by the authors.) Note: (1) Autopsy
prevalence rate for North
American Indians includes
several southwestern tribes
and is less than the true prevalence of gallstones in the
Pima (see Fig. 2); (2) the gallstone prevalence rate in Poland is an estimate based on
the known high prevalence
rate in eastern Europe (e.g.,
Czechoslovakia, Fig. 6.)*

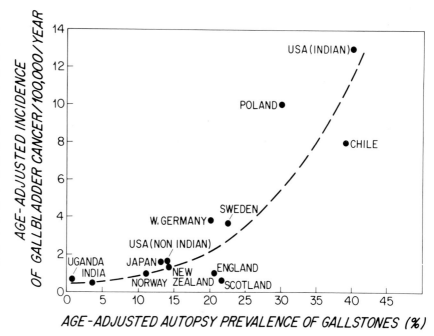

gallstone prevalence rates, gallbladder cancer is relatively rare. The incidence of gallbladder cancer increases slightly in the western industrial societies in concert with an increased prevalence of gallstones. Extraordinarily high incidence rates of gallbladder cancer in association with epidemic prevalence rates of gallstones are found in Poland and Chile and in North American Indians. It can only be conjectured as to whether this epidemiological relationship is one of cause and effect; for example, it is not known whether lithogenic bile and/or gallstones cause gallbladder cancer in humans. Nevertheless, there is persuasive evidence from animal studies that certain experimental carcinogens, which normally do not attack the biliary tree, induce gallbladder cancer when the gallbladder sequesters lithogenic bile or is filled with diet-induced or surgically implanted gallstones.

The evidence is highly controversial as to whether the risks of developing colonic cancer are increased following cholecystectomy. To many physicians, such a risk makes plausible teleological sense, since in the absence of a gallbladder, there is increased bile secretion, increased recycling of the bile salt pool, and increased exposure of bile to colonic bacterial flora. Many low-grade dietary cocarcinogens and promoters are secreted as polar metabolites into bile, and bacterial metabolites of bile salts may also be promoters of colonic carcinogenesis. Similar hypotheses for the role of bile in causation of gastric stump carcinoma have been proposed. These arguments may be specious to some extent. There are elevated levels of secondary bile salts in bile of gallstone patients with functioning gallbladders and markedly elevated levels in bile of gallstone patients who have lost normal gallbladder function following cholecystitis. Both of these observations suggest that increased exposure of bile to the colonic bacterial flora is an inevitable association with gallstone disease.

NATURAL HISTORY OF GALLSTONES

Rational management of patients with gallstones is predicated on an accurate knowledge of the natural history of gallstones. A large literature exists, but in our opinion published work on the clinical outcome of gallstones is, in the main, inaccurate and misleading. Evaluation of the natural history of gallstones requires careful definition of the population at risk, a large cohort of subjects, prolonged periods of surveillance, and unequivocal characterization of what is being measured. Most studies fail to fulfill these stringent requirements.

In the early part of the century, the prevailing views on the management of gallstones were based solely on anecdotal experience rather than on scientifically acquired information. Thus, Kehr in 1901 stated that "quiet-lying gallstones are no subject for treatment, for a persistent latent stage is almost as good as a cure." Osler, in his textbook (1909 edition), was of the same opinion and stated that "most gallstones are symptomless." However, Mayo in 1911 promulgated what now appears to be a biased management policy with the bold statement "[the] innocent gallstone is a myth." Mayo's dictum had wide and enduring influence and most surgeons and physicians adhered to Mayo's approach to gallstones until quite recently. In an attempt to glean a more scientific perspective, a number of studies carried out since World War II have attempted to define the natural history of gallstone disease. Unfortunately, most of these studies had unrecognized flaws and lacked full documentation: (1) various clinical subgroups of patients with cholelithiasis where neither identified nor categorized; many authors failed to differentiate between totally asymptomatic (silent or quiescent) gallstone patients and those who were "mildly" symptomatic. (2) It was not generally recognized that "dyspeptic" symptoms, such as fatty food intolerance, flatulence, bloating, and postprandial discomfort, were nonspecific symptoms that were more likely to have causes other than gallstones; in many studies, "symptomatic" patients were often studied as a group with no distinction between patients with biliary pain ("colic") and those with flatulent dyspepsia. (3) Many studies were retrospective and depended upon mailed questionnaires and clinical chart analyses to determine the clinical outcome of documented gallstones.

For all of these reasons, some of the often quoted high risks of symptoms and complications of gallstones in the literature suffer from a lack of definition of the population subgroups and historical outcomes under study. Based on a collation of the most critical literature, we believe that clinical gallstone disease falls logically into three subgroups:

1 The asymptomatic (silent or quiescent) gallstone patient

2 The "mildly" symptomatic gallstone patient

3 The truly symptomatic gallstone patient and/or the patient with complications of gallstones

The asymptomatic gallstone patient

By definition, the asymptomatic gallstone patient has no history whatsoever of biliary pain (colic) or complications and is commonly discovered to have gallstones incidentally, at a comprehensive medical examination, ultrasonography of the upper abdomen, oral cholecystography carried out in the evaluation of some vague abdominal discomfort, or by a routine plain x-ray of the abdomen. As shown in Table 3, we have collected 440 patients from four studies in the literature who, at time of diagnosis, had asymptomatic gallstones and who were followed for periods of 5 to 30 years. While all of these studies provide important information, not one of the studies was ideal. The studies of Comfort et al. and of Ralston and Smith were retrospective evaluations; the study of Newman et al. is sparse in information on the characteristics of the patients, and that of Gracie and Ransohoff consisted mainly of white American males. Nevertheless, in terms of clinical outcome, there are both consistency and concordance among the four studies. These results support the conclusion that the truly asymptomatic gallstone patient runs a relatively benign course. This is particularly the case in the male-dominated study (Gracie and Ransohoff), where the percentage that remained free of symptoms or complications for 24 years was 87 percent, a figure similar to the percentage (81 percent) of asymptomatic male Pima Indians

with gallstones (Fig. 2). Taken as a whole, both retrospective and prospective studies indicate that about 86 percent of asymptomatic gallstones in both sexes remain quiescent. This conclusion is further supported by the high ratio of autopsy prevalence rates of gallstones compared with the prevalence rates of cholecystectomy in the general population. The prospective studies in our compilation suggest that the risk of developing symptoms from stones diminishes with time after diagnosis and that the rare complication is usually preceded by warning symptoms. From these data we calculate that the cumulative chance of an asymptomatic male gallstone patient developing symptoms within 5 years of diagnosis is less than 10 percent. In the case of females, this figure probably needs a small upward adjustment.

The mildly symptomatic gallstone patient

The precise definition of what constitutes the *mildly* symptomatic gallstone patient is difficult. For the purposes of this discussion, we define this subgroup, crudely, as those patients with at least one episode of "mild" biliary pain (colic) which was not frequent, did not disrupt life-style, and did not require hospitalization. Obviously, patients with a history of nonspecific dyspeptic symptoms or with a history of complications such as acute cholecystitis, choledocholithiasis,

TABLE 3
Natural history of asymptomatic ("silent" or "quiescent") gallstones

	Comfort et al. (1948)*	Ralston and Smith (1965)†	Newman et al. (1968)‡	Gracie and Ransohoff (1982)§
Total number of subjects	112	14	191	123
Male	NR¶	2	NR	110
Female	NR	12	NR	13
Age range	NR	18–89	NR	29–87
Average age at diagnosis	48.2	NR	NR	54
Duration of follow-up years	10–20	15–30	5	11–24
Developed symptoms "Biliary pain" or "colic"	21 (18.7%)	1 (7%)	20 (10.4%)	16 (13%)
Developed complications Generally cholecystitis or pancreatitis	5 (4.4%)	NR	NR	3 (2.4%)
Required cholecystectomy	24 (21.6%)	2 (14%)	10 (5.2%)	14 (11.3%)
Remained asymptomatic	91 (81.3%)	11 (78.5%)	171 (89.6%)	107 (86.9%)

* *MW Comfort et al, Ann Surg 128:931, 1948.*
† *DE Ralston and LA Smith, Minn Med 48:327, 1965.*
‡ *HF Newman et al, Am J Gastroenterol 50:476, 1968.*
§ *WA Gracie and DF Ransohoff, N Engl J Med 307:798, 1982.*
¶ *NR = not recorded.*

TABLE 4
Natural history of "mildly" symptomatic gallstones

	Lund (1960)*	Ralston and Smith (1965)†	Wenckert and Robertson (1966)‡	Thistle et al. (1982)§
Total number with biliary pain or "colic"	87	60	781	305
Male	22 (25.2%)	6 (10%)	NR¶	129 (42.3%)
Female	65 (74.7%)	54 (90%)	NR	176 (57.7%)
Age range	10–90	18–89	NR	21–79
Mean age	NR	NR	NR	54.7
Duration of follow-up years	5–20	15–30	1–11	2
Developed severe frequent pain	26 (30%)	~ 25–35 (41–58%)	254 (33%)	136 (44.6%)
Developed complications (Acute cholecystitis, jaundice, pancreatitis)	43 (49%)	NR	144 (18%)	65 (18.5%)
Required cholecystectomy	18 (20%)	38 (63.6%)	173 (22.1%)	12 (3.9%)

* *J Lund, Ann Surg 151:153, 1960.*
† *DE Ralston and LA Smith, Minn Med 48:327, 1965.*
‡ *A Wenckert and B Robertson, Gastroenterology 50:376, 1966.*
§ *JL Thistle et al, Gastroenterology 82:1197, 1982* (Abst.)
¶ *N.R. = not recorded.*

and jaundice or pancreatitis are excluded. We have collected information from four studies in the literature in which duration of follow-up varied from 2 to 30 years (Table 4). An examination of these data clearly indicates that the mildly symptomatic patient runs a less benign course than the asymptomatic patient. Biliary pain recurs and becomes more frequent, the risk of developing complications increases with time, and the longer these patients are followed, the more frequent cumulative cholecystectomy rates become (Table 4). We have estimated from these results that the cumulative chance of developing severe symptoms and/or complications from mildly symptomatic gallstones is 20 percent at 5 years for males and about 30 percent at 5 years for females.

The symptomatic gallstone patient

All retrospective or prospective studies of symptomatic patients, regardless of biliary complications, clearly indicate that the disease runs an ominous course. Table 5 summarizes the results of a classic study on a large cohort of patients (392) who, for diverse reasons, did not initially undergo surgery; all were symptomatic and necessitated hospitalization at the time of diagnosis. Recurrence of biliary pain is the rule, complications are frequent and increase cumulatively with time, and most importantly, a nonfunctioning gallbladder approximately doubles the risk of complications. We have estimated from these

and other data that the cumulative chance of developing severe recurrent symptoms or complications within 5 years is 30 percent for males and about 40 to 50 percent for females, the latter values being similar to clinical prevalence rates of gallstones in female Pima Indians (Fig. 2).

TREATMENT OF GALLSTONES

Three potential choices are now available for managing patients with gallstones: (1) expectant management ("observe"); (2) medical management with gallstone-dissolving bile acids ("obliterate"); and (3) surgical management by cholecystectomy with bile duct exploration when necessary ("operate"). Our discussion of the role of each therapeutic modality in the modern management of gallstones will rely predominantly on the natural history of the three patient subgroups with gallstones summarized above. We will also emphasize the crucial role of modern radiologic practice in aiding preoperative and intraoperative surgical management, and we will indicate the restricted but nonetheless important role of medical dissolution therapy with chenodeoxycholic or ursodeoxycholic acids based on their efficacy and safety as inferred from controlled clinical trials.

Expectant management

Based on the data summarized in Table 3, it is our conclusion that the vast majority of otherwise healthy patients with asymptomatic (silent, quiescent) gallstones should be treated expectantly. Since the small percentage of these patients who develop symptoms do so during the first 5 years following diagnosis, the patients should be advised that they have an approximately 1:10 risk of developing manifest clinical disease. If symptoms occur, the decision should be reevaluated at that time. The decision to proceed to surgery would then seem appropriate, since the rare complication in these patients is usually heralded by biliary pain.

In order to rationalize management of asymptomatic gallstones and place clinical decisions on a more quantitative basis, Ransohoff and colleagues performed a decision analysis in which they compared prophylactic cholecystectomy at the time of diagnosis with expectant management, in which a cholecystectomy was performed only after the development of biliary pain or a complication. Probability values were derived from their natural history study of a predominantly male patient population with asymptomatic gallstones (Table 3), published cholecystectomy mortality rates, and U.S. life tables. Their results suggest that overall survival is decreased slightly by prophylactic cholecystectomy: for a 30-year-old man who chooses prophylactic cholecystectomy instead of expectant management, approximately 4 days of life are lost; for a 50-year-old man who makes the same choice, 18 days of life are lost. As will be discussed later, consideration of monetary costs argues further against prophylactic cholecystectomy. Nevertheless, sensitivity analysis that

took into account a broad range of probability values demonstrated that the differences in survival for the two strategies, in both men and women, remained small. In view of the similarities in the outcome of all four studies on the natural history of asymptomatic gallstones (Table 3), we believe that this decision analysis supports the recommendation that prophylactic cholecystectomy should not be employed for patients of either sex with asymptomatic gallstones.

We believe that expectant management should also be the therapy of choice in patients with asymptomatic pigment gallstones, particularly those associated with chronic hemolytic anemia syndromes (hereditary spherocytosis, thalassemia, and sickle cell disease). The known high prevalence rates of cholelithiasis in such patients and the unexpectedly high prevalence rates even below the age of puberty (Fig. 4), coupled with the low incidence of clear-cut symptoms at all ages, raise strong doubts regarding the justification of prophylactic surgical intervention. The higher rates of complications from surgery and anesthesia in patients with either congenital or acquired chronic hemolytic syndromes indicate that the conservative approach should be strongly considered.

Another subset of patients who should be treated by expectant management are patients with asymptomatic gallstones and cirrhosis of the liver. In both alcoholic and (primary) biliary cirrhosis, the incidence of gallstones is twice that of the general population and increases with age. Pigment stones account for the increased inci-

TABLE 5
Natural history of severely symptomatic gallstones

	Severe symptoms, no complications	*Severe symptoms plus complications*
Total number	183	209
Males	43 (23.4%)	55 (26.3%)
Females	140 (76.5%)	154 (73.6%)
Age range	10–90	10–90
Duration of follow-up years	5–20	5–20
Continued to have severe symptoms	53 (29%)	46 (22%)
Subsequent complications (Acute cholecystitis, jaundice, pancreatitis)	46 (25%)	82 (39%)
Total with severe symptoms and complications	99 (54%)	128 (61%)

SOURCE: *J Lund, Ann Surg 151:153, 1960.*

dence of stones in alcoholic cirrhosis, but cholesterol stones are predominant in primary biliary cirrhosis. The documented morbidity plus mortality risks for both elective cholecystectomy and emergency cholecystectomy in such patients are formidable. In one study these rates were 9.3 and 26 percent, respectively, for cirrhotics whose prothrombin times were prolonged < 2.5 s and 83 and 100 percent, respectively, in cirrhotics whose prothrombin times were prolonged > 2.5 s. As in the general population, most cirrhotics do not have either symptoms or complications from their stones and jaundice per se is, as might be expected, no criterion for the presence of choledocholithiasis. Fruitless exploration of the common bile duct adds to the hazards of surgery in such patients. If severe symptoms or a biliary complication develops in cirrhotics with gallstones, biliary tract surgery should be deferred as long as possible and only employed as the very last resort. Many of these patients can be managed conservatively or by nonsurgical approaches such as a trial of medical dissolution and endoscopic papillotomy for choledocholithiasis during coverage with plasma transfusions. When gallbladder surgery is required on an emergency basis, cholecystostomy and drainage may be the procedures of choice.

What, then, are the specific clinical or epidemiological considerations where expectant management would not be advisable for patients with asymptomatic gallstones? This question is not easily answered, but clearly certain subsets can be singled out for individualized treatment. One subset would be otherwise healthy individuals with asymptomatic gallstones who are forced by occupational necessity to spend long periods of time in environments where medical facilities would be substandard or simply not available. Missionaries, explorers, astronauts, field meteorologists, and long-distance sailors could all be included in this category. When faced with a rational evaluation of the small but definite risk of developing symptoms or complications and the relatively minimal risks of surgery when performed under ideal circumstances, many of these patients and their physicians would probably decide on prophylactic cholecystectomy for asymptomatic gallstones.

The question of whether the patient with asymptomatic cholelithiasis is at risk for gallbladder cancer is still uncertain. In the general population, the risk of gallbladder cancer is small (0.5 percent of autopsies); in gallstone patients in the west, this risk is somewhat higher (about 1 percent), as inferred from pathological examination of gallbladders removed for stones. Hence, in populations with low prevalence rates of gallbladder cancer (Fig. 7), prophylactic cholecystectomy is not justified on this basis, despite large variations (1 to 22 percent) in the age-adjusted autopsy prevalence of gallstones, since average surgical mortality rates far outweigh the risks of developing gallbladder cancer. A more aggressive surgical approach should perhaps be adopted in such countries and racial groups (Poland, Chile, and North American Indians) where autopsy prevalence rates of gallstones reach epidemic proportions. This is particularly the case among females in these populations in whom prevalence rates of gallbladder cancer are four- to sevenfold greater than in average western populations (Fig. 7). An analysis of the regression curve in Fig. 7 suggests that in these high-risk populations, for every 100,000 new patients with gallstones per year, about 2000 to 4000 will eventually develop gallbladder cancer.

Unless contraindicated for other reasons, prophylactic cholecystectomy would appear to be the only logical choice for three other subgroups: (1) diabetic patients with asymptomatic gallstones; (2) patients with calcinosis of the gallbladder (porcelain gallbladder); and (3) *Salmonella typhosa* carriers.

Whether or not there is an association between diabetes and the prevalence of gallstones is not clear. This relationship was not found to be statistically significant in the Pima Indian study (Fig. 3). Autopsy prevalence rates, which suggest such an association, are of questionable relevance since many diabetics die in hospital. It is also uncertain whether diabetics have a higher incidence of symptoms and complications from gallstones compared with nondiabetic subjects. Gallbladder hypotony is more frequent in diabetic patients, and diabetics with autonomic neuropathy frequently have a "neurogenic gallbladder syndrome" characterized by an enlarged gallbladder (often three to nine times normal), poor contraction, and/or poor visualization of the gallbladder, often in the absence of symptoms due to gallstones or gallbladder disease. Possibly for the latter reasons, many diabetics with gall-stones remain asymptomatic until an abdominal catastrophe occurs. When a complication, particularly acute cholecystitis, supervenes, it follows a more fulminant course in diabetics than in the average patient with rapid progression of infection and necrosis. Therefore, diabetics with acute cholecystitis have a much graver prognosis; the associated mortality rates vary from 11 to 22 percent. In one series of diabetics with acute cholecystitis, the incidence of gallbladder necrosis was greater than 70 percent and either gallbladder perforation or gangrene occurred within 24 h of the onset of symptoms.

It is not entirely clear why bacterial overgrowth and invasion progress so rapidly in diabetic bile. Most diabetics with gallstones do not have evidence of vascular insufficiency or neuropathy of the gallbladder, and in contrast to urine, there is no glucose in human bile. Because of the high incidence of acute cholecystitis without pain, gangrenous perforation, and fistula formation, cholecystectomy should be recommended as soon as is convenient for diabetic patients with asymptomatic gallstones. For these reasons, it is advisable that all diabetics should undergo routine ultrasonographic surveillance of the gallbladder annually. In contrast to the portentous risks of cholecystitis in diabetics, these patients, if well prepared, in good control, and free of infection, tolerate elective surgery for gallstones as well as do the general population.

Patients with porcelain gallbladders and those who are chronic gallbladder carriers of *S. typhosa* are both at high risk for developing gallbladder cancer. Once the condition has been diagnosed, prophylactic cholecystectomy should also be performed. The former condition represents a deposition of calcium phosphate in the wall of the gallbladder and is associated with a 30 to 60 percent risk for developing carcinoma of the gallbladder; the chronic typhoid carrier has a sixfold increased risk of developing (hepato) biliary cancer. In contrast, patients with the rare "milk of calcium" bile syndrome (i.e., gallsand composed of calcium carbonate and oxalate) appear to have the same risks of developing symptoms and complications as do the general gallstone population and are not at a greater risk of developing gallbladder cancer.

We would like to emphasize that patients with cholesterolosis or adenomyomatosis (hyperplastic cholecystoses) are not at greater risk than the general population for developing cholelithiasis, cholecystitis, or gallbladder cancer. These disorders are detected with considerable frequency on ultrasonography and oral cholecystograms and are found in 25 to 40 percent of gallbladders removed at surgery or at autopsy. Cholesterolosis is the end result of the accumulation of triglycerides and sterol esters in macrophages of the lamina propria, imparting a "strawberry" appearance to the gallbladder mucosa. Adenomyomatosis involves hyperplasia of the tissues of the gallbladder wall with outpouches of the mucosa (Rokitansky-Aschoff sinuses). While cholesterolosis can potentially give rise to biliary pain from detachment of a cholesteryl ester polyp, adenomyomatosis is symptomless. Neither condition requires treatment unless asymptomatic gallstones are present; then expectant management should be planned.

Surgical management

General considerations   In 1867 and 1878, respectively, Bobbs in the United States and Tait in England independently performed the first successful operations on the gallbladder. This operation was a cholecystostomy with decompression, removal of gallstones, and drainage. In 1882 Langenbuch introduced cholecystectomy for treating gallstone-associated cholecystitis. Three years later, cholecystectomy had a mortality rate of 50 percent but in the same year, Tait reported 15 cases of cholecystostomy without death. Why was cholecystectomy so strongly upheld and widely adopted over the ensuing years? Simply answered, cholecystectomy cures the disease and generally prevents stone recurrence in the biliary tree. With cholecystostomy, an abscess of the gallbladder can be drained and the tension of cholecystitis relieved, but it will not always enable the removal of an impacted stone. Recurrent abscesses and mucus fistulae are common and, even in the successful case, gallstones may recur within a few years. In this century, advances in anesthesia, radiology, antibiotic therapy, and fluid and electrolyte regulation have made cholecystectomy an extremely safe operation. At the present time, there is still no question that cholecystectomy is the treatment of choice for the vast majority of gallstone patients with symptoms and/or complications.

One million new cases of gallstones are diagnosed in the United States each year, and a cholecystectomy is performed on approximately 500,000 of these new cases. It has been estimated that 4 to 7 percent of these operations are performed on persons with neither symptoms nor stones, approximately 25 percent of operations are performed on patients with stones and no symptoms, and excess surgery is performed on patients with nonspecific dyspeptic symptoms that are not necessarily due to their gallstones. Recent prevalence rates for common surgical procedures suggest that cholecystectomy is the fifth most frequently performed operation in western industrialized societies. This operation is performed three times more frequently in the United States than elsewhere, despite gallstone prevalence rates that are intermediate with respect to geographic variation (Fig. 1).

Morbidity and mortality The mean nationwide (United States) mortality rate of cholecystectomy for cholelithiasis is 1.7 percent. The factors responsible for this astonishingly high mortality rate are related to the heterogeneous nature of the population at risk and the diverse quality of the surgical settings. For example, this statistic includes patients with and without symptoms; patients with complications, such as acute cholecystitis, acute pancreatitis; choledocholithiasis with obstructive jaundice with and without cholangitis; and patients with preexisting medical and surgical problems. It includes ideal and nonideal surgical, anesthetic, and postoperative conditions; operations carried out electively and on an emergency basis. In patients under 65 years of age, the baseline mean mortality rate for general anesthesia is 0.2 percent. The excess mortality rates of cholecystectomy are associated with shock from hemorrhage, cardiac failure, electrolyte imbalance, infection, thromboembolic disease, acute respiratory failure, the result of intraoperative drugs, specific biliary tract complication such as surgical misadventure, retained common duct stones and their treatment, bile peritonitis, biliary fistula, and liver failure.

Ransohoff and colleagues compiled age- and sex-related mortality rates for cholecystectomy from United States, Canadian, and French medical sources and divided the results on the basis of surgery for gallstones in patients with and without preoperative biliary complications. These results are displayed in Fig. 8 and show that the age-specific mortality rates are initially very low but increase 8 to 10 percent per year from ages 30 to 75 and are much greater (by extrapolation) thereafter. In all age groups, mortality rates for males are twice those for women, and mortality rates for cholecystectomy performed for a biliary complication of stones quadruple those for an elective operation (i.e., before a biliary complication has occurred). Because of excessive mortality rates in persons 75 years and older, these data would tend to favor prophylactic cholecystectomy for asymptomatic gallstones at a younger age. However, average life expectancy, even in individuals with gallstones, is approximately 72 years for males and 76 years for females. Other reasons why this strategy is not advocated have been presented earlier in this chapter.

What these data do support is a recommendation that, if the patient is truly symptomatic or has a complication and is under the age of 65, cholecystectomy is clearly the therapeutic procedure of choice. The operation is obviously extremely safe, especially in patients with symptomatic gallstones and no biliary complications, being associated with a mean mortality rate of 0.3 to 0.5 percent. If acute cholecystitis or another complication has supervened, the operative mortality is about 1 to 2 percent higher. When intervention is necessary and the age of the patient is greater than 65, we believe that treatment should be individualized. If the patient with gallstones has a preoperative biliary complication, but is otherwise healthy, surgery is also the most reasonable choice. If a patient older than 65 years is symptomatic but has no biliary complication, then the risks of surgery should be weighed against other options: one could either temporize and treat symptoms conservatively in the belief that life expectancy is limited or, if the patient is a suitable candidate, proceed to a trial of medical dissolution therapy with a gallstone-dissolving bile acid.

When age is not a factor and the patient is otherwise healthy, surgery within 72 h of the

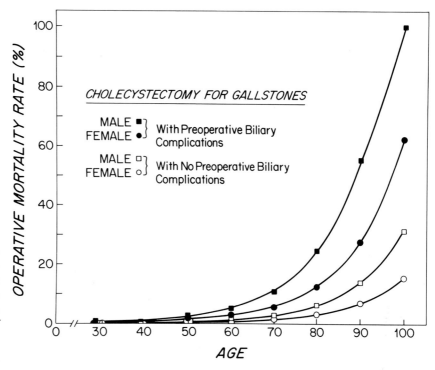

FIGURE 8

Age- and sex-related operative mortality rates for cholecystectomy in patients with and without preoperative biliary complications of gallstones. (After WF Ransohoff et al, Ann Intern Med 99:199, 1983.)

onset of a biliary complication should be recommended. It is relatively easy to remove the gallbladder within the first 3 days of the onset of the most common complication, acute cholecystitis. In fact, edema which occurs around the inflamed gallbladder does not impair, but rather assists, surgical dissection and removal. Once the patient has been stabilized and hydrated, and complicating medical conditions have been ruled out, the operation should be scheduled routinely. Surgery may be an ominous undertaking if the patient's general medical condition is not amenable to acute therapy. Expectant management with hydration, analgesia, nasogastric suction, and antibiotics and close surveillance is then desirable. In 80 percent of such patients the acute cholecystitis subsides, and in many does not recur. If it becomes obvious during the first 24 h that the patient's condition is deteriorating, then cholecystostomy and drainage under local anesthesia may be lifesaving. This should only be entertained when the patient is unfit for a prolonged and difficult dissection but requires immediate relief from a tense, inflamed gallbladder. Prior to surgery, an intravenous infusion of an inhibitor of prostaglandin synthesis such as in-

domethacin has been suggested as a possible measure to reduce gallbladder tension and pain and to prevent rupture. In such cases cholecystectomy must eventually be performed when the patient's medical condition is suitable. Cholecystectomy, carried out between the third day and third week following onset of acute cholecystitis, is a most difficult and dangerous procedure and should not generally be entertained.

Finally, with regard to the overall safety of the surgical management of gallstones, the results of over 7000 cholecystectomies for cholelithiasis with and without preoperative complications performed over a 30-year period by a single experienced surgical team in a major New York teaching center are illustrative. In patients under the age of 50 years, the operative mortality rate was 0.08 percent; older than 50 years, 0.8 percent. Perioperative morbidity for the cohort as a whole was only 7 percent.

Choledocholithiasis: Common duct stones and retained stones The common bile duct is explored in nearly 25 percent of the 500,000 cholecystectomies performed annually in the United States. In approximately 60 percent of these explorations, common duct stones are discovered and removed. The incidence of choledocholithotomy is therefore at least 75,000 cases per year. Despite recent surgical advances, retained stones occur in 2 to 6 percent of patients after common bile duct exploration. Since duct exploration and retained stones increase morbidity and mortality, a major surgical challenge is to decrease the frequency of retained common duct stones and, at the same time, to avoid unnecessary choledochotomy.

STONE TYPES AND PREVALENCE Common duct stones may be primary, that is, stones which form de novo in any part of the biliary tree; or secondary, when stones result from the passage of gallbladder stones through the cystic duct. The latter are by far the most frequent and are, therefore, usually cholesterol stones. Migration of multiple gallbladder stones from the gallbladder through the cystic and common bile ducts into the duodenum is more common than is generally appreciated. In patients with multiple asymptomatic stones who have been followed by oral cholecystography for nearly 20 years, about 7 percent have evacuated their gallbladders completely only to reform gallbladder stones at a later time. Further, it has been reported that 10 to 20 percent of patients with common duct stones have no stones in their gallbladder at the time of surgery. When low-grade stasis and infection are caused by choledocholithiasis, the stones grow within the duct by the deposition of a soft brown "earthy" shell of calcium bilirubinate. By this means a small stone from the gallbladder may serve as a nidus to which adhere sludge, pigment, and in some cases cholesterol, giving the outward appearance of a primary rather than a secondary stone.

Controversy over the relative frequency of primary as opposed to secondary stones continues, but little research on their pathogenesis and incidence has been carried out. As in the gallbladder, it is likely that primary stones are a manifestation of the interaction between cholesterol- or pigment-saturated bile, nucleating and antinucleating agents, other solubilizing factors, and stasis. For example, in cholecystectomized animals, stones form above experimental strictures of the common bile duct, and bile duct strictures in human beings frequently result in biliary sludge and stones proximal to the obstruction. In the oriental hepatolithiasis syndrome, intrahepatic stones are often present without involvement of the gallbladder. In a large series (47) of symptomatic patients with congenital absence of the gallbladder, 20 patients (43 percent) had common duct stones.

The following criteria for the diagnosis of primary duct stones have been suggested. At reexploration for choledocholithiasis, the patient should have had (1) a previous cholecystectomy, (2) a 2-year asymptomatic period following cholecystectomy, (3) ductal stones of a soft-brown earthy appearance, and (4) no evidence of a stricture or a long cystic duct remnant. Of 758 patients undergoing choledochotomy at Johns Hopkins Hospital, 30 (4 percent) satisfied these criteria for primary common duct stones. Since removal of the gallbladder reduces the cholesterol lithogenic potential of ductal bile, most of these stones are predominantly calcium bilirubinate with much less cholesterol than gallbladder or secondary ductal stones. Curiously, the majority of patients with primary ductal stones, in accordance with the above criteria, do not have any indication of partial biliary obstruction other than from the stone itself. It has recently been suggested that a motor disorder of Oddi's sphincter may have induced functional stasis in these patients. Only one study has focused on the chronological incidence of ductal stones following cholecystectomy. This was a retrospective analysis of 91 patients presenting with common duct stones over a 10-year period. If the majority of ductal stones had been simply overlooked at prior surgery, then the incidence of symptomatic stones versus time after cholecystectomy should have been defined by a single exponential curve. What was found was that there was an exponential decline during the first 2 postoperative years, as expected, but this was interrupted by a rise in incidence which peaked at the third to fourth postoperative year. In the entire cohort of patients, 26 percent presented with ductal stones 10 or more years following cholecystectomy. While not conclusive, this study suggests that an appreciable number of primary stones form in the ducts following removal of the gallbladder.

There is persuasive evidence that the inci-

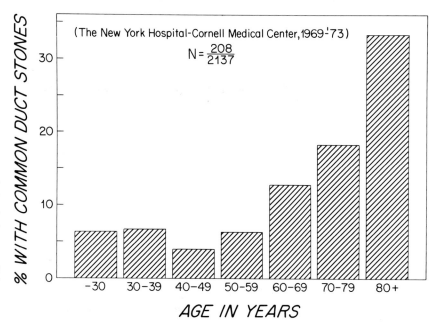

FIGURE 9
Age-related incidence of common duct stones at primary surgery for gallstones from The New York Hospital–Cornell Medical Center Series, 1969–1973. [After F Glenn, CK McSherry, in Current Problems in Surgery, MM Ravitch et al (eds), June 1975, pp 3–38.]

dence of secondary ductal stones increases according to the age of the patient (Fig. 9). In this series of 2137 choledochotomies at a primary exploration for calculous biliary tract disease from 1969 to 1973, Glenn and colleagues at the New York Hospital–Cornell Medical Center found that 208 (10 percent) of these patients had common duct stones. Up to the age of 60, the incidence was about 6.5 percent, but in the elderly patients incidence increased markedly. This suggests that the longer the presence of stones in the gallbladder, the greater the risk of choledocholithiasis.

NATURAL HISTORY The natural history of choledocholithiasis is unpredictable. As a rule, small gallstones can pass spontaneously into the duodenum without causing symptoms. However, a large number of small stones can accumulate simultaneously and cause obstruction, particularly if the ampulla is narrow. Both small and large stones may temporarily obstruct the pancreatic duct and induce acute pancreatitis; spontaneous expulsion is the rule with relief of symptoms. In several studies, more than 80 percent of patients with gallstone pancreatitis had stones ranging in size from 1 to 12 mm in their feces; approximately 10 to 15 percent of the control population (with gallbladder stones) were also shown to have fecal gallstones, attesting to the frequency

of silent stone migration. Stones that do not pass spontaneously can reside in the common duct for long periods. Eventually, about 50 percent, without warning symptoms or signs, precipitate an episode of jaundice or cholangitis. The presenting clinical features of choledocholithiasis are, in order of decreasing prevalence, (1) an unanticipated finding at routine cholecystectomy; (2) a history of a single episode of hyperbilirubinemia, acute pancreatitis, or biliary pain; (3) intermittent jaundice without fever or chills; (4) intermittent jaundice with fever and chills (Charcot's triad); (5) asymptomatic protracted jaundice without superinfection; (6) jaundice with refractory sepsis, hypotension, and mental confusion due to acute suppurative cholangitis; and (7) neglected protracted jaundice with biliary cirrhosis, hepatic failure, and portal hypertension.

MANAGEMENT OF CHOLEDOCHOLITHIASIS Evidence of fever, chills, jaundice, and profound leukocytosis suggests choledocholithiasis and cholangitis until proved otherwise. About 80 percent of patients exhibiting these symptoms will respond to antibiotics and supportive therapy, thus allowing time for a complete diagnostic evaluation. Refractory sepsis with developing signs of suppurative cholangitis demands immediate operation before definitive diagnostic evaluation is completed. Prompt operation with biliary decompression, stone evacuation, and drainage of purulent bile will rescue 50 to 70 percent of these patients. Many endoscopists would argue that, if a patient has a stone impacted at the ampulla of Vater and has cholangitis, an endoscopic papillotomy should be done immediately. Without formal or endoscopic operation, the mortality from shock, septicemia, and abscess formation approaches 100 percent. In the absence of sepsis, the preoperative evaluation of the patient with possible choledocholithiasis can proceed at a more measured pace. The extent of preoperative evaluation depends principally on whether or not the patient is jaundiced. In the nonjaundiced patient, even if there is a past history of transient jaundice or acute pancreatitis, the routine use of endoscopic retrograde cholangiopancreatography (ERCP) or transhepatic cholangiography (THC) is unwarranted. In most patients, the accuracy of intraoperative assessment with routine intraoperative cholangiography and careful inspection and palpation of the duct system is greater than 95 percent.

In the jaundiced patient the problem is different and more difficult since it is necessary to ascertain (1) that the extrahepatic duct system is indeed obstructed, (2) that the obstruction is due to a stone and not to some other etiology, and (3) the site of obstruction and the anatomy of the duct system. The older technique of intravenous infusion cholangiography (IVC) with tomography is now considered obsolete for this purpose. Bilirubin levels greater than 3 mg/dl and allergy to the contrast agents preclude its use. The procedure fails in 50 percent of patients even when bilirubin levels are less than 3 mg/dl, and in the successful cases the diagnostic accuracy rate is less than 40 percent. Ultrasonography may be employed as a primary screening examination in the diagnosis of common duct stones, although its sensitivity is extremely low ($\sim$ 25 percent). It is helpful if it detects dilatation of the biliary tree, suggesting obstruction, whether or not the actual stones are visualized. The accuracy of ultrasonography of the duct system is further questionable since biliary duct size does not appear to be a useful predictor of biliary duct disease, and an adequate examination is often difficult due to overlying bowel gas.

The primary modalities in the preoperative evaluation of the jaundiced patient are ERCP and THC. The diagnostic effectiveness of each depends on many factors, and the choice of which procedure to use will be influenced by technical competence, anatomic constraints, necessity for therapeutic intervention, the status of liver function, and the need to visualize the pancreas. Because THC is simpler, less expensive, and frequently more available, this technique probably commands priority when ultrasonography demonstrates dilated biliary ducts. THC using the Okuda-Chiba needle visualizes $\sim$ 100 percent of dilated ducts but only 60 percent of undilated ducts. However, contraindications are many, prior evaluation is extensive, and complications such as bleeding and bile peritonitis are often unpredictable and occult. ERCP appears to be of greater value in the patient with undilated ducts or who has findings suggestive of other pathology in the stomach, duodenum, or pancreas requiring endoscopic evaluation. Contraindications are few, prior evaluation is minimal, complications are rare and obvious, and the pancreas is usually well demonstrated. However, anatomic constraints are prominent, the technique is complex and costly, but therapeutic potential is great in that endoscopic papillotomy can be performed. Obviously, the selection of the preferred technique to evaluate the jaundiced patient will depend on local availability of skilled operators experienced in the use of the techniques and their interpretation, and the specific nature of each patient's presentation.

Skilled intraoperative management of choledocholithiasis is aimed at the detection and extraction of all ductal stones, the avoidance of ductal injury, and the avoidance of unnecessary choledochotomy. While in the past liberal use of choledochotomy was practiced to minimize the incidence of retained stones, this procedure, whether positive or negative, is not benign. One study reported a 2.4 percent mortality rate for negative choledochotomy, and a 3.9 percent mortality rate for choledocholithotomy. These data indicate that the avoidance of unnecessary duct exploration is the single most important factor influencing overall mortality from biliary surgery. The most important radiologic advance in the management of choledocholithiasis is routine intraoperative cholangiography. This procedure clearly decreases the incidence of negative common duct exploration without increasing the incidence of retained stones. High-quality x-rays, meticulous technique, and an experienced surgeon and radiologist are critical to reliable cholangiography. False-negative and false-positive results are all too common from incomplete or overfilling of the ducts and the introduction of air bubbles, respectively. Further, for optimal performance, the operating suite should be equipped for intraoperative fluoroscopy, image intensification, and video monitoring. Under these conditions, constant visualization can take place during infusion of contrast material, and multiple spot x-rays can be taken. The most recent innovation is for the surgeon to scan the entire duct system intraoperatively with a sterile hand-held real-time ultrasonographic probe. Whether this procedure is superior to, or only an adjunct to, intraoperative cholangiography and whether it will reduce the incidence of retained stones remain to be evaluated.

The most accurate cholangiographic indicators for duct exploration are intraductal filling defects; the diagnostic accuracy is about 98 percent, but figures vary widely. The presence of a dilated bile duct (> 10 mm) and diminished or no flow of contrast into the duodenum are only 75 and 80 percent accurate, respectively. The time-honored "relative indications" for duct exploration (prior history of jaundice or pancreatitis, faceted stones in the gallbladder, common bile duct > 15 mm) should now be considered "absolute indications" for greater care in the performance and scrutiny of intraoperative cholangiograms. However, there are absolute indications for common duct exploration, and all of these indications are associated with high diagnostic accuracy (given in brackets): (1) palpable ductal stones [97 percent], (2) jaundice with cholangitis [97 percent], and (3) jaundice with conjugated hyperbilirubinemia > 7 mg/dl together with ERCP or THC evidence of an impacted stone [> 95 percent]. However, despite these absolute indications, most surgeons consider that an intraoperative cholangiogram should also be performed. This will verify that the stones are still present and will facilitate the determination of their size, location, and number. In addition,

the procedure visualizes the ampullary region in the untraumatized state and gives a clear picture of the biliary anatomy. Intraoperative manometry of the duct system and choledochoscopy and a "completion" cholangiogram are being proposed as methods to improve diagnostic accuracy and diminish the incidence of retained stones. The first of these is still being evaluated, the second has been proved beneficial but adds appreciably to the manipulation of the duct system with the risks of trauma, and the "completion" cholangiogram clearly has been shown to be highly beneficial in reducing the incidence of retained stones.

RETAINED STONES   Despite the greatest operative and radiologic precautions, a rare patient will harbor a ductal stone undetected by preexploratory and completion cholangiography, manometry, and choledochoscopy. The prevalence of retained stones correlates negatively with the expertise and facilities available to the surgeon and radiologist and positively with the number of stones lodged in the biliary duct system. Occasionally, an impacted stone cannot be extracted at operation. Approximately 5000 patients will have retained postoperative common duct stones yearly in the United States. This is approximately 1 retained stone per 100 cholecystectomies and between 2 to 4 percent and 4 to 15 percent of common duct explorations carried out in specialized or nonspecialized medical centers, respectively. This problem occurs even more frequently in countries where routine operative cholangiography is poorly done or not practiced at all.

The management of retained common duct stones is now less serious a problem than it was, since percutaneous extraction and retrograde papillotomy have practically eliminated the need for reoperation. Repeated common duct explorations are associated with a higher morbidity and mortality than the original operation; furthermore, the danger of injury to the biliary ductal system with later stricture formation increases with each operative procedure. About 7 days following surgery, a T-tube cholangiogram is obtained to verify the absence of stones and free flow of contrast media into the duodenum. If the cholangiogram reveals a retained stone, the T tube is left in place for 6 to 12 weeks to allow formation of a mature sinus tract. If the stones have not passed spontaneously during this period, the plan of management should be to proceed to direct percutaneous extraction of the stone within a well-equipped radiologic suite. A cholangiogram is first performed to locate the stone(s), the T tube then is removed, and under fluoroscopic control a steerable catheter is passed beyond the stone and opened distally; by this means the stone is caged and removed with the catheter through the T-tube tract. In skilled hands this procedure is successful in more than 90 percent of cases, and morbidity and mortality are negligible. In the failures, the physician should then proceed to ERCP, with endoscopic papillotomy and transphincteric stone removal. The ideal outcome is for the operator to snare the stone with a Dormia basket passed through the endoscope. If this fails, a generous papillotomy will frequently allow a stone located higher in the ducts to pass spontaneously into the duodenum during the ensuing days to weeks. The mortality from this procedure varies from 0.5 to 1.5 percent. In the unlikely event that all of these measures fail, and if the patient is not obstructed or infected, the patient should be placed in oral medical dissolution therapy with ursodeoxycholic acid (see ''Medical Management'' section below), provided the original stones from the gallbladder contain > 40 percent cholesterol. If the patient is obstructed and infected, early reoperation is required.

We believe that transductal perfusion of cholesterol solvents such as the unconjugated bile salt, sodium cholate, or the monooctanoin enriched oil, Capmul, has little place in the clinical management of retained common duct stones. No controlled trials have been published, and review of the literature suggests that infusions of saline alone are as effective as either cholate or Capmul (~ 60 percent). Both agents have a number of toxic effects on the liver, the biliary duct system, the pancreas, and the small and large intestines. For example, there is an unacceptably high incidence of cholangitis, pancreatitis, hemobilia, duodenal erosions, and often intolerable diarrhea. A number of patients have died from upper gastrointestinal hemorrhage, cholangitis, and dehydration, and long-term chemical injury

to the ducts with stricture formation is a real possibility.

Finally, a note about surgical misadventure. Cholecystectomy and common bile duct exploration are major surgical procedures; the anatomy is often anomalous and the operation is frequently performed in settings that are far from ideal. The duct is directly injured by inadvertent ligation, transsection, and other trauma in 1:4000 cholecystectomies with or without common bile duct explorations. Even with the most expert remedial efforts, about 30 percent of these patients will die from the injury, usually from chronic obstruction and secondary biliary cirrhosis, with its sequelae of portal hypertension and hepatic failure.

Prophylactic cholecystectomy in the absence of stones Most surgeons and physicians who take care of patients on long-term TPN for small intestinal failure (massive resection, Crohn's disease, collagenous sprue, and other causes) are becoming increasingly aware of the dangers to the gallbladder and biliary tree from sludge (gallsand) and gallstones. As discussed earlier, nearly 100 percent of patients on long-term TPN acquire gallbladder sludge and mainly calcium bilirubinate gallstones. Animal models have been developed but, while the pathogenesis is attributed to gallbladder hypotony and stasis, other as yet poorly defined factors are undoubtedly involved. For example, many patients on TPN develop subclinical or even clinical cholestasis and secondary bile acids; in particular, lithocholic acid increases markedly in bile. Further, amino acid infusions lead to sustained somatostatin release into the portal and systemic circulations. What is peculiar and as yet unexplained is that biliary pain, acute cholecystitis, jaundice, and pancreatitis are much more frequent hazards of sludge and gallstones in this population than in otherwise healthy individuals with cholelithiasis. It is now advocated that these patients should undergo prophylactic cholecystectomy (of normal gallbladders) at the time of the primary laparotomy if it involves a major intestinal resection. In fact, many would advocate that, if a patient is on TPN for 3 months and if this plan of management cannot be discontinued, the patient should be considered at high risk for a biliary tract complication and an elective cholecystectomy should be performed.

Cost considerations   In the United States, the financial costs of an uncomplicated cholecystectomy are higher than in any other developed country and are increasing exponentially. Figure 10 depicts Blue Cross/Blue Shied (United States) estimates for the average total charges levied on patients for an uncomplicated cholecystectomy between the years 1950 and 1982. Each estimate takes into consideration the charges for 10 to 11 days in a modern semiprivate hospital room, special hospital and operating room costs, and the anesthesiologist's and surgeon's fees. Charges in each category vary widely throughout the United States; Blue Cross/Blue Shield has estimated that in 1980 and 1982, the range of the mean was ± $1800. Cholecystectomy charges doubled between 1950 (~ $300) and 1960 (~ $600). The increases were exponential in the following decades and, in 1982, the latest year for which figures are available, the mean cost was a little over $5600. On the basis of the exponential trend that became apparent between 1965 and 1975, earlier estimates suggested that the average cost of a cholecystectomy would be close to $6000 by 1985. With the inclusion of the latest data, our extrapolation (Fig. 10) now suggests that a cholecystectomy will cost approximately $8000 in 1985. In 1985, eastern- and western-coast urban medical centers will probably charge $10,000 for the operation, whereas the "cheapest" cholecystectomy that may be available in the United States will cost $6000. It is estimated that surgery on the biliary tree which precedes or follows a biliary complication of gallstones will possibly cost twice these amounts.

A further element that must be considered in a cost analysis of gallstones is the overall burden to the economy of prophylactic cholecystectomies versus expectant management for asymptomatic gallstones. According to estimates derived from the Framingham Study and autopsy prevalence rates, at least 20 million Americans have gallstones. Every year in the United States, over 2 million oral cholecystograms and ultrasound examinations of the gallbladder are performed; about 1 million patients are found to have cholelithiasis, and of these, according to

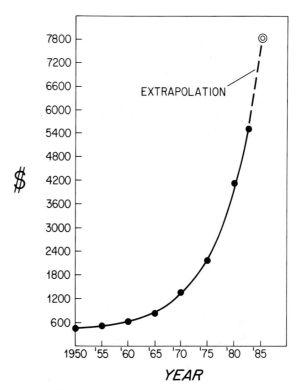

FIGURE 10

Total cost of an uncomplicated cholecystectomy: U.S. national average. (After Blue Cross/Blue Shield USA data, Time, November 15, 1976, with additions from Blue Cross/Blue Shield.)

present estimates, 50 percent undergo biliary tract surgery. A conservative assumption suggests that 20 percent of the patients who have a cholecystectomy are in the 30 to 40 year age group and have asymptomatic stones. Based on our 1985 estimate ($8000), the aggregate cost of these operations will be $800 million. On the contrary, expectant management of these 100,000 patients suggests that only 20,000 cholecystectomies will eventually be necessary, resulting, for this group, in a total cost of $160 million. If we factor in the annual reduction in costs for 30- to 40-year-old individuals by discounting survivors at 5 percent per year, this will decrease average cholecystectomy costs to approximately $80 million.

Medical management

At the present time it appears that medical management of cholelithiasis with the cholelitholytic bile acids, chenodeoxycholic acid (CDCA) and ursodeoxycholic acid (UDCA), represents only a small, but important, "window" in the therapeutic armamentarium. It has been estimated that, if all gallstone patients were to be treated actively, then perhaps only 10 to 20 percent of patients would be suitable candidates. Obviously, this percentage could be scaled upward considerably by careful selection of the patient population, that is, if the size of the denominator were reduced. In our opinion, conventional dissolution therapy should, at present, be reserved for cholesterol gallstone patients with biliary pain that necessitates intervention but who are poor surgical candidates or who refuse surgery. As we have discussed earlier in detail, we believe that the natural history of asymptomatic gallstones is relatively benign (Table 3) and that these patients should be treated neither medically nor surgically unless symptoms develop. The most suitable patients for medical dissolution therapy would probably fall in the older age groups, possibly patients older than 60 to 65 years of age. As we have discussed earlier, therapy for this group as a whole should be reserved for those with biliary pain or complications and should be individualized. The risks, failures, and recurrences associated with medical therapy should be weighed against the increased mortality of elective cholecystectomy in these age groups and of emergency surgery in patients with complications.

What of the efficacy and safety of CDCA and UDCA? Despite the results of the National Cooperative Gallstone Study (Schoenfield et al.) and a multitude of controlled and uncontrolled trials with CDCA and UDCA carried out in many parts of the world, we are still left with incomplete answers to these questions. It is reasonably certain that overall efficacy (as a percentage of unselected patients that would normally be treated by cholecystectomy) is low, possibly no more than 3 to 10 percent. The reasons for this are several: (1) many patients must be excluded from treatment; for example, neither CDCA nor UDCA is effective in patients with pigment gallstones, large gallstones, or calcified gallstones; cystic duct obstruction and failure of gallbladder contractile function preclude therapy; (2) other patients may be excluded for relative contraindications such as severe obesity, asymptomatic

choledocholithiasis, chronic liver disease, chronic inflammatory bowel disease, and women in the reproductive age groups; (3) patients with gallstone complications such as cholecystitis, cholangitis, and pancreatitis are excluded since these complications constitute absolute contraindications to chronic management; (4) patients with recurrent and severe symptoms coupled with the slow rates of dissolution and the requirements for regular medical observation lead to high drop-out rates; (5) the relatively low success rates of "complete" dissolution (~ 25 percent) among those thought to be ideal candidates; and (6) the high recurrence rate after successful dissolution, possibly greater than 50 percent within 5 to 7 years. Other considerations are the fact that the natural history of the stone disease (i.e., frequency of colic and complications) and the rates of cholecystectomy are not diminished during dissolution with CDCA, and when CDCA is employed in an optimal dose (15 mg/kg per day), the drug is associated with a high rate of hypertransaminasemia and diarrhea (40 to 50 percent), infrequent mild and reversible hepatotoxicity (~ 3 percent), and a 10 percent elevation in LDL cholesterol. There are also animal data which suggest that chronic CDCA therapy may be a promoter of amyloidosis and colonic carcinogenesis. In our view, suitable patients should be treated with CDCA for a limited period of time, certainly no longer than 2 to 3 years, and when therapy is successful, as judged by negative ultrasonography, then dietary or other interventions (such as low-dose UDCA) should be employed in the hopes of forestalling recurrence of stones.

A vast number of studies suggest that UDCA is as effective as CDCA and is a safer drug when employed in optimal doses (8 to 12 mg/kg per day). Diarrhea and hypertransaminasemia are rare, and serum lipid abnormalities do not occur. Further, UDCA appears to exert a salutary effect on the natural history of stone disease because biliary pain, complications, and the indications for cholecystectomy appear to be lessened during therapy. In highly selected cases, especially patients with very small floating stones, its efficacy may be higher than that of CDCA. Further, there exists in vitro evidence that low-dose UDCA may be more promising than low-dose CDCA in preventing stone recurrence in vivo.

For a trial of either therapy, the stones should be radiolucent and less than 15 mm in diameter, the gallbladder should function on an oral cholecystogram, and the patient should not be overly obese. The best predictor of success is partial dissolution evaluated by oral cholecystography and ultrasonography after therapy for 6 to 9 months. The degree of cholesterol saturation of duodenal bile in an individual patient is not particularly helpful as a pre- or posttreatment indicator of success.

Dissolution therapy with bile acids costs approximately $1500 per year. This figure includes the cost of the drug, diagnostic monitoring procedures, plus visits to the physician and radiologist. If dissolution is successful, medical therapy will, in 1985, be much less expensive than a cholecystectomy. If unsuccessful, or if the stones recur, then this cost may have to be added to that for a cholecystectomy (total cost: $11,000 to $12,000 in 1985). Because the physicochemical control of gallstone dissolution depends principally on the stones' surface area/volume ratios, small gallbladder stones dissolve much faster than do larger stones. Adjuvant measures such as low cholesterol diets and bedtime CDCA or UDCA have been shown to accelerate the rate of gallstone dissolution but overall efficacy is not appreciably increased.

What's on the horizon?

Basic research on the origin, composition, and functions of bile and on the pathobiology of the enterohepatic circulation has played a central role in the development of medical dissolution therapy for gallstones. For multiple reasons, as discussed in the last section, this therapeutic modality as presently practiced has only a small role to play in the management of patients with gallstones. Developments in the field of medical technology have resulted in the deployment of extracorporeal high-energy shock waves to fragment kidney stones. Studies currently in progress are attempting to refine this technique for the safe destruction of gallstones in situ. Although the management of biliary tract stone disease is still largely surgical, technological, biochemical, and pharmaceutical advances may make the noninvasive approach a more feasible option in the future.

References

ALLEN B et al: Sludge is calcium bilirubinate associated with bile stasis. Am J Surg 141:51, 1981

ARANHA GV et al: Cholecystectomy in cirrhotic patients: A formidable operation. Am J Surg 143:55, 1982

BATES GC, BROWN CH: Incidence of gallbladder disease in chronic hemolytic anemia (spherocytosis). Gastroenterology 21:104, 1952

CHASSY F et al: First clinical experience with extracorporeally induced destruction of kidney stones by shock waves. J Urol 127:417, 1982

CLASSEN M, OSSENBERG FW: Nonsurgical removal of common bile duct stones. Gut 18:760, 1977

DENBESTEN L, DOTY JE: Pathogenesis and management of choledocholithiasis. Surg Clin North Am 61:893, 1981

DEWEY KW et al: Cholelithiasis in thalassemia major. Radiology 96:385, 1970

DOYLE PJ et al: The value of routine preoperative cholangiography: A report of 4,000 cholecystectomies. Br J Surg 69:617, 1982

FILLY RA et al: In vitro investigation of the origin of echoes within biliary sludge. J Clin Ultrasound 8:193, 1980

GADOMSKA H, ROMEJKO M: Epidemiology of hepatic and gallbladder carcinoma in the population of Warsaw in the years 1963–1972. Pol Tyg Lek 31:23, 1976

GLENN F, MCSHERRY CK: Calculous biliary tract disease, in *Current Problems in Surgery,* MM Ravitch et al (eds). Chicago, Year Book, 1975, pp 3–38

GROSS BH et al: Ultrasonic evaluation of common bile duct stones: Prospective comparison with endoscopic retrograde cholangiopancreatography. Radiology 146:471, 1983

JORDAN RA: Cholelithiasis in sickle cell disease. Gastroenterology 33:952, 1957

MARINOVIC I et al: Incidencia de lithiasis biliar en material de autopsias y analysis de composicion de los calculos. Rev Med Chil 100:1320, 1972

MAYO WJ: "Innocent" gallstone a myth. JAMA 56:1021, 1911

MCPHERSON K et al: Small area variations in the use of common surgical procedures: An international comparison of New England, England and Norway. N Engl J Med 307:1310, 1982

NEWMAN HF et al: Complications of cholelithiasis. Am J Gastroenterol 50:476, 1968

RANSOHOFF DF et al: Prophylactic cholecystectomy vs. expectant management for silent gallstones: A decision analysis to assess survival. Ann Intern Med 99:199, 1983

ROSLYN JL et al: Gallbladder disease in patients on long-term parenteral nutrition. Gastroenterology 84:148, 1983

SALVIOLI G et al: Oral ursodeoxycholate therapy for biliary duct stone dissolution. Gut 24:609, 1983

SCHOENFIELD LJ et al: Chenodiol (chenodeoxycholic acid) for dissolution of gallstones: The National Cooperative Gallstone Study: A controlled trial of efficacy and safety. Ann Intern Med 95:257, 1981

SHAFFER EA, SMALL DM: Gallstone disease: Pathogenesis and management. Curr Probl Surg 13:1, 1976

SIEVERS ML, MARQUIS JR: The southwestern American Indian's burden: Biliary disease. JAMA 182:570, 1962

TINT GS et al: Ursodeoxycholic acid: A safe and effective agent for dissolving cholesterol gallstones. Ann Intern Med 97:351, 1982

VERNICK LJ et al: Relationship between cholecystectomy and ascending colon cancer. Cancer 45:392, 1980

WOLPERS C: Relapses after spontaneous dissolution of gallstones, in *Bile Acids in Human Diseases,* P Back and W Gerok (eds). Stuttgart–New York, E.K. Schattauer, 1972, pp 171–174

APPLICATIONS OF PROTON NUCLEAR MAGNETIC RESONANCE IMAGING IN NEUROLOGY

F. S. BUONANNO, J. P. KISTLER, and J. B. MARTIN

Since its first description in 1946, nuclear magnetic resonance (NMR) has been applied to the study of molecular structure and, more recently, to biochemical investigations in tissue. The demonstration in 1973 that NMR signals could be rendered spatially dependent and utilized to generate images fostered the development of numerous NMR-imaging techniques currently being introduced into clinical practice. Most NMR images have been generated using characteristics of proton (^{1}H) resonance. In this article we review briefly the principles of NMR spectroscopy and the extension of these techniques into NMR-imaging procedures, and we discuss initial results of observations made in neurological disorders.

NMR SPECTROSCOPY

The principles of NMR spectroscopy can be illustrated best by examining the properties of hydrogen atoms (protons, ^{1}H), the nuclei most commonly used in NMR-imaging studies (Fig. 1). The hydrogen atom, which contains one unpaired proton, serves as a paradigm of those atomic nuclei that possess a nuclear magnetic moment, a property which is generated by an unpaired proton or a neutron within the nucleus (Table 1). Because a proton has mass and electric charge, its spinning creates an angular momentum which produces a small magnetic field. In the earth's weak magnetic field, the individual magnetic moments of a group of protons in tissues orient randomly (Fig. 2); under these circumstances there is no net macroscopic magnetization vector (**M**) generated. However, if the

tissue sample is placed within a strong, external, constant, and homogeneous magnetic field, the spin axes of protons tend to align either with or against the field, occupying one of two energy levels allowed by the principles of quantum mechanics (Fig. 3) and thereby producing a net nonzero magnetization.

The energy level of nuclei with spin aligned in the direction of the externally applied field is lower than that of nuclei aligned against it. The energy difference between the two levels is proportional to the strength of the externally applied magnetic field strength and is determined by the relation

$$\Delta E = \mu H_o = \gamma \frac{h}{2\pi} H_o$$

where ΔE = energy difference
μ = nuclear magnetic moment
H_o = homogeneous magnetic field
h = Planck's constant
γ = gyromagnetic ratio

The unit of magnetic field strength is called a gauss (G). The earth's magnetic field is 0.6 G as measured at Washington, D.C. The other unit used to express magnetic field strength is tesla; one tesla (T) is equal to 10 kG.

Each NMR-sensitive atom has a particular gyromagnetic ratio and a specific spinning frequency in the radio frequency (RF) range (Table 1). For example, in a magnetic field of 1 T, protons have a spinning ("resonance") frequency of 42.58 MHz; ^{31}P, 17.24 MHz; and ^{23}Na, 11.26 MHz. Planck's constant is independent of any

TABLE 1
Nuclear magnetic resonance characteristics of certain clinically relevant nuclei

Isotope	Spin, units of H/2	NMR frequency, MHz at 1 T	Natural abundance,* percent	Sensitivity at constant frequency for equal number of nuclei	Molar concentration†
^1H	½	42.5759	99.98	1	99
^{31}P	½	17.237	100	0.405	0.35
^{13}C	½	10.705	1.108	0.251	0.1
^{23}Na	³⁄₂	11.262	100	1.32	0.078
^{19}F	½	40.055	100	0.941	0.0066

* *Percent of isotope normally present in tissues.*
† *Assumes that 75 percent of tissue mass and volume is water.*

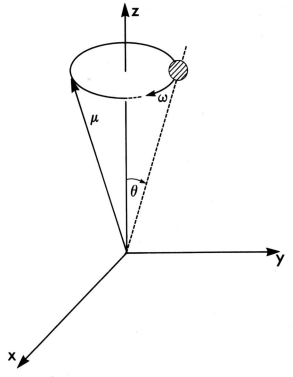

FIGURE 1
A spinning proton with magnetic moment (μ) at an angular velocity (ω) and at an angle (θ) with the external magnetic field directed in the z direction.

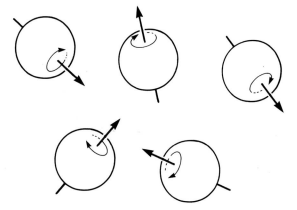

FIGURE 2
In the absence of any externally applied magnetic field, individual nuclear magnetic dipoles within a sample are randomly oriented.

given nuclear species. The nuclei aligned with the externally applied magnetic field can be flipped between energy states, causing a different alignment by application of an RF pulse at the appropriate frequency ν_0 (determined by $\Delta E = H\nu_0$). It is possible, therefore, to "tune-in" to a specific nuclear species by virtue of its unique magnetic properties. This potential can be exploited both to "image" the nuclear species as well as to measure its "biochemical" concentration.

To pass from one energy level to the other after delivery of an RF pulse, the nuclei have to absorb and then release energy in the amount ΔE. The difference in the number of nuclei populating the various energy levels, and hence the overall magnetization, is proportional to the number of nuclei present, to the gyromagnetic ratio squared, and to the strength of the field (Curie's law). Magnetic fields of greater strength produce a greater energy difference and, accordingly, a larger signal amplitude. Protons, with the largest gyromagnetic ratio and highest biological

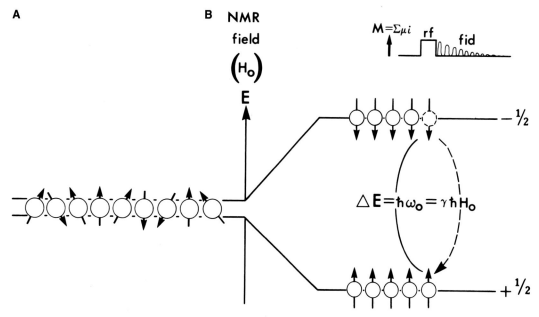

FIGURE 3

Behavior of spin ½ nuclei in a magnetic field, H_o.
A. In the absence of an external magnetic field, the individual magnetic moments (μ_i) comprising a sample (e.g., of tissue protons) are randomly oriented. B. On placing the sample in a strong, static, external magnetic field (H_o), the spinning nuclei orient either parallel (+½) or antiparallel (−½) to the field. ΔE is the energy separation between the two energy levels. A net magnetic moment (M) is generated because of the slight excess of parallel (Np) to antiparallel (Nap) nuclei, by the ratio $Np/Nap = 1.0000007$. C. The

nature of the nuclear magnetic resonance experiment is to induce transitions between the levels by absorption or emission of the requisite energy. Transitions between the high- and low-energy levels can be induced by applying radio frequency energy satisfying the equation $\Delta E = \hbar\omega_o = \gamma\hbar H_o = \gamma(\hbar/2\pi)H_o$ (see text). The emitted energy is detected as a free-induction decay (FID) RF signal. By the mathematical process of Fourier transformation, the FID signal can be analyzed in terms of a frequency-vs.-amplitude plot (spectrum).

concentration, are the nuclei most readily observable by NMR (Table 1).

When energy in the form of an RF pulse is applied to the sample via a coil surrounding it, the macroscopic, or bulk, magnetization vector is displaced away from its equilibrium position (i.e., to an alignment parallel to the magnetic field) (Figs. 3 and 4). The changes that occur can be described by reference to a set of orthogonal **x, y,** and **z** vectors situated in three-dimensional space, where the **z** vector is defined along the homogeneous magnetic field. Because of the torque that a magnetic field exerts on a magnetic moment, the nucleus spins, or precesses, at an angle about H_o, in a manner analogous to that of a spinning top or a gyroscope which precesses in the earth's gravitational field. The precessional or angular frequency is called the *Larmor* or *resonance frequency* and is defined by

$\omega_o = H_o$, where $\omega_o = \pi \cdot \nu_o$. By properly imposing an RF pulse at the same resonance frequency, a second magnetic field is created perpendicular to the external field generated by the magnet. The effect of the RF pulse is to add another precessional movement along an axis at right angles to the magnetic field.

After application of an RF pulse of a duration and strength which tips the magnetization into a position at right angles to H_o (defined as the *xy* plane), an alternating voltage is generated in the *xy* plane. This voltage signal, called the *free-induction decay,* is recorded by a receiving RF coil (which is usually the same coil which is used to transmit RF pulses). Following appropriate detection and amplification, the induced signal may be monitored, digitized, and Fourier-transformed into a signal-vs.-amplitude plot (spectrum) (Fig. 5).

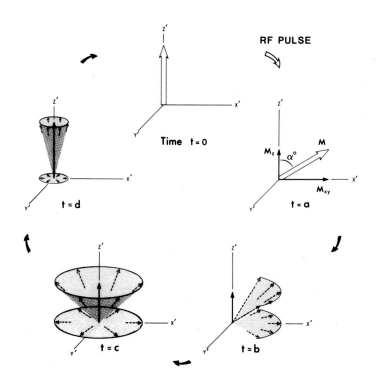

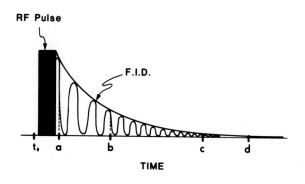

FIGURE 4

*Relaxation behavior of the macroscopic magnetization vector (**M**) in the rotatory frame of reference, and free-induction decay of the nuclear signal. Before the radio frequency pulse, the magnetic moment is aligned with the z axis. The z axis conventionally defines the direction along the lines of induction of the static, external magnetic field. Immediately following an α° pulse, **M** makes an angle α with the z axis. The vector component in the xy plane (**M**xy) generates the nuclear signal. The vector then relaxes back to its equilibrium position, and the z component of magnetization (**M**z) increases exponentially with a time constant T_1. T_2 relaxation occurs simultaneously with T_1 relaxation. Internuclear magnetic interactions and field heterogeneities slightly alter the local magnetic fields experienced by the various nuclei, and some begin to precess at different rates: The components of magnetization in the xy plane disperse (t_1 and t_2), the FID signal begins to decay with a time constant T_2. Stated more simply, T_1 is the time required to complete the cycle from t = 0 to t = 0 (see arrows). T_2 is the time elapsed from t = o to t = c. Thus, the termination of the FID corresponds to T_2. Eventually, the components of magnetization in the xy plane will be randomly distributed (tc, td) and the FID amplitude approaches zero. (From Pykett et al.)*

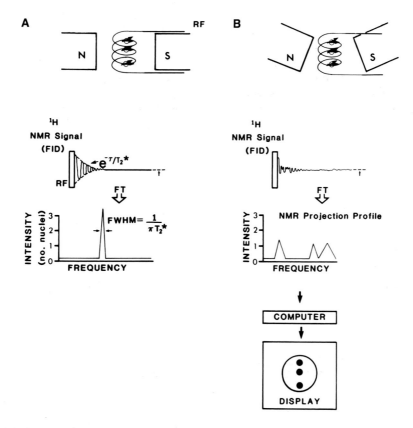

FIGURE 5

A, top. Schema of a nuclear magnetic resonance spectroscopy experiment. A hypothetical sample containing three protons is placed within a homogenous magnetic field, represented here by equidistant north and south magnetic poles. The individual magnetic moments are aligned (straight arrows) with the lines of force of the magnetic field. The sample is surrounded by a radio frequency coil which alternatively functions as a transmitter or a receiver antenna. Upon application of an RF pulse at an appropriate (resonant) frequency, the magnetic moments are displaced by an α° angle. After the RF pulse is terminated, the magnetic moments tend to realign with the field, and reemit RF energy, detected by the coil as a free-induction decay (FID) signal (center panel). The oscillating behavior of the FID within the signal-decay envelope reflects the alternating nature of the signal induced in the receiver coil. In a hypothetical, perfectly uniform magnetic field, the FID decays with a time constant T_2; because of slight imperfections in real magnetic fields, however, the time constant of decay of the FID occurs more rapidly, and is denoted T_2^* (bottom): By subjecting the FID to the mathematical process of Fourier transformation, a frequency-vs.-intensity plot (spectrum) is obtained. The single peak in the spectrum indicates that the nuclear signal essentially contains only a single resonant frequency; this occurs because the same magnetic field is experienced by all nuclei. There is no spatial information in such an NMR spectrum. B. NMR imaging. A linear magnetic field gradient (shown schematically by the unequal distances between the magnetic poles) is superimposed on the static magnetic field. Nuclei in one position within the graded field experience a different field than nuclei elsewhere; hence, they resonate at different frequencies. Repeating the NMR experiment now yields an FID signal with a complex decay envelope containing different frequencies. Fourier transformation of this FID yields a spectrum characterized by three peaks, each of proportionally reduced intensity and each at the frequency corresponding to the spatial location of the given nucleus within the graded magnetic field. The resultant spectrum can be considered a one-dimensional projection profile of the nuclear-signal strength. Computer processing of a series of such projections obtained over at least 180° around the sample allows reconstruction of an image.

When the RF field which has disturbed a sample of protons is terminated, the protons return gradually (relax) to their state of equilibrium with magnetization parallel to the external magnetic field. The detected free-induction decay signal gradually diminishes. The nature of this relaxation process can be characterized by two distinct parameters. The *spin-lattice relaxation time* (T_1) is the time constant of return to the equilibrium state after termination of the RF pulse; this re-equilibrium occurs when the absorbed energy is dissipated to the surrounding environment (the lattice) and occurs over a period of 0.1 to 2 s for protons in biological samples. T_1 is also known as the longitudinal relaxation time because it describes the time required for the vector component of macroscopic magnetization along the longitudinal axis (M_z) to return from a submaximal value at the instant the RF pulse is terminated to its full equilibrium magnetization value (Fig. 4). The *spin-spin relaxation time* (T_2) characterizes the rate of signal decay after the RF pulse is applied (i.e., the disappearance of the transverse or right-angled component of the magnetization vector). T_2 reflects the exchange rate of absorbed energy among neighboring nuclei in the sample, and occurs over 10 to 1000 ms for protons in biological tissues. After excitation by the RF pulse, each nucleus experiences not only the external static field but also local fields associated with the magnetic properties of neighboring nuclei and their electron clouds; the nuclei will therefore exhibit a range of slightly different precessional frequencies, and the net magnetization in the *xy* plane (and, thus, the NMR signal) will also be reduced (Fig. 4). The same mechanisms are also responsible for another effect, called the chemical shift, discussed in greater detail below.

The two relaxation times differ depending upon the chemical state of the sample and upon the conditions under which the experiment is performed. Nuclei in solids are essentially static, making T_2 very short; in liquids, the nuclei move about more freely and rapidly, and T_2 is much longer. T_1 relaxation times in solids or at low temperatures can be very long; in liquids the opposite is the case, and T_1 relaxation occurs much more rapidly. It should be noted that T_2 can never exceed T_1, since no net transverse component of magnetization can exist after complete longitudinal (T_1) relaxation has occurred.

In proton NMR imaging, only the signal from "liquidlike" regions is observed; rigidly bound protons give essentially zero signal. Thus, in proton NMR images, the ^1H nuclei in compact bone are NMR silent and yield no signal observable with current NMR-imaging methods; in contrast, the marrow within long bones and cancellous bone is visualized. By selecting appropriate RF pulse sequences, NMR imaging can be performed with a view toward detecting or highlighting such in vivo variations in relaxation times.

Proton relaxation times in tissues are also affected by a variety of mechanisms such as water-membrane and water-protein interactions, paramagnetic effects (see below), and influences of molecular motion (such as diffusion and flow) across local magnetic field gradients. It is generally agreed that the water-protein interaction has the most important effect on tissue-proton relaxation times. All mechanisms associated with T_1 have a corresponding effect on T_2. Some low-frequency transitions (such as intra- and intermolecular chemical exchanges) may have a greater effect on T_2 than on T_1. Therefore, measurements of T_2, while similar to those of T_1, nevertheless represent a different NMR parameter and may provide different information of clinical importance.

NMR IMAGING

Since the observed free-induction decay represents a summation of the signal response from the entire sample, no spatial information is obtained from a conventional NMR spectroscopy experiment (Fig. 5*A*). However, if a linear magnetic field gradient is superimposed on the static field, nuclei at one position within the sample will experience a slightly different total magnetic field and will resonate at slightly different frequencies than nuclei elsewhere in the sample. A linear distribution of resonant frequencies across the sample is produced whereby a given frequency corresponds to a known position in space. The resultant frequency spectrum can be used as a one-dimensional projection profile of the nuclear-signal strength (Fig. 5*B*). By varying electronically the orientation of the linear gradients, a series of projection profiles is obtained. Computer analysis of these multiple projections allows an image of the whole sample to

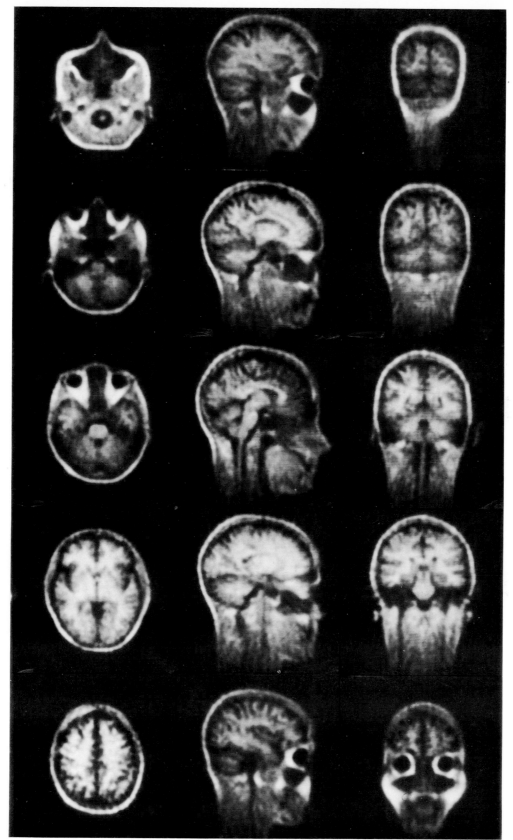

FIGURE 6

Inversion-recovery images reconstructed from a true three-dimensional data set. The 3-mm-thick planes can be reconstructed at any desired orientation, including transaxial (left column), parasagittal (center), *or coronal (right). Areas of low proton density or short T_1 relaxation times appear bright, areas of high proton density or long T_1 appear dark. Bone, containing only rigidly bound protons, gives essentially no signal and appears dark.*

be reconstructed. Other spatial-encoding techniques and image-generation methods are also used in NMR imaging.

In most currently used clinical imaging systems, information is acquired from either one plane or a set of planes at a time (planar or multiplanar imaging). Information can also be acquired simultaneously from the whole volume enclosed within the transmitter-receiver coil system. At the Massachusetts General Hospital, NMR data are usually collected from the total volume of the head using a true three-dimensional method which allows subsequent reconstruction of any arbitrary plane through the head (Fig. 6). The three-dimensional technique appears optimal for volumetric studies of the brain. It also permits comparison with the exact planes obtained from other studies (e.g., CT scanning, autopsy sections). However, single-plane techniques may be advantageous in certain circumstances, as in scanning uncooperative patients who require very short imaging time.

RF PULSE SEQUENCES

The image created by the application of NMR techniques can be varied by changing the timing and type of RF pulse sequences that are applied to the tissues. Three RF pulse sequences are commonly used in NMR spectroscopy: (1) saturation-recovery (SR), (2) inversion-recovery (IR), and (3) Carr-Purcell-Meiboom-Gill (CPMG) spin-echo techniques (Fig. 7). Both SR and IR pulse sequences yield T_1-weighted images, whereas the CPMG sequence gives a series of T_2-weighted images, each corresponding to one echo from the series. The results of these manipulations produce strikingly different images, as illustrated in Fig. 8.

In actual practice, NMR images are frequently derived from modified pulse sequences which introduce T_2 effects into SR and IR images. Nevertheless, by appropriate manipulation of data obtained from two imaging-data sets generated at different pulse repetition rates, it is possible

NMR Pulse Sequences

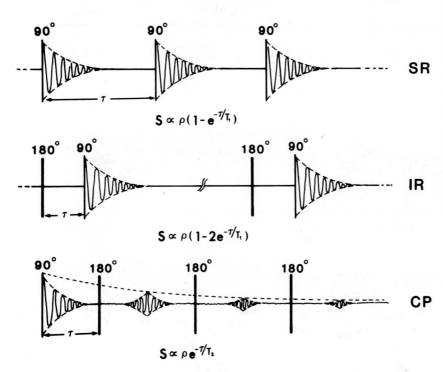

$$S \propto \rho(1 - e^{-\tau/T_1})$$

$$S \propto \rho(1 - 2e^{-\tau/T_1})$$

$$S \propto \rho\, e^{-\tau/T_2}$$

SR

IR

CP

FIGURE 7
Schematic representation of three pulse sequences commonly used for nuclear magnetic resonance imaging. Saturation-recovery (SR) and inversion-recovery (IR) sequences yield T_1-weighted images, whereas spin-echo sequences, such as the Carr-Purcell-Meiboom-Gill (CPMG), produce T_2-weighted images. In all cases, the influence of relaxation times on the resultant signal (S) depends on the time value chosen for the interpulse interval (τ).

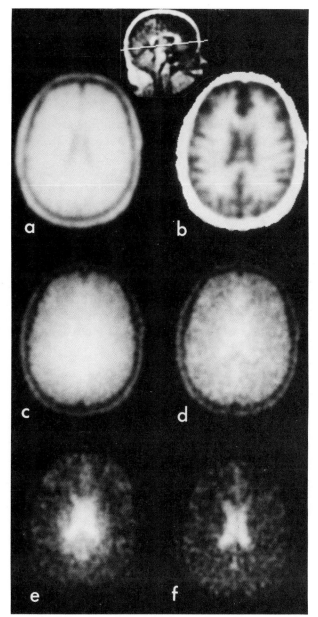

FIGURE 8

Image information content varies with the particular radio frequency pulse sequence used. An approximation of a proton spin-density image (a) can be obtained concomitantly with inversion-recovery data and a corresponding T_1 rate map (b) generated. There is a homogeneous distribution of protons within neural tissue (a). In (b), areas of low T_1 appear bright, images of longer T_1 darker; by simple region-of-interest programs, T_1 can be measured with high spatial selectivity in such quantitative tomographic "maps". Spin-spin relaxation time (T_2) can be qualitatively assessed from spin-echo images obtained at 61 (c), 122 (d), 183 (e), and 244 (f) ms after the initial 90° RF pulse in a Carr-Purcell-Meiboom-Gill pulse sequence; in this sequence, more solidlike areas of short T_2 exhibit rapid decay of signal intensity, whereas more liquidlike areas of longer T_2, such as cerebrospinal fluid, exhibit a slower rate of signal decay and appear brighter in later echoes. (From FS Buonanno et al, DM 29:1, 1983.)

to elminate the terms depending on T_2 and to calculate in vivo T_1 values on a regional basis. A T_1-rate ($1/T_1$) map (Fig. 8*B*) can thus be generated.

CLINICAL APPLICATIONS

Studies of the central nervous system in normal volunteers and patients show that pulse sequences of the IR type provide particularly high-contrast resolution. An interpulse interval of 400

ms appears adequate for most routine imaging applications, enabling sharp differentiation of the cerebrospinal fluid from the brain parenchyma while maintaining adequate demarcation of gray and white matter (Fig. 6). The brain is easily distinguished from the ventricles and subarachnoid space because cerebrospinal fluid, with a low oxygen tension and high water content, has relatively long T_1 and T_2 relaxation times, yielding a relatively weak signal as it recovers slowly between pulse repetitions. Gray matter possesses a longer T_1 than white matter because of its higher water content and fewer lipids. Differentiation of subcortical structures (such as the caudate, thalamus, or certain brainstem nuclear masses) from surrounding white matter or cerebrospinal fluid is usually possible. The area around the Sylvian fissure is clearly delineated. Computer ripple ("overshoot") artifacts are not a problem as they were in early computerized tomography (CT) scans.

In the posterior fossa, the cerebellum and brainstem are easily recognized, and the ventricular system is again sharply demarcated. The marrow within bone is evident, but bone itself—containing only rigidly bound protons—appears dark. No streak artifacts are seen extending from bone, which is a common problem in x-ray CT scans. However, it is sometimes difficult to separate bone from cerebrospinal fluid using pulse sequences which produce T_1-weighted images.

On the exterior of the cranium, soft tissues are well delineated. The subcutaneous fat stands out brightly, as does fat in the orbits. The ocular globes, their internal structures, and the ocular muscles are visible. Nasal and paranasal sinuses can be seen. With the appropriate pulse sequence and timing parameters, major blood vessels that contain flowing blood appear as tubular structures with dark lumens; by appropriate alterations in the timing of various RF pulse sequences, flow may be measured in vessels lying parallel to the z axis of the magnetic field.

CPMG sequences may provide additional information confirming or complementing the results of IR scans since the range and variations of T_2 in different tissues do not necessarily parallel those of T_1, as discussed above. In addition, data obtained using CPMG sequences appear to provide a high index of detection sensitivity for edema. SR scans obtained at various repetition rates may highlight regions with long T_1, may demonstrate the presence of fluid, or may furnish indications as to motion and flow. Only extensive clinical trials will establish which pulse sequences and which instrumental settings are optimal for the detection, differentiation, and monitoring of various disease processes.

Cerebrovascular disorders

In studies of experimental ischemic infarction, we have reported that brain changes occur promptly and are sharply demarcated from the surrounding nonischemic parenchyma. Image alterations in the form of areas of focal brightening are evident within 3 h, and sometimes as early as 30 min, after symptomatic carotid ligation in gerbils; the proportion of positive cases increases to more than 90 percent when symptomatic animals are allowed to survive for 24 h. Similar changes are frequently noted by 4 h after middle cerebral artery occlusion in cats. Refinement of the techniques used, emphasizing either T_1 or T_2 relaxation times preferentially (such as IR or CPMG sequences), will likely reveal changes at even earlier times, since alterations of relaxation times have been documented in NMR-spectroscopy studies of brain within 30 min of induction of ischemia. Unfortunately, to date it has not been possible to study human cerebrovascular disorders at such early times after onset.

No systematic study has documented the time of onset of NMR-imaging changes compared, in particular, to CT scanning in human ischemic infarction. However, experience indicates that infarction of less than 24-h duration is easily detected on IR images as areas of decreased image intensity signifying prolongations in T_1 values. In contrast, CT-scan changes in comparably sized infarcts are often not apparent for 48 to 72 h. In some reports, the acute prolongations in T_1 are said to be accompanied by increases in mobile proton density, and may reflect, among other processes, the well-known increases in water content (brain edema) commonly found in particular stages of the evolution of cerebral ischemic insults.

In our initial clinical experience we compared the results of NMR imaging and conventional CT scanning in 25 patients with clinical diagnoses of cerebral infarction of various durations. All patients underwent CT scans in close temporal proximity to the NMR-imaging study. In each of 20 patients with abnormalities on the CT scan, there were similar lesions noted on NMR imaging. No lesions detected by CT scan failed to be visualized on NMR using the IR pulse sequence. Three patients had both a normal CT and NMR study. NMR imaging demonstrated lesions in two patients who had a negative CT scan: in one patient, IR NMR was positive at 18 h, while an initial CT scan was negative at 12 h but positive at 48 h; in the second patient, IR NMR was positive at 1 week while CT was negative at both 2 and 7 days.

The anatomic location and extent of ischemia-related changes are usually well delineated in the NMR study, although it is not possible with current imaging techniques to separate definitively regions of infarction from surrounding edema. Embolic or thrombotic infarctions (Figs. 9 and 10) produce areas of decreased IR-image intensity, usually corresponding to well-known anatomic and vascular distributions.

In some instances only loss of contrast between gray and white matter is noted in peripherally located infarcts. In some cases the mass effects induced by the infarct produce noticeable displacements or deformities of intracranial structures. Watershed infarcts can be easily documented in the border zones between the anterior, middle, and posterior cerebral arteries (Fig. 11). Lacunar infarcts can be seen as small, usually circular defects located in the territory of a deep penetrating vessel; in some patients they are multiple (Fig. 12). Infarctions in posterior fossa structures are particularly well visualized because of the lack of signal from bone (Fig. 9). In a series of 16 patients with infarcts in the territory supplied by the posterior circulation, NMR imaging was performed between 36 h and 2 months after onset of symptoms; in each case the infarcted zone was identified as an area of decreased image intensity (signifying prolonged T_1 relaxation times) on the IR scan and as areas of increased intensity in images of later echoes from the CPMG sequence (signifying prolonged T_2 values) (cf. Figs. 7 and 9). However, not all infarcts demonstrated equivalent prolongations in T_1 and T_2 relaxation times. On occasion, and especially in cases of multiple lacunar infarcts, lesions are noted with unequal T_1 and T_2 prolongations. Only further study will determine whether such findings can be correlated with either the age of the infarct or the relative amount of edema or ischemia within such lesions.

Some intracranial or intracerebral hemorrhages, hemorrhagic infarcts, or blood clots within giant aneurysms appear as areas of increased image intensity on IR scans, probably reflecting shortened T_1 values (Fig. 13). Some cases of acute hemorrhages and blood clots appear to have a shortened T_2, whereas the remainder of the hemorrhagic lesions mentioned above appear to possess lengthened T_2 relaxation

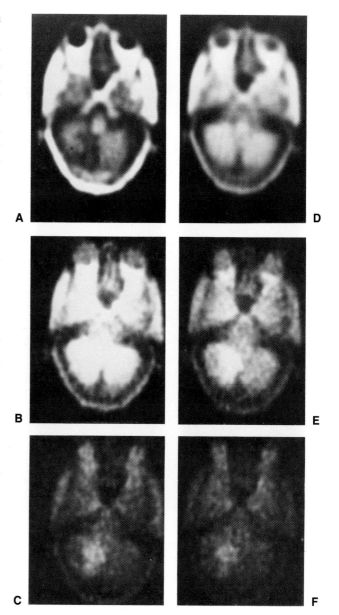

FIGURE 9

Cerebellar infarction. Inversion-recovery image (a), at 36 h after onset of symptoms, demonstrates decreased image intensity, compatible with prolonged T_1 in mesial and posterior portions of the left cerebellar hemisphere. The proton spin-density image (b) did not show the lesion. In the Carr-Purcell-Meiboom-Gill (CPMG) pulse sequence, four consecutive spin-echo images obtained at 61 (c), 122 (d), 183 (e), and 244 (f) ms after the initial 90° pulse show an area of slower signal decay (i.e., progressive relative brightening in the latter spin-echo images). This is suggestive of moderately prolonged T_2 values in the same area, compatible with infarction. (From Kistler et al.)

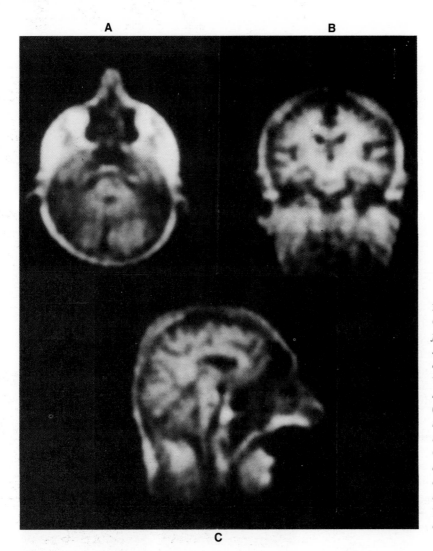

A

B

C

FIGURE 10
Orthogonal views reconstructed from a three-dimensional inversion-recovery data set. A 4-day-old, right basis pontis infarct is well seen in the transverse (a) section; in the parasagittal view (c), the orocaudal extent of the infarct occupying the caudal third of the pons is appreciated. On the coronal section (b), the area of abnormality is seen to extend into the midcentral left basis pontis, the significance of which is unknown. (From Kistler et al.)

times. Our experience is in accord with the scanty published clinical and experimental evidence which suggests that the relaxation times of some acute hemorrhages may be insignificantly different from those of normal white matter; although these characteristics would diminish the probability of detecting such lesions, most, if not all, intraparenchymal hemorrhages are separated from normal brain by surrounding zones of decreased IR and increased CPMG signal intensities, thought to represent edema. Nevertheless, it may be difficult or impossible to demonstrate small hemorrhages restricted solely to, or embedded in, normal white matter, if this rim of edema is lacking (e.g., acute hemorrhage) or when the lesion produces no, or minimal, distortion of normal anatomy.

Various groups have reported other examples of cerebral vascular pathology, including the vasculitides and changes in the controversial Binswanger's disease; as in our experience with radiation-induced vasculitis, no pathognomonic characteristics have been noted on either IR or CPMG images. On the other hand, arteriovenous malformations are visualized as tangles of serpiginous, tubular structures, if the vessels contain flowing blood. If the arteriovenous malformation is embedded in edematous brain tissue, which also appears dark on IR images, differentiation of the malformation from the surrounding parenchymal changes may be difficult (Fig. 14). However, CPMG images often clarify the issue: edematous brain stands out brightly, and patent blood vessels are negatively outlined.

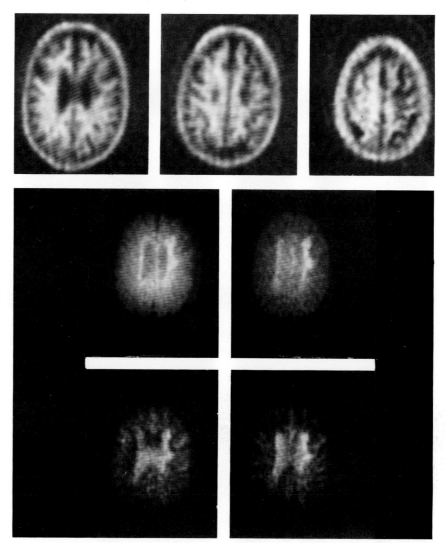

FIGURE 11
Inversion-recovery ^1H nuclear magnetic resonance images (top panel) show ventricular dilatation and a right anterior cerebral-middle cerebral artery watershed infarction, which has prolonged T_1 values; parietal regions are spared. Spin-echo ^1H NMR images from a four-buffer Carr-Purcell-Meiboom-Gill T_2 sequence (lower set), at the same midventricular level, demonstrate periventricular edema and slower rate of signal decay in areas of infarction, suggesting prolonged T_2 values. (From FS Buonanno et al, Neurol Clin NA 1:243, 1983.)

Neoplasia

The study of neoplasia was one of the initial biomedical applications of NMR. Using traditional NMR spectroscopy of tissue samples obtained by biopsy, Damadian was able to differentiate neoplastic from normal tissues on the basis of prolonged T_1 relaxation times. This work was confirmed and extended by several others to include observations of prolonged T_2 relaxation times. Such studies have helped stimulate the development and clinical application of proton NMR imaging.

The mechanisms underlying prolongation of relaxation times in tumors are poorly understood, and remain a subject of controversy.

Many studies have demonstrated that cancerous tissue has a higher total water content than normal tissue, and many investigators believe this to be a sufficient explanation; others, studying both normal and malignant tissues, failed to demonstrate a direct correlation between tissue-proton T_1 and T_2 relaxation times and the total tissue-water content. Studies aimed at characterizing and differentiating various normal and abnormal tissues on the basis of their proton NMR parameters are currently in progress.

Early studies using prototype imaging systems and various RF pulse sequences reported that normal brain tissue could be differentiated from neoplasia. Although the features of several types of malignant or benign intracranial tumors have

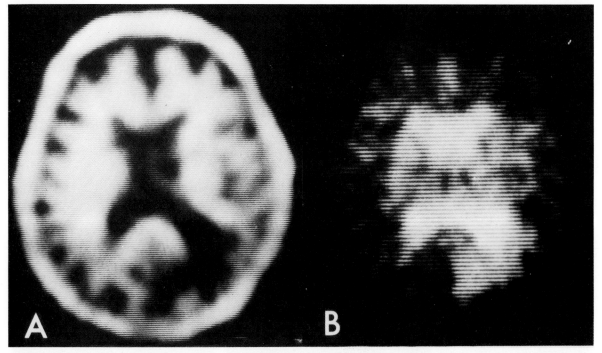

FIGURE 12
¹H Nuclear magnetic resonance images in a patient with embolic infarction in the right posterior cerebral artery territory, well seen as a dark region (prolonged T_1) in the inversion-recovery image (A). Older infarcts are seen also in the left caudate and right subcortical white matter. The right posterior cerebral artery infact is seen as a region of increased image intensity (prolonged T_2) in a later buffer from the Carr-Purcell-Meiboom-Gill (CPMG) T_2 sequence. The left caudate exhibits a more extensive abnormality in the spin-echo images.

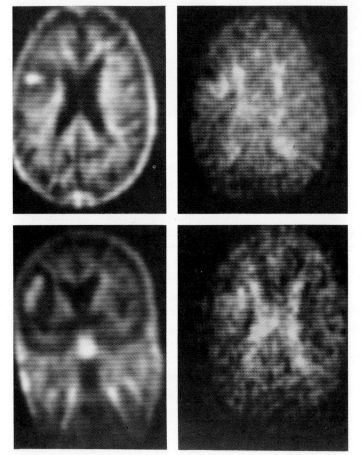

FIGURE 13
Transverse (upper left) and coronal (lower left) inversion-recovery ¹H nuclear magnetic resonance sections demonstrate a cerebral hemorrhage and surrounding edema. The hemorrhage is composed of two parts, one with very short T_1 (bright), probably representing thrombus surrounded by a prolonged T_1 (dark), probably representing serum; the latter is confounded with the rim of prolonged T_1, representing edema. Images from a four-buffer Carr-Purcell-Meiboom-Gill spin-echo sequence (upper and lower right) at the same transverse level as in upper left also show the hemorrhage to be composed of two parts: a small anterior area of short T_2 (dark), probably representing thrombus, and a subjacent area of prolonged T_2 (increased relative brightness), probably representing serum. The latter has T_2 values similar to those of edematous brain and approaches the T_2 values of cerebrospinal fluid. (FS Buonanno et al, Neurol Clin NA 1:243, 1983.)

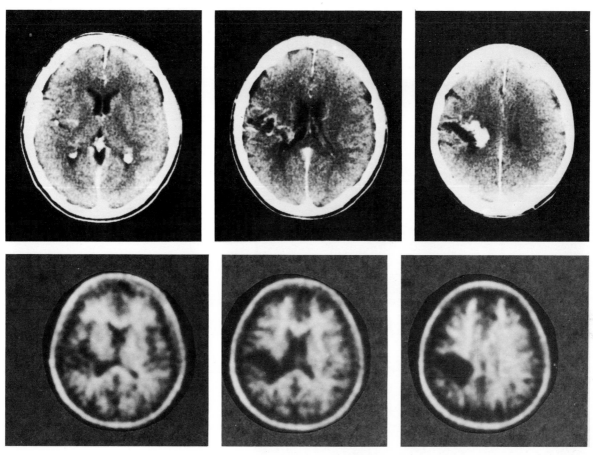

FIGURE 14

Patient 6. Contrast enhanced computerized tomography scan (upper row) clearly shows an arteriovenous malformation and associated changes in brain tissue.

Inversion-recovery ¹H nuclear magnetic resonance study (bottom row) adds no additional information. (From Buonanno et al.)

been reported, few have had detailed histopathological confirmation.

Gliomas appear as regions of bright signal intensity on steady state free-precession or CPMG images or as dark areas on IR studies (Fig. 15). In one case of a pathologically proved low-grade astrocytoma, the image characteristics were not different from those of tumors of higher malignancy (Fig. 16). It has been suggested that benign tumors such as meningioma have T_1 values intermediate between those of normal brain and those of highly malignant gliomas and thus should have intermediate intensity on NMR images produced by appropriate pulse sequences. In some tumors, rims of altered image intensity are noted, which are thought to represent edema. In the limited experience accumulated so far,

NMR imaging has not been proved to be capable of differentiating various types of tumors.

It is not clear whether the use of different imaging techniques will provide a means to differentiate reliably tumor from surrounding edema. In our experience with IR scans using an interpulse spacing of 400 ms and a repetition interval of 900 ms, edema has been difficult to distinguish from tumor. Maintaining the same interpulse spacing of 400 ms, but with a longer repetition interval of 1400 ms, Bydder et al. reported that they were able to provide differentiation in 5 of 14 patients with primary or secondary malignancy. Further prolongation of the pulse intervals to 800 and 2400 ms, respectively, resulted in better definition in a few cases. However, with the steady state free-precession pulse

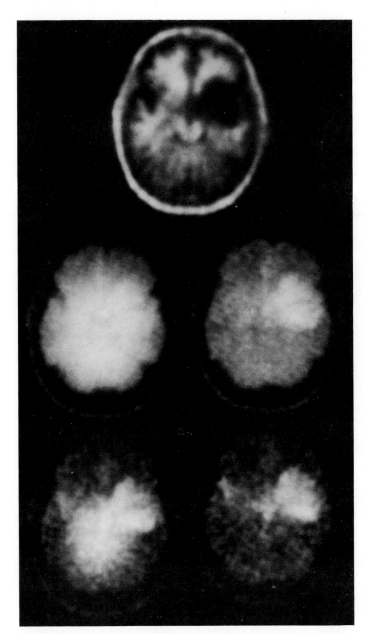

FIGURE 15
In a patient presumed to have a glioma, inversion-recovery image (top) shows a large zone of decreased image intensity in the right frontotemporal area, suggesting prolonged T_1. Images from a Carr-Purcell-Meiboom-Gill sequence demonstrate prolonged T_2. It is not possible to differentiate tumor nidus from surrounding edema in the images. (From FS Buonanno et al, DM 29:1, 1983.)

sequence, benign or malignant tumors, as well as edema, all appear bright.

The additional information obtained by CPMG techniques has not given better delineation of tumor from edema; the T_2 values obtained from the tumor may be either shorter or longer than the T_2 values in the surrounding edema. However, CPMG techniques have been proved useful in the detection and sizing of tumors adjacent to bone, such as meningioma or acoustic neuroma.

In these circumstances, both the tumor and bone appear dark on the IR image, but on the CPMG images, the tumor appears bright whereas bone remains dark.

We studied 10 patients with pituitary neoplasms (one growth hormone, seven prolactin, and two nonhypersecretory adenomas. Three small tumors (less than 200 mm^3 as measured by CT scan) were not clearly identified. Tumors of moderate or large dimensions (Fig. 17) were vi-

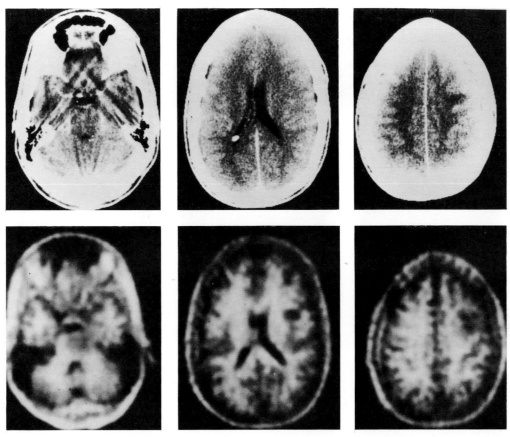

FIGURE 16
Low-grade astrocytoma. Postcontrast computerized tomography scan (top row): no parenchymal abnormality is seen at pontine level (left) albeit posterior fossa artifacts are present; section through ventricular bodies (center) reveals subtle mass effect with downward displacement of right hemisphere and right ventricular enlargement; over the convexity (right) there is an ill-defined area of decreased x-ray attenuation separating the right posterior frontal and parietal gyri.

Inversion-recovery nuclear magnetic resonance images (bottom) at levels corresponding to the CT scan reveal a rounded zone of decreased image intensity occupying the left pons and extending across the midline. A well-defined circular area of decreased intensity is also noted in the right insular region. A less sharply demarcated abnormality is evident in the frontoparietal region. Biopsy of the right insular lesion revealed a low-grade astrocytoma. (From FS Buonanno et al, J Comput Assist Tomogr 6:529, 1982.)

sualized as masses of altered image intensity by SR scans in 7 of 9 cases, by IR in 6 of 9, and by CPMG in 2 of 4. In these 10 patients, CT scan failed to reveal an adenoma in only 1 case: that of a woman with a prolactinoma documented by CT scan 4 months prior to NMR study, who subsequently was treated with bromocriptine, and developed a partially empty sella within which no tumor could be identified either by NMR or by a second CT scan.

In these preliminary qualitative studies of pi-

tuitary tumors, no correlation was found between tumor type and alterations in image intensity. Most (7 of 10) pituitary adenomas exhibited a bright appearance on IR and/or SR scans, suggesting shortened T_1 relaxation times; this finding contrasts with the increases in T_1 (and of T_2) relaxation times commonly noted in neoplasia. In one case, we observed a heterogeneously increased image intensity on both IR and SR scans (suggesting shortened T_1 values) and an increased image intensity on all four echo images

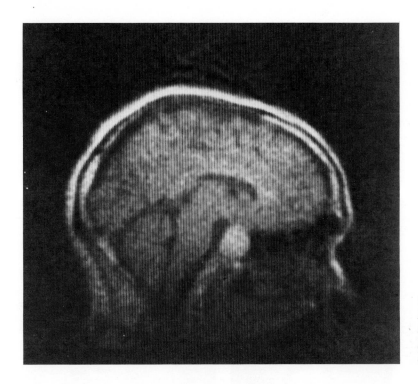

FIGURE 17
High-resolution, midline sagittal saturation-recovery image of a large pituitary adenoma. (From Oot et al.)

from the CPMG study (suggesting increased proton density and prolonged T_2 values); at operation, an old hemorrhage was found.

Multiple sclerosis

Visualization of plaques in multiple sclerosis has been difficult by CT scanning, although the resolution is improved with the use of new-generation scanners combined with high-dose contrast infusions and delayed imaging. A number of reports have demonstrated that IR NMR techniques reveal numerous abnormalities in patients with advanced multiple sclerosis (Fig. 18). Although there has been no anatomical-pathological verification that the NMR lesions correspond to multiple sclerosis plaques, the evidence offered in the various reports is strongly convincing. Hence, NMR imaging has been proposed as a highly sensitive method for the detection of multiple sclerosis plaques and for the asessment of their sequelae (cerebral atrophy, hydrocephalus ex vacuo).

In our earliest experience, using only quantitative IR techniques, four patients with clinically definite multiple sclerosis exhibited 22 clearly delineated lesions in white matter. T_1 relaxation times were significantly prolonged in those lesions (439 ± 32 ms) when compared to values obtained in controlateral normal areas (349 ± 14 ms). In one patient with acute vertigo, ataxia, and nystagmus, the single posterior fossa lesion had a T_1 value of 486 ms; three "silent" paraventricular lesions, probably corresponding to two previous attacks 2 and 3 years before, had T_1 values of 415 ± 13 ms. On the basis of these findings it was suggested that quantification of NMR parameters for individual plaques may provide a useful gauge for staging and monitoring disease activity, which may prove useful in judging the effects of therapy.

In some patients, T_2 techniques appear to improve the identification of certain plaques, leading some investigators to propose a greater sensitivity with this pulse sequence. Visualization of areas with prolonged T_2 appears more efficient because with the general decay in brain signal during the course of a CPMG study, lesions tend to stand out brightly; it is visually easier to note a bright spot against a black background than a dark-gray spot within a full-range white-to-black background. However, these early studies which touted a superiority of T_2-weighted images over

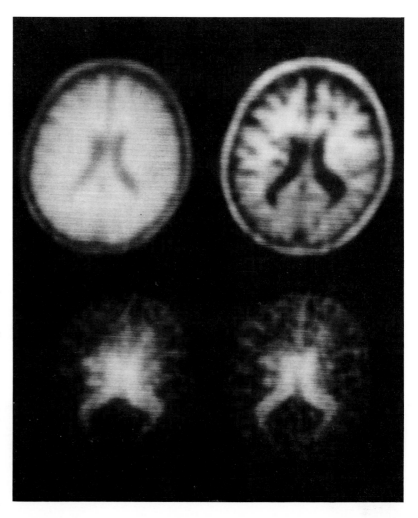

FIGURE 18

Multiple sclerosis. Proton density (upper left) is essentially featureless; areas containing cerebrospinal fluid, such as the ventricles and the cystic residuum of a left frontal plaque, appear dark because of partial saturation effects. Numerous paraventricular and subcortical white matter plaques are evident on the inversion-recovery image (upper right) as are areas of prolonged T_1 (dark). Many plaques also possess prolonged T_2 and appear as focal areas of relative brightening in images of later echoes from a Carr-Purcell-Meiboom-Gill (CPMG) sequence (bottom row). (From Buonanno et al.)

T_1-weighted images for the detection of multiple sclerosis plaques did not evaluate patients falling into the clinically possible multiple sclerosis category, and did not convey an appreciation of the possibility that multiple sclerosis plaques may in fact possess various combinations of T_1 and T_2 values.

Our subsequent experience has been extended in 18 patients to an analysis of both T_1 and T_2 techniques. The clinical gamut of possible, probable, and definite multiple sclerosis was studied. NMR imaging revealed 54 lesions in 12 of the 18 patients; in 6 patients, no lesions could be demonstrated in the cerebral hemispheres, cerebellum, or brainstem. Of the 54 lesions detected, 38 were seen by both T_1 and T_2 techniques; however, in 16 (~30 percent) of the remaining lesions, the CPMG-T_2 study was normal when the

IR study was clearly abnormal. The discrepancy between the results of the two imaging techniques supports the hypothesis that relaxation times within multiple sclerosis plaques may vary depending on the activity of the disease at that location. Thus, in 10 acute lesions (less than 12 weeks), both T_1 and T_2 were prolonged, while in about 40 percent of lesions of undertermined age and prolonged T_1, the T_2 study was normal. Our findings suggest that, with the passage of time, both T_1 and T_2 relaxation times may return to normal. From these initial observations we believe that normalization may occur in both parameters within 1 to 7 months after the acute attack.

NMR imaging appears to be an important and useful adjunct in the evaluation of patients with multiple sclerosis. In most patients with definite or probable multiple sclerosis, cranial NMR imaging detects a large number of lesions, many of which are presumably "asymptomatic." However, if the disease is restricted to the spinal cord or optic nerves, cerebral NMR scans may persist in being normal. In patients wtih chronic myelopathy and suspected multiple sclerosis, cerebral NMR imaging may reveal abnormalities even when, as occurred in four of our patients, there was no clinical, electrophysiological, or CT-scan evidence of central nervous system abnormality above the spinal cord level. The potential usefulness of whole-body NMR-imaging techniques, which holds promise for visualization of the spinal cord in multiple sclerosis, has yet to be determined.

Other conditions

NMR findings in disparate clinical conditions affecting the nervous system have been given in various communications from NMR centers.

These have included results on NMR imaging of the following conditions:

Malformations (Arnold-Chiari, syringomyelia, hemiatrophy, agenesis of the corpus callosum)

Atrophic-degenerative diseases of the central nervous system (late-onset cerebellar atrophy, Friedreich's ataxia, motor neuron disease, senile and presenile dementia)

Infections (neurosyphilis, tuberculosis, herpes simplex, brain abscess, other meningitides, septicemia)

Various types of hydrocephalus (noncommunicating or communicating posttraumatic hydrocephalus or normal pressure hydrocephalus)

Basal ganglia diseases (Parkinson's, Huntington's, or Wilson's)

Other neurological conditions (benign intracranial hypertension, Behcet's disease, Steele-Richardson-Olszewski syndrome, suspected encephalitis; and methotrexate encephalopathy)

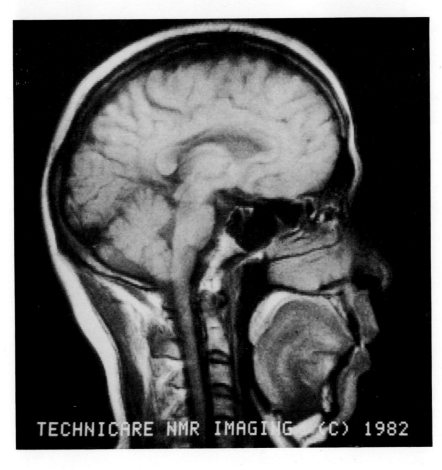

FIGURE 19
Sagittal section demonstrating normal cranial, facial, and cervical anatomy. Image obtained by a saturation-recovery pulse technique at a 5.0-kG-magnetic-field strength. (Courtesy of Technicare Corporation, Solon, Ohio.)

Various affects on other cephalic structures (bony involvement in Paget's disease, nasopharyngeal carcinoma, chronic sinusitis)

No attempt is made here to discuss critically these findings; they are simply mentioned to illustrate the rapidly accumulating experience in the NMR assessment of structural diseases of the central nervous system. Such efforts will undoubtedly continue to expand at a rapid pace. At the present time it appears that NMR is capable of visualizing lesions in the brain with the same accuracy and sensitivity as fourth-generation CT scans; further improvement in the clinical usefulness of NMR imaging may accompany the introduction into clinical practice of higher-field, whole-body imaging systems furnishing high-resolution, high signal-to-noise images such as those shown in Figs. 19 and 20.

PARAMAGNETISM AND NMR IMAGING

Paramagnetic species are substances (ions or small molecules) that increase the ability of another substance to become magnetized. They are currently being studied in NMR imaging as tracer or "contrast-enhancing" agents. Paramagnetic effects enhance the applied magnetic field experienced by nuclei neighboring on, or interacting with, paramagnetic species; in contrast, diamagnetic substances produce decreases of the magnetic field. Typically, a paramagnetic substance possesses an unpaired electron. The magnetic moment of an electron spin is 657 times larger than that of a proton and produces not only chemical-shift effects (see below) but also very marked changes in relaxation times. The presence of a paramagnetic species may provide the dominant relaxation mechanism within a sample, since an unpaired electron has a relaxation mechanism about 500,000 ($\sim 657^2$) times more efficient than that of a proton.

Most divalent transition-metal ions and trivalent lanthanide ions are paramagnetic, as are stable free radicals. Some molecules of biological interest naturally contain paramagnetic species such as Cu^{2+}, Fe^{3+}, and Mn^{2+} ions; in other cases, paramagnetic probes may be added to a system (e.g., by replacing Mg^{2+} with Mn^{2+} in certain enzyme reactions). In chemistry and physics, such paramagnetic probes have been

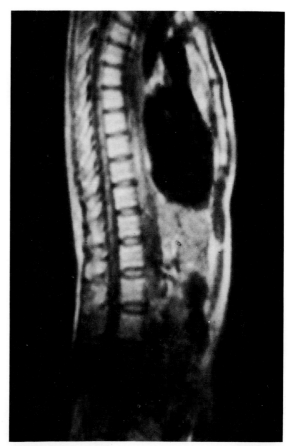

FIGURE 20
Sagittal section of the dorsolumbar spine area. Image obtained in a 3.0-kG system, using a two-dimensional acquisition and a saturation-recovery pulse technique. (Courtesy of Technicare Corporation, Solon. Ohio.)

quite useful in studies of molecular structure and kinetics; in NMR imaging, a small quantity of a paramagnetic substance has potential to enhance the visibility of a given molecular species in a magnetic field.

Most diseases tend to be associated with prolongations of T_1 relaxation times. Diseases in which there is an excessive accumulation of copper or iron would be expected to produce shortened T_1 relaxation times in the affected organs. Although Lawler et al noted morphological abnormalities in livers and brains of patients with Wilson's disease, measurements in vivo of T_1 relaxation times in affected regions were within normal limits, suggesting that the increased liver content in copper reflects an NMR-insensitive form (e.g., copper tightly bound in a protein complex). In some cases, but not all, of biliary cirrhosis, hemochromatosis, or hemosiderosis, liver T_1 relaxation times have been slightly shorter than those of normal liver.

Although used extensively for in vitro biochemical studies, the Mn^{2+} ion has had limited in vivo applications. NMR images of excised hearts from dogs in which 0.5 M solutions of $MnCl_2$ had been administered prior to experimental induction of myocardial infarction, have demonstrated an observable contrast differential between normally perfused and hypoperfused areas which permitted accurate quantification of infarct size. Mn^{2+} has also been used to label antimyosin monoclonal antibodies with high affinity for circumscribed areas of ischemic myocardial damage.

A major disadvantage of paramagnetic inorganic ions such as Fe^{3+}, Cu^{2+}, or Mn^{2+} is their toxicity. Furthermore, the relative lack of chemical versatility of these ions in forming magnetically active yet rapidly excreted and nontoxic compounds is likely to retard or prevent in vivo use of such ions as contrast media. Some researchers are actively investigating nitroxide-stable free radicals for potential applications in NMR imaging.

The oxygen molecule is a paramagnetic substance that is nontoxic and potentially of great biological interest. Chiarotti and Giulotto measured the effect of dissolved oxygen on the relaxation times of water protons and found that change in relaxation rate was indeed proportional to the concentration of oxygen molecules. In blood with an oxygen tension of 100 torr there is an oxygen concentration of about 4 parts per million. The results of manganese studies suggest that concentrations on the order of 1 part per million of paramagnetic metal ion in tissue can change tissue-proton relaxation rates. In tissues at normal oxygen tensions, paramagnetic oxygen would contribute only 1 to 2 percent of the bulk relaxation rate. But Gore et al. have demonstrated both in rabbits and in humans (Fig. 21) that breathing 100% oxygen for 15 min produced not only marginal increases in myocardial-pro-

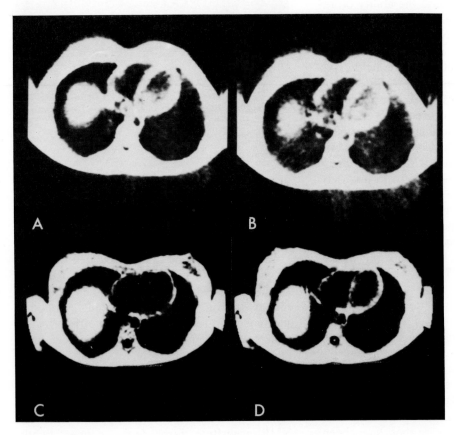

FIGURE 21

Inversion-recovery images transversely through the level of the human heart, with the subject breathing room air (A, C) and 100% oxygen (B, D). Note enhancement of the left-ventricular blood pool in B and, after appropriate windowing, also of the myocardium (D). (From JC Gore et al, in Nuclear MagneticResonance(NMR) Imaging, CL Partain et al (eds), Philadelphia, Saunders, 1983.)

ton-MNR-image intensity, but also a major reduction in T_1 relaxation times of the left (but not the right) intraventricular blood pool. The feasibility of applying similar techniques to enhance NMR imaging of the brain is currently undergoing investigation.

BIOCHEMICAL APPLICATIONS

The application of a magnetic field induces electronic currents in atoms and molecules resulting in an additional field at the nucleus (H_o σ), so that the total effective field at the nucleus is equal to $H_o(1 - \sigma)$, where σ is the shielding or screening constant. The local variations in the effective field are responsible for the separation of resonance frequencies (Fig. 22) from a suitably chosen reference for nuclei of a given species (e.g., ^{31}P); this phenomenon is called the *chemical shift*

(δ) and is expressed in terms of "dimensionless" units (viz., parts per million). The separation of resonance frequencies is, of course, proportional to the strength of the magnetic field; larger fields produce greater separations and hence improve the spectral resolution (Fig. 22).

High-resolution NMR spectroscopy relies on chemical-shift information to study the presence, amounts, and relationships of different chemical forms containing a given nuclear species, such as phosphorus. Important information on the structure of molecules has accumulated over the past 30 years; more recently, high-resolution spectroscopy has been applied to the in vitro and in vivo study of complex, heterogeneous biological samples. Recent technological and conceptual advances now allow direct clinical evaluation of certain biochemical processes in the human.

FIGURE 22

In complex samples, similar atomic nuclei occupying different chemical sites in a molecule may have slightly different resonance frequencies (chemical shift) depending on the detailed chemical structure of the molecule. These effects are also field dependent, as demonstrated by the low- (A) and high- (B) resolution ^1H spectra of ethyl alcohol. Similarly, an ide- *alized ^{31}P spectrum in the region of the high-energy phosphates (C) will typically show five or six clearly identifiable peaks: 1 to 3 = β, α, γ phosphates of ATP; 4 = phosphocreatine; 5 = inorganic phosphate; 6 = sugar phosphate. The three peaks from ATP are also shown at higher resolution as observed at the much higher field of 23.3 kG (D). (Cf. Figs. 23 and 24.)*

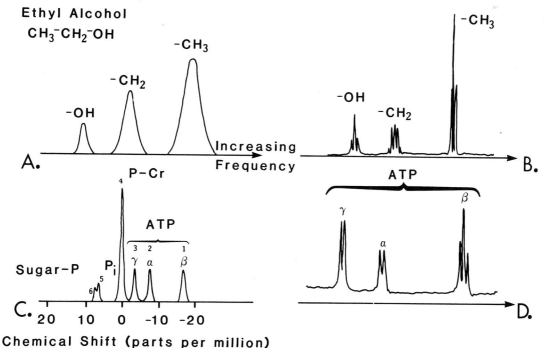

Because of the underlying physical phenomena, the chemical shift is small, only a few parts per million, and is observed only in magnetic fields with homogeneity exceeding 1 part in 10^6, which is usually obtainable only with high-field superconducting magnets. At present, most NMR-imaging magnets have homogeneities of only a few parts in 10^4 or 10^5 and are inadequate to resolve the small chemical-shift effects that occur in vivo. Since the absolute magnitude of the chemical shift is field dependent, it can be detected optimally by systems that utilize high-strength magnets (1.5 T). Most resistive magnets currently in use have field strengths less than 3.5 kG (0.35 T); superconductive magnets of 15 kG (1.5 T) field strength are currently in development for potential clinical use.

Several biologically relevant nuclei can theoretically be investigated in vivo by NMR spectroscopy (Table 1). Natural isotopic abundance, sensitivity to NMR detection, and physiological concentration are important in determining the potential clinical utility of such biological studies. The three nuclei that hold the greatest promise are ^{31}P, ^{13}C, and ^{23}Na.

A detailed review of the numerous in vitro studies or of various aspects of metabolism that have been investigated by NMR is beyond the scope of this article; interested readers are referred to any of several excellent current references. A few examples which illustrate the far-reaching potential of in vivo NMR-imaging metabolic studies will be given.

From a biological point of view, perhaps the most interesting nuclear species is phosphorous. ^{31}P NMR has been used to study several biochemical species and enzymatic reactions involving phosphocreatine and high-energy phosphates. Such experiments furnish information concerning the activity of enzymes, allow chemical identification and quantitation of products, permit determination of dissociation constants, and provide data for calculation of exchange rates in phosphorylation reactions. In 1960 Cohn and Hughes showed that the ^{31}P resonances of phosphates of adenosine are sensitive to pH. Shulman and coworkers have determined the concentration of phosphorylated metabolites such as ATP, ADP, and P. Measurement of the latter can be used, for example, to determine

intracellular pH and its changes directly by a noninvasive technique (Fig. 23).

By using surface coils, significant changes in phosphocreatine and ATP have been noted in regions affected after regional cardiac or cerebral ischemia. Similar variations have been reported in the process of altering a tissue from an aerobic to an anaerobic state or in ischemic muscles of rats; in the latter, pretreatment with verapamil and, to a lesser degree, with chlorpromazine tended to maintain levels of cardiac phosphocreatine and ATP near normal after coronary ischemia. Related studies have been performed on the brains of living animals and in human limbs. Thus, tetanic contractions of muscle over 1 min reveal total loss of phosphocreatine, with a marked increase in P_i and a pH shift a few tenths of a unit toward acidity, changes which recover over approximately 20 min. Further technological advances have permitted the study of similar changes in internal organs. Topical magnetic resonance utilizes a high-field (e.g., 1.9 T) superconductive magnet and high-order field gradients to produce a defined volume of a homogeneous magnetic field, 1 part in 10^7 or better, from which to record a high-resolution spectrum.

The logical extension of topical magnetic resonance and surface coil studies to the in vivo demonstration of abnormal metabolic pathways and processes was recently reported. In a case of McArdle's syndrome evaluated during aerobic and ischemic exercise, ^{31}P studies revealed a paradoxical increase in the P_i peak (Fig. 23), consistent with the underlying inability of such patients to break down glycogen. Similar studies have also been reported in cases of phosphofructokinase deficiency.

Another example of a potential clinical application of in vivo NMR spectroscopy is the assessment of the viability of kidneys harvested for transplantation. Screening of human kidneys has been undertaken with the rationale that a kidney able to maintain a high tissue pH would have suffered minimal ischemic damage and would have a better chance of being successfully transplanted. Tissue pH as measured from the P_i shift in ^{31}P NMR studies is only one aspect of the potential usefulness of biochemical studies of organs.

Bottomley and collaborators have recently

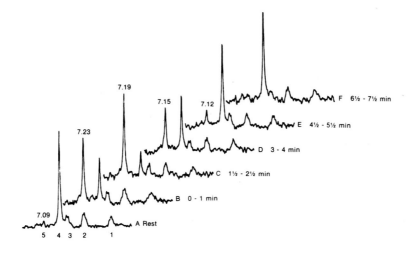

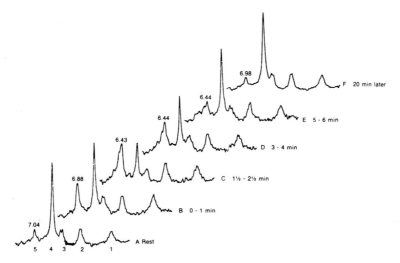

FIGURE 23

In vivo phosphorus (³¹P) NMR spectra in a control subject (upper set) and in a patient with McArdle's disease (lower set), showing the effects of ischemic exercise. Peak assignments as in Fig. 22C. Values of pH are given above each inorganic phosphate peak. The first spectrum in each set (A) was recorded at rest before exercise; subsequent spectra (B to F) were recorded during the periods shown. Exercise was maintained during the period from zero to 1½ min in the normal subject and from zero to ¾ min in the patient, but arterial occlusion was maintained for up to 3 min before arterial flow was restored. Ischemic exercise produced a greater decrease in phosphocreatine (peak 4) in the patient than in the normal subject and was accompanied with a decrease in intracellular pH; there were no changes in ATP (peaks 1 to 3) concentrations. (From Ross et al.)

demonstrated the feasibility of proton imaging coupled with surface coil ³¹P for in vivo spectrometry of the human brain. High-resolution spatial images were obtained in a 1.5-T, whole-body superconducting magnet. The images were used to guide placement of the surface coils (Fig. 24). The technique shows great promise for potential applications to study biochemical changes in the brain, although, at present, the relatively large volume sampled by surface coils limits their useful application mainly to organs or tissues close to the body surface.

High-resolution NMR spectroscopy, by virtue of its noninvasive nature and absence of radia-

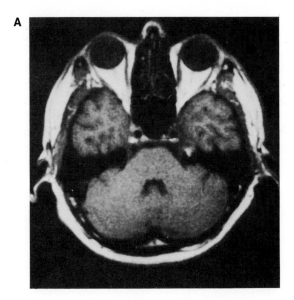

A

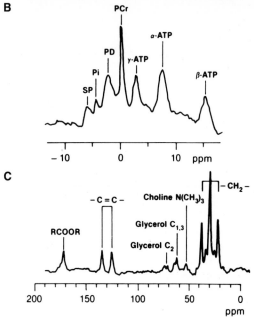

B

C

FIGURE 24

Nuclear magnetic resonance imaging and spectroscopy studies of the human head. (A) 4-mm-thick, high resolution portion of an NMR image of the human head obtained at 1.5 T. (B) ^{31}P NMR spectrum from temple with a 6.5-µm surface coil applied within the same system. The coil samples a volume surrounded by the coil circumference and one radius deep. As in previous figures, chemical shifts are in parts per million relative to phosphocreatine. PD = phosphodiesters. The spectrum includes a subjacent broad hump deriving from phospholipids and mineral phosphates in bone. (C) ^{13}C NMR spectrum recorded from the same areas as in (B). Chemical shifts are relative to tetramethylsilane. CH_2 = alkyl carbons; RCOOR = carboxyl groups; —C≡C— = double-bonded carbons; glycerol $C_{1,2,3}$ = triglyceride carbons. (From Bottomley et al, Lancet 2:273, 1983.)

tion exposure, can be anticipated to provide exciting new methods for in vivo study of metabolism, adding new dimensions to the frontiers of clinical medicine.

SAFETY

One of the attributes of NMR techniques that has made it appealing for clinical use is the apparent lack of a significant health hazard. A major advantage is the absence of operator or patient exposure to ionizing radiation. However, it must be recalled that subjects undergoing NMR studies may be exposed for up to a few hours to both strong static and dynamically changing magnetic fields, as well as to frequently repeated pulses of RF energy. Numerous articles, chapters, symposia proceedings, and books have reported studies concerning the potential biological hazards in NMR applications. At best, the reported results have been contradictory or not replicated despite fastidious attempts to follow previously published experimental conditions. The reader is referred to the recent critical reviews by Budinger and by Saunders and Orr for their detailed expositions and extensive bibliographies. The current state of knowledge is briefly summarized below.

Three possible sources of biohazards associated with NMR can be envisioned: effects associated with (1) RF fields, (2) strong static magnetic fields, and (3) rapidly changing magnetic fields which may produce induced currents in tissues.

The known biological hazards associated with RF fields are related to heating effects produced by absorbed power, diathermy being a common example. Threshold values of 1.5 W per kilogram of body weight for long-duration studies, and of 4 W/kg for studies lasting 10 min or less, have been proposed as being safe from the point of view of tissue heating. Most heating occurs at the surface of the body, and, due to body shape and to the heterogeneity of tissues, hot spots are expected to occur. Thus, heating around the ribs, groin, or axillae was noted to be increased sixfold relative to the very small whole-body heating. In the worst-case situation of surgical clips or metallic prostheses (uncooled by blood flow), no significant heating has been noted in NMR studies. Budinger has calculated that the expected temperature increase [in soft tissue assumed to have a specific heat of 0.83 (kcal/kg)/°C] is less than 0.7°C for a specific absorbed power of 4 W/kg for ten min. In biological tissues such effects would be expected to be maximized where heat dissipation (e.g., by blood flow) is poorest (e.g., in testes or lens oculi). Pathological changes have been induced in mouse testes by acute exposure producing absorbed power in excess of 20 W/kg. It can be concluded that no evidence exists to suggest a substantial risk by virtue of RF effects.

The issue of detrimental effects from strong static magnetic fields remains sub judice: conflicting evidence has been reported in a vast literature regarding cellular, animal, and human studies, and—with the exception of certain electrocardiographic abnormalities discussed below—no reproducible, conclusive evidence has been offered to substantiate the various purported harmful effects. As summarized by Budinger, mechanisms whereby magnetic fields

might influence biological processes include (a) changes in macromolecular orientation altering chemical kinetics or membrane permeability, (b) changes in enzyme kinetics, (c) reductions of nerve-conduction velocity, and (d) superposition of induced-flow electropotentials on natural biopotentials. Thresholds for the first three mechanisms are 1 to 20 T or above and are not likely to play a significant role in clinical NMR-imaging studies.

Changes in magnetic fields produce electric field changes. In tissue, this may occur either when the magnetic field changes in relation to tissues or when tissue is in motion in relation to the magnetic field. Measurable flow potentials of a few millivolts may be induced by fields above 0.2 T. Flow of blood perpendicular to a static magnetic field will generate a potential across the diameter of the vessel. The magnitude of the flow potential is proportional to the blood vessel diameter and to blood velocity. For humans placed in the most commonly used magnet designs (i.e., with the field parallel to the long axis of the body), a major flow potential would be generated up to 5 cm into the aortic arch and theoretically would be on the order of a few millivolts per tesla. It is unlikely that these small flow potentials have any physiologic effect. In our experience with over 400 subjects studied up to 2 h in a 0.147-T system, no symptoms have been reported by these individuals and there have been no clinically detectable changes in blood pressure or pulse. Moreover, infants treated at the Massachusetts General Hospital for esophageal atresia by electromagnetic bouginage have been exposed for many weeks to high-intensity magnetic fields without adverse effects.

Rapidly changing, dynamic magnetic fields induce electric currents in tissue in direct proportion to the rate of change of the magnetic field. Thus, the induction of sensation of flashing lights ("magnetophosphenes") or of a metallic taste, or the stimulation of peripheral nerves in animals and humans, has been reported. However, the conditions required to produce these effects involve much higher fields and time-varying magnetic-field gradients than those used in clinical NMR imaging. For example, to stimulate peripheral nerves in limbs of humans, 180-ms pulsed magnetic fields of circa 10^4 T are required. According to guidelines issued by the U.S. Bureau of Radiological Health in February 1982, time-varying magnetic fields of 3 T/s do not present an unacceptable risk; the National Radiological Protection Board of the United Kingdom Guidelines suggest that the rate of change should not exceed 20 T/s for pulse of 10 ms or longer.

The above discussion should not be interpreted to mean that anyone may safely approach or enter a large magnetic field. Certain types of pacemakers may become reprogrammed or converted from demand-mode to fixed-rate mode after exposure to a high-intensity magnetic field; furthermore, the pacemaker electrode may potentially conduct induced currents. Similarly, patients with metallic implants (e.g., surgical or vascular clips) must not be exposed. The longitudinal forces and torques exerted on certain clips may be sufficient to risk dislodgement of the clip or injury to surrounding tissue. For these reasons, patients with pacemakers or metallic implants should not enter strong magnetic fields, the fringes of which may extend for 10 to 15 feet from the magnet core. System operators and staff may also find that magnetically encoded cards (such as bank and charge cards and magnetic keys) will be erased by exposure to a large magnetic field.

CONCLUSIONS

This brief overview of ^{1}H NMR imaging in neurological disorders confirms the widespread excitement regarding the potential of this new approach. It is apparent already that NMR imaging has several advantages over conventional x-ray CT scans: NMR imaging does not rely on ionizing radiation; it presents few, if any, biological hazards; it exploits inherent tissue-biophysical characteristics to provide superior contrast resolution; and it is intrinsically a whole-volume-imaging technique. Furthermore, its accuracy and sensitivity for detecting lesions in the brain are equal to or better than that of CT scans in many areas.

Because the information contained in an ^{1}H-NMR-imaging study depends on proton physicochemical characteristics, it provides the exciting capability, already reported from nonimaging experiments, of noninvasive in vivo biochemical studies of tissue. Further research is required to determine the role and impact of this new methodology in the practice of clinical neurology.

References

BUDINGER TF: Potential medical effects and hazards of human NMR studies, in *Nuclear Magnetic Resonance Imaging in Medicine,* L Kaufman et al (eds). New York, Igaku-Shoin, 1981, pp 207–231

BUONANNO FS et al: ^{1}H nuclear magnetic resonance imaging in multiple sclerosis, in *Neurologic Clinics Symposium on Multiple Sclerosis,* J Antel (ed) Philadelphia, Saunders, 1983, pp 757–764

—— et al: Proton NMR imaging in experimental ischemic infarction. Stroke 14:178, 1983

—— et al: Proton (^{1}H) NMR imaging in cerebral infarction in *Cerebral Vascular Disease 4,* JS Meyer et al (eds). Amsterdam, Excerpta Medica, 1983, pp 71–75

—— et al: Proton NMR imaging of normal and abnormal brain: Experimental and clinical observations, in *NMR Imaging,* RL Witcofski et al (eds). Winston-Salem, NC, Bowman Gray School of Medicine Press, 1982, pp 147–157

BYDDER GM et al: Clinical NMR imaging of the brain: 140 cases. AJR 139:215, 1982

CHIAROTTI G, GIULOTTO L: Proton relaxation in water. Physiol Rev 93:1241, 1954

COHN M, HUGHES TR JR: Phosphorus magnetic resonance spectra of adenosine di- and triphosphate: I. Effect of pH. J Biol Chem 235:3250, 1960

DAMADIAN R (ed): *NMR in Medicine.* New York, Springer-Verlag, 1981, pp 1–16, 59–80

EDWARDS RHT et al: Clinical use of nuclear magnetic resonance in the investigation of myopathy. Lancet 1:725, 1982

GADIAN DG: *Nuclear Magnetic Resonance and Its Applications to Living Systems.* Oxford, Clarendon Press, 1982

GOLDMAN MR et al: Quantification of experimental myocardial infarction using nuclear magnetic resonance imaging with paramagnetic ion contrast enhancement in excised canine hearts. Circulation 66:1012, 1982

HUTCHISON JMS, SMITH FW: Human imaging, in *Nuclear Magnetic Resonance Imaging in Medicine,* L Kaufman et al (eds). New York, Igaku-Shoin, 1981, pp 101–127

KISTLER JP et al: Vertebral basilar territory stroke: Delineation by proton nuclear magnetic resonance imaging, Stroke (in press)

LAI CM, LAUTERBUR PC: True three-dimensional image reconstruction by nuclear magnetic resonance zeugmatography. Phys Med Biol 26:851, 1981

LAWLER GA et al: Nuclear magnetic resonance (NMR) imaging in Wilson Disease. J Comput Assist Tomogr 7:1, 1983

LUKES SA et al: Nuclear magnetic resonance imaging in multiple sclerosis. Ann Neurol 13:592, 1983

MANSFIELD P, PYKETT IL: Biological and medical imaging by NMR. J Mag Res 29:355, 1978

OOT R et al: Preliminary assessment of ^{1}H NMR imaging of pituitary adenoma. Am J Neuroradiol (in press)

PYKETT IL et al: Techniques and approaches to proton NMR imaging of the head. Comp Radiol 7:1, 1983

ROSS BD et al: Examination of a case of suspected McArdle's syndrome by ^{31}P nuclear magnetic resonance. N Engl J Med 304:1338, 1981

SAUNDERS RD, ORR JS: Biological effects of NMR, in *Nuclear Magnetic Resonance (NMR) Imaging,* CL Partain et al (eds). Philadelphia, Saunders, 1983

SHULMAN RG et al: Cellular applications of ^{31}P and ^{13}C nuclear magnetic resonance. Science 205:160, 1979

SINGER JR, CROOKS LE: Nuclear magnetic resonance blood flow measurements in the human brain. Science 221:654, 1983

SMITH FW et al: Nuclear magnetic resonance tomographic imaging in liver disease. Lancet 1:963, 1981

YOUNG IR et al: Nuclear magnetic resonance imaging of the brain in multiple sclerosis. Lancet 2:1063, 1981

CONSERVATIVE MANAGEMENT OF CHRONIC RENAL FAILURE

RALPH A. KELLY and WILLIAM E. MITCH

Chronic renal failure (CRF) is defined as an irreversible loss of kidney function leading to accumulation of the products of protein metabolism and, ultimately, to symptoms of uremia. There are two prominent characteristics of CRF. First, after initial damage to the kidney, CRF is progressive and the rate of loss of residual renal function can be estimated reliably. In virtually all patients, this rate of loss is constant (Fig. 1). Second, the development of uremic symptoms is closely linked to the accumulation of waste products derived from protein catabolism.

It has been commonly assumed that patients with CRF will inevitably require dialysis and that therapy should be directed solely at minimizing uremic symptoms. Thus, "conservative" management previously had consisted of dietary potassium and phosphate restriction when hyperkalemia or hyperphosphatemia was found, modest limitation of dietary protein when uremic symptoms such as nausea and fatigue became apparent, control of hypertension, and treatment of infections and other reversible causes of renal dysfunction so as to minimize complications during the inexorable descent to dialysis. In occasional patients, attempts have been made to treat certain diseases affecting the kidney, using immunosuppressive drugs or corticosteroids. However, since dialysis has always been considered inevitable, common wisdom has held that conservative management should not include placing more restrictions on the patient than dialysis itself would necessarily impose, especially since too vigorous protein restriction might lead to malnutrition. Indeed, it has been suggested that

asymptomatic patients with CRF require no specific treatment. However, we intend to detail the therapeutic principles by which uremic symptoms can be controlled. In addition, we will show that protein restriction and careful medical management might alter the constant rate of deterioration of renal function and therefore should probably be initiated early in the course of renal failure. Specifically, we will discuss nutritional therapy of patients with CRF and the impact of this therapy on the progression of the disease. For a more extensive discussion of the other goals in Table 1 and the pathophysiology of CRF, see Kelly and Mitch, and Schrier and Anderson.

NITROGENOUS WASTE PRODUCTS AND UREMIA

The syndrome of uremia is due to complex metabolic consequences of a decrease in functioning renal mass. The predominant biochemical result is the retention of waste products of nitrogen metabolism. Although the precise nature of the

TABLE 1
Goals of conservative management of chronic renal failure

Reverse factors adversely affecting renal function
Correct electrolyte abnormalities
Minimize alterations in calcium and phosphate
  homeostasis
Reduce symptoms caused by accumulation of waste
  products
Maintain protein nutrition
Retard the progression of renal insufficiency

199

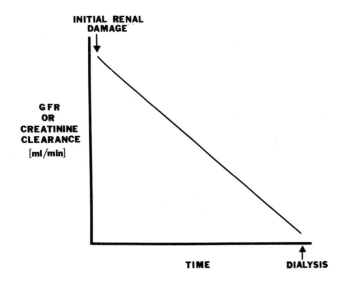

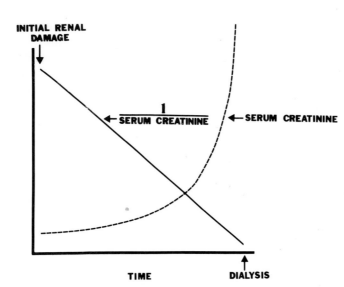

FIGURE 1
The course of chronic renal failure (CRF) in an individual patient is represented in the upper panel as a constant rate of loss of glomerular filtration rate (GFR) (or creatinine clearance) with time. The lower panel indicates that the constant rate of loss of renal function can be estimated by plotting the decline in the reciprocal of serum creatinine with time; analyzing the rise in serum creatinine with time is more difficult. Time is in months or years depending upon the rapidity of the loss of renal function in an individual patient (see Fig. 3).

putative toxins of uremia is unknown, uremic symptoms correlate closely with the serum urea nitrogen concentration (SUN). This is because changes in the SUN closely parallel the degree of retention of all nitrogenous waste products in the body. In addition, there is evidence that urea itself may be toxic. For example, when the SUN of stable, well-dialyzed patients was maintained at a level greater than 150 mg/dl for more than a week by adding urea to the dialysis bath, uremic symptoms including nausea, gastrointestinal distress, and fatigue occurred even though other waste products were effectively removed by maintaining an otherwise regular dialysis schedule. This does not mean necessarily that urea itself is the only uremic toxin. It may be that a metabolite of urea (e.g., ammonia) or a combination of urea and other waste products produces uremic symptoms. Regardless, the rate of accumulation of urea always is directly related to the quantity of protein ingested, and hence can be used as an index of the accumulation of other protein-derived toxins. This relationship also permits the SUN to be used in measuring the urea appearance rate. This rate provides an easily calculated and reliable means of monitoring compliance with the different low-protein diets we will discuss.

Urea nitrogen appearance

The urea nitrogen appearance rate or the net rate of urea nitrogen production is equal to the quantity of urea nitrogen "appearing" in urine and body water each day. Because gut bacteria degrade urea contained in gastrointestinal secretions to ammonia which is reabsorbed, there is essentially no urea nitrogen in the stool. There is a close correlation between the urea nitrogen appearance rate and total nitrogen intake or excretion because protein nitrogen is converted almost completely to urea nitrogen in both normal and uremic subjects. Moreover, the quantity of dietary nitrogen not ultimately converted to urea remains remarkably constant at 2 to 3 g of nitrogen per day in spite of large changes in dietary protein. Thus, if nitrogen intake is known, nitrogen balance can be estimated easily from the urea nitrogen appearance rate (Table 2).

An important potential error in calculating the

urea nitrogen appearance rate and nitrogen balance of the CRF patient is to disregard changes in the urea nitrogen pool. There is little fluctuation in the size of the urea pool of normal subjects because the kidneys rapidly excrete urea formed. In the CRF patient, however, a small change in the SUN can mean that a large change in the urea nitrogen pool has occurred, thereby significantly affecting the estimation of nitrogen balance. In calculating the size of this pool, it is fortunate that urea is distributed equally throughout body water so that its volume of distribution can be estimated reliably as 60 percent of body weight (i.e., total body water) of nonedematous subjects. This estimate of body water (in liters) multiplied by the SUN (expressed as mg/liter) gives the size of the urea pool in milligrams of urea nitrogen. In the measurement of nitrogen balance, changes in the amount of nitrogen in this pool are calculated as the difference in the urea nitrogen pool size over time. To calculate the urea nitrogen appearance rate, this daily rate of accumulation (which may be either positive or negative) is added to the average daily rate of urea nitrogen excretion measured during the same period (Table 2). When weight and the SUN are stable, the urea nitrogen appearance

TABLE 2

Use of urea kinetics to estimate nitrogen balance

$$B_N = I_N - U - NUN \tag{1}$$

$$B_N = I_N - (U_U V + \Delta) - 2.5 \text{ gN/day}$$

where B_N = nitrogen balance in grams of nitrogen (gN) per day
I_N = nitrogen intake in gN per day (16% of protein intake)
U = urea nitrogen appearance excretion in gN per day
Δ = change in urea nitrogen pool in gN per day
SUN = serum urea nitrogen concentration in mg/dl
C_{Urea} = urea clearance
NUN = nonurea nitrogen excretion in gN per day

$$SUN = \left(\frac{I_N - 2.5}{C_{Urea}} \right) \times 100 \tag{2}$$

Example: Urea clearance 6 ml/min or 8.64 liters/day
(creatinine clearance about 10 ml/min)

Dietary protein, g	*I_N − 2.5 gN per day*	*Steady state SUN, mg/dl*
40	3.9	45
60	7.1	83
80	10.3	120

The relationships between the urea nitrogen appearance rate, nitrogen balance, and urea clearance in Eq. (2) allow estimation of the steady state SUN that should be observed for a given protein intake rate equals the daily rate of urinary urea nitrogen excretion.

Nonurea nitrogen excretion

There are changes in the metabolism of nonurea nitrogen-containing compounds in uremic subjects, although the clinical importance of these changes depends upon the degree of imbalance between production and elimination of each of the products. For example, it has been shown that uric acid is degraded extensively by gastrointestinal bacteria of uremic patients and that this partially compensates for the lower capacity of the kidney to excrete uric acid. Consequently, the rise in serum uric acid levels is limited. The biological importance of this extrarenal clearance of uric acid and of other nitrogenous waste products might at first seem considerable. However, since the compounds are simply converted to another retained product that may be no less toxic, an increased extrarenal clearance does not reduce the quantity of retained waste nitrogen.

The quantity of nitrogen in the stool of CRF patients usually is not increased, though it occasionally may be higher because of low-grade, occult gastrointestinal bleeding. It may vary, however, because prolonged, severe dietary protein restriction, or intravenous hyperalimentation, can decrease fecal nitrogen to very low levels.

In patients with the nephrotic syndrome, the amount of protein in the urine must be included in the calculation of nitrogen balance and the dietary protein requirement. This is especially important when protein-restricted diets are used to treat these patients because 1.2 g per day of "high-quality" protein should be added to the diet for every gram of protein lost each day. The higher amount is necessary because protein synthesis is not 100 percent efficient; if this higher amount is not provided, negative nitrogen balance and protein wasting will occur.

As we have noted, the rate of nonurea nitrogen excretion varies only slightly from day to day. This rate, which is the difference between total nitrogen excretion and the urea nitrogen appearance rate, averages 2 to 3 g of nitrogen per day. Using this average value and the calculated urea nitrogen appearance rate that must result from a given amount of dietary protein,

the steady state SUN for a patient can be predicted, assuming that the patient is in nitrogen balance (Table 2). If the measured SUN is substantially higher than the calculated SUN, either dietary compliance is poor, or less commonly, urea nitrogen is being produced from another source of protein such as hemoglobin resulting from gastrointestinal bleeding or accelerated catabolism of endogenous protein. For most patients, this simple calculation also can be used to monitor compliance with the dietary regimen or to estimate nitrogen balance (Table 2).

DESIGNING A DIET FOR THE RENAL FAILURE PATIENT

In order to limit waste-product accumulation in patients with CRF, it is universally acknowledged that protein intake must be reduced. However, unresolved questions remain. When should dietary protein restriction be instituted? To what level should protein intake be reduced? Can the progressive loss of renal function be slowed or reversed by nutritional therapy? The following guidelines seem reasonable and prudent. Subtle symptoms of uremia usually can be detected when the SUN has reached 60 mg/dl. Therefore, dietary protein should be restricted at this level of SUN to avoid developing more obvious symptoms. If this is done using the principles discussed below, malnutrition will be avoided and uremic symptoms reduced; in addition, the progressive loss of renal function may be slowed. It should be emphasized that when these principles are followed, protein depletion and loss of lean body mass will not occur.

Protein requirement

A major factor limiting the degree to which dietary protein can be restricted in both normal subjects and uremic patients is the necessity for a dietary source of utilizable nitrogen for synthesizing body protein. This means that there is a requirement for dietary protein containing a high proportion of essential amino acids (EAA) (i.e., high-quality protein). For healthy young adults, a mixture of as little as 7 g per day of the nine EAA can maintain nitrogen balance if there is an additional 2.5 g per day of dietary nitrogen.

Larger amounts of EAA are required for growing children. If EAA requirements are provided solely in the protein available in foods, at least 0.5 to 0.6 g of protein per kilogram body weight per day of high-quality protein (e.g., eggs or lean meat) is necessary to ensure neutral nitrogen balance. In catabolic (infected or traumatized) subjects, the protein requirement rises sharply.

Early studies suggested that patients with CRF were different from normal subjects and could achieve neutral nitrogen balance at a substantially lower intake of high-quality protein such as that supplied in the Giordano-Giovannetti diet. This apparently different requirement for EAA of CRF patients led to the postulate that they could synthesize amino acids from the ammonia nitrogen derived from their circulating urea. However, this biochemical reaction actually directs ammonia nitrogen toward resynthesis of urea rather than toward amino acid synthesis. Indeed, detailed, quantitative studies have failed to confirm the hypothesis that urea reutilization contributes significantly to the protein nutrition of CRF patients. For example, it has been shown that no more than 2 to 6 percent of the nitrogen in albumin of uremic subjects can be derived from urea degradation. In fact, when urea degradation was suppressed in such patients using oral, nonabsorbable aminoglycoside antibiotics, analysis of urea kinetics revealed that ammonia derived from urea degradation was simply recycled to urea. Importantly, studies have shown definitively that the minimum protein requirement of CRF patients does not differ from that of normal subjects; it is about 40 g per day, of which at least 24 g should be high-quality protein. Thus, a diet of 40 g of protein per day (Table 3) will maintain neutral nitrogen balance and will prevent loss of lean body mass while diminishing uremic symptoms. As pointed out in Table 2, the SUN will be maintained below 60 mg/dl with a diet of 40 g of protein per day as long as the creatinine clearance exceeds 10 ml per minute. It should be emphasized that this diet restricts the variety of foods that can be eaten because of the requirement that a high proportion of the protein be of high quality. Therefore, compliance can be a major obstacle to using this diet.

To assess the nutritional status of patients on this and other protein-restricted diets, plasma proteins, weight, and mid upper arm circumference, in addition to other anthropometric indexes, should be measured repetitively. The best indications of adequate protein nutrition are maintenance of weight and normal values of serum albumin and transferrin.

Essential amino acid supplements

When creatinine clearance is less than 10 ml per minute, dietary protein must be restricted below the level of 40 g per day in order to maintain a reasonable SUN. This can be accomplished by giving a supplement of EAA or their nitrogen-free analogues. By supplying EAA, the variety of foods from which the patient can choose is greater, despite the lower total protein intake. Representative diets containing 40 and 25 g protein per day are presented in Table 3. The greater flexibility with the 25 g protein per day diet has been a major factor in achieving compliance with the supplemented regimens. In addition, because the requirements for EAA are being met at a lower nitrogen intake, there is less accumulation of waste products.

There have been several studies of the acceptability and efficacy of a regimen of 15 to 25 g of protein per day (about 0.35 g/kg per day) of unrestricted quality given with an EAA supplement provided in capsules or tablets. Generally, at least 14 g of EAA including histidine has been prescribed. In early studies metabolic acidosis developed occasionally because certain EAA were given as their acid salts, but lysine is now given as the acetate salt and histidine is given as the free base and this complication rarely occurs. In most subjects, institution of this regimen promptly improved uremic symptoms and promoted neutral nitrogen balance. Even though protein intake was so limited, muscle strength increased and serum albumin and transferrin levels were maintained in spite of severe renal insufficiency (i.e., serum creatinine greater than 10 mg/dl). Without such a regimen, the patients would have developed anorexia, nausea and vomiting, loss of muscle mass, and low plasma proteins because of the catabolic effects of severe uremia. Thus, there is good evidence that a low-protein diet supplemented with EAA is an effective method of maintaining lean body mass and decreasing uremic symptoms. This reg-

TABLE 3

Sample diet of 40 g per day of predominantly high-quality protein and the 25 g per day of mixed-quality protein diet to be supplemented with essential amino acids or their nitrogen-free analogues

40 g per day	*25 g per day*
BREAKFAST	
3/4 cup Cream of Wheat with sugar	1 cup cornflakes
1/2 cup whole milk	1/2 cup nondairy creamer*
1/2 grapefruit with sugar	1 slice rye toast with margarine
2 slices pumpernickel toast with margarine and jelly	1 cup mixed fruit
	8 oz fruit juice
Coffee with nondairy creamer*	1 cup coffee with nondairy creamer*
LUNCH	
1 fried egg	Large green salad (with tomatoes, cucumbers, and radishes)
2 slices pumpernickel toast with margarine and jelly	2 tbsp French dressing
1 can ginger ale	1 slice rye bread with margarine
2 sugar cookies	1 cup mixed fruit
3/4 cup canned peaches	8 oz fruit juice
SUPPER	
2 oz steak	1 oz lamb chop
1 baked potato with margarine	1/4 cup corn
1 cup asparagus with margarine	1/2 cup green beans
Tossed green salad (with tomatoes)	2 tbsp margarine
2 tbsp French dressing	1/2 cup cranberry sauce
Jello	1 slice rye bread with margarine
1 can ginger ale	1 cup sliced fresh pears
1 cup coffee with nondairy creamer* and sugar	8 oz fruit juice
3/4 cup canned pears	1 cup coffee with nondairy creamer*
SNACK	
1 can ginger ale	Coffee with nondairy creamer*
50 g hard candy	4 oz hard candy
TOTALS FOR DAY	
Calories	
2422	2520
Protein	
40 g	25 g
Sodium	
1766 mg	1290 mg
Potassium	
2389 mg	3598 mg
Phosphorus	
761 mg	465 mg

* *Coffeemate or Polyperx*

imen generally is more acceptable than a 40 g per day predominantly high-quality protein diet, presumably because a greater variety of foods is permitted.

The proportions of EAA usually prescribed for patients with CRF are identical to those recommended for normal subjects. However, it is likely that these proportions are not optimal for the following reasons: (1) plasma and intracellular concentrations of amino acids in uremic patients differ markedly from those of normal subjects; (2) there are specific defects in amino acid metabolism in patients with renal failure; (3) during dietary restriction of one or more amino acids, plasma amino acid levels change in a pattern different from that observed in normal subjects.

Recent studies have used different proportions of amino acids to treat patients with CRF in order to normalize the amino acid patterns. For example, the nonessential amino acid, tyrosine, has been added since inadequate amounts of this amino acid in the diet could limit protein synthesis. Other changes have included increasing the content of several of the EAAs, specifically, valine, lysine, and threonine, above the level recommended for normal subjects. This supplement has been found to normalize the concentrations of amino acids in plasma and in muscle cells during long-term therapy. During clinical trials, it appears that overall nitrogen metabolism is improved with this supplement, at least compared to a supplement based simply on the minimum daily requirements of EAA for normal subjects.

Nitrogen-free analogues of essential amino acids

Nitrogen intake can be reduced even further than with EAA supplements if the carbon skeletons of EAA (ketoanalogues, Fig. 2) are prescribed. These compounds, in which the alpha amino group is replaced by a ketone, can be transaminated to form the respective EAA. Seven ketoanalogues of the nine EAA have been used successfully to replace the respective EAA in the diet of experimental animals. The ketoanalogues of the other two EAA, lysine and threonine, do not undergo transamination and, therefore, these EAA must be provided in the diet. There also have been studies demonstrating that ketoanalogues can replace the corresponding EAA in the diet of humans. The importance of these compounds for conservative therapy of patients with CRF is that their use allows a further reduction in dietary nitrogen and hence will reduce the accumulation of nitrogenous waste products. Studies of a regimen consisting of ketoanalogues added to a diet of 25 g of protein per day indicate that nitrogen balance will remain neutral and serum protein levels will be maintained, indicating conservation of body protein. It should be pointed out, however, that neither the amino acid analogues nor an EAA supplement

FIGURE 2

The conversion of the α-ketoanalogue of an essential amino acid to the corresponding amino acid. The source of NH_2 is glutamate. Excess ketoacids are used as an energy source and metabolized to CO_2 and H_2O.

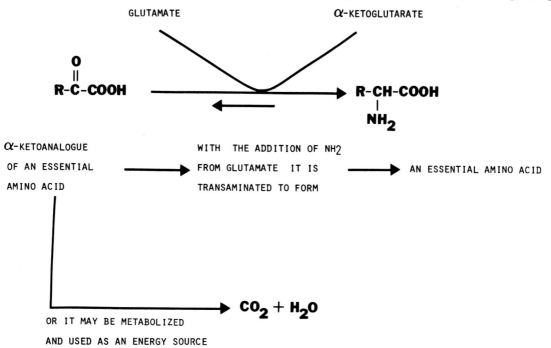

had any substantial nutritional benefit for uremic subjects who were eating more than the minimum daily protein requirement of 40 g per day. In this case, the excess EAA or ketoanalogues were presumably degraded rather than used for synthesis of new protein.

When effectiveness of isomolar proportions has been compared in subjects with CRF, protein nutrition appeared to be improved as judged by the somewhat higher levels of serum transferrin and other proteins achieved with the analogue supplement than with the EAA supplement despite the lower nitrogen intake and, consequently, the lower SUN achieved. In other studies, analogue supplements have reduced the rate of urea nitrogen appearance more than an almost isonitrogenous mixture of EAA and also appeared to have a more beneficial effect on nitrogen balance. The reason for this apparent advantage over EAA supplements is unknown, but the results suggest that the analogues affect overall protein metabolism in some manner beyond their capacity to substitute for the respective EAA. The metabolic basis for this is becoming clearer since the ketoanalogue of leucine (α-ketoisocaproate) has been shown to reduce endogenous protein catabolism. This effect not only would reduce the accumulation of waste products derived from breakdown of endogenous protein, it also would lower the amount of new protein that would have to be synthesized each day in order to maintain neutral nitrogen balance.

In most early studies of amino acid analogues in patients with CRF, it was noted that occasional patients developed gastrointestinal distress, perhaps related to the high calcium content of the supplement because the analogues were given as calcium salts. As a result, about 5 percent of patients developed hypercalcemia during long-term therapy. In addition, the regimen frequently lowered serum phosphorus sharply, possibly because of increased tissue anabolism and because dietary phosphate was lower as a consequence of the lower protein intake. This decrease in plasma phosphorus may explain why ketoacid therapy can ameliorate the secondary hyperparathyroidism of CRF which is presumably a consequence of hyperphosphatemia.

A new ketoanalogue supplement which does not include extra calcium was designed to provide more optimal proportions of ketoacids and amino acids based on the considerations detailed previously. In this supplement, ketoacids of the branched-chain amino acids are given as salts of basic amino acids (ornithine, lysine, and histidine); in addition, tyrosine, threonine, and small amounts of the hydroxyanalogue of methionine are given but the analogues of phenylalanine and tryptophan are omitted. At least some phenylalanine and tryptophan are provided in the diet when this supplement is given with 25 g per day of dietary protein. During long-term evaluation of this regimen in patients with severe CRF [average estimated glomerular filtration rate (GFR) is 4.8 ml per minute], there were several encouraging findings: nitrogen balance was neutral or positive, the urea nitrogen appearance rate was lowered, and normal plasma concentrations of albumin and transferrin were maintained in some patients for 2 years or more. (Since the supplement plus the dietary protein did not provide the quantities of all EAA required for normal subjects, it must be concluded that EAA requirements of CRF patients are different from those of normal subjects.) In summary, ketoanalogue therapy has been shown to be successful in maintaining protein nutrition while effectively reducing uremic symptoms even in patients with advanced CRF. We suggest that the impact of nutritional therapy might be far greater if it were initiated at an earlier stage of CRF, since the toxic effect of excessive dietary protein on residual renal function might be avoided (see below).

Protein requirement for dialysis patients

We should emphasize that patients being treated by dialysis have markedly different protein requirements than nondialyzed patients. The protein requirement of patients undergoing maintenance intermittent hemodialysis is at least 1 g of protein per kilogram body weight per day containing a large proportion of high-quality protein. Since the minimum daily protein requirement for patients with CRF not being dialyzed (0.5 to 0.6 g/kg per day) is the same as that of normal subjects, the higher requirement of dialysis patients suggests that the dialysis procedure, rather than uremia, causes catabolism. A possible explanation for this is that the amino acid pool is depleted by nonselective removal of plasma amino acids in addition to nitrogenous waste products by the dialysis process. This, in turn, would increase protein catabolism. The daily protein requirement for patients being treated by intermittent peritoneal dialysis is at least as high as that of hemodialysis patients (1 g/kg per day); for patients treated by chronic ambulatory peritoneal dialysis (CAPD) the protein requirement is even higher (1.4 kg per day). The higher requirement of CAPD patients is due almost certainly to the protein lost (40 to 62 g per week) into the peritoneal cavity during dialysis. Although theoretically possible, the potential for reducing the frequency of dialysis by using protein-restricted diets supplemented with either EAA or nitrogen-free analogues of EAA has not been explored fully.

Energy requirements

The caloric requirement of patients with renal insufficiency has received attention for two reasons. First, when adults with CRF eat very low protein diets, their nitrogen balance can improve as calorie intake increases. However, this should not be interpreted as meaning that a very high calorie intake, as suggested for the Giordano-Giovannetti diet, would enable the patient to achieve neutral or positive nitrogen balance when dietary protein remains below 0.5 to 0.6 g/kg per day. Indeed, if protein intake is less than 0.4 g/kg per day, nitrogen balance will be negative even at a very high calorie intake. On the other hand, if sufficient nitrogen as EAA is given, nitrogen balance can be achieved readily. Moreover, it should be emphasized that very high calorie diets that are low in protein are unpalatable and poorly tolerated. If EAA requirements are met and nitrogen intake is adequate, it is not necessary to exceed the recommended daily allowances for healthy men and women (age 23 to 50 years, 38 and 36 kcal/kg; more than 50 years, 34 to 33 kcal/kg for active men and women respectively). Any additional "nitrogen-sparing" effect of prescribing excess calories may be counterproductive because of reduced compliance with the diet. Second, there is controversy surrounding the means by which calorie requirements are met because of the influence of dietary carbohydrates on insulin resistance and

hyperlipidemia in patients with CRF. The metabolism of carbohydrates and lipids by patients with CRF will be reviewed briefly to provide a background for understanding currently recommended intakes of foods providing energy.

Carbohydrate metabolism

Patients with CRF are characterized by an inability to metabolize normally an oral or intravenous glucose load. Although the maximum blood glucose concentration seen during a glucose tolerance test rarely exceeds 210 mg/dl in nondiabetic subjects, the glucose disappearance phase is prolonged and the initial insulin response is excessive. In addition, the rate of decline of circulating insulin after a glucose challenge is prolonged. Since blood glucose decreases more slowly than normal in spite of higher plasma insulin levels, peripheral tissues must be insensitive to the hypoglycemic action of insulin. In addition, the delayed disappearance of endogenous insulin in uremia is caused by decreased renal clearance of the hormone. Excessive ketosis and hyperglycemia are unusual in nondiabetic CRF patients and rarely require specific treatment. It is interesting that the degree of the abnormality in glucose metabolism is not correlated closely with the degree of uremia, though a uremic toxin probably produces the defect since adequate hemodialysis therapy usually results in marked improvement in the glucose tolerance test.

Lipid metabolism

Abnormal lipid metabolism is common in both acute and chronic renal failure. With the exception of patients with the nephrotic syndrome, hypertriglyceridemia is the most common abnormality regardless of the etiology of kidney failure. However, the plasma lipoprotein profile may change during progression of renal insufficiency or with the institution of various treatments.

In nonnephrotic patients with renal failure, the total content of cholesterol and triglyceride in very low density lipoprotein (VLDL) particles is increased as is the concentration of the late pre-β particles consisting of intermediate density lipoproteins. Nevertheless, in these patients both serum total cholesterol and low-density lipoprotein (LDL) cholesterol are usually normal, and high-density lipoprotein (HDL) cholesterol is decreased. In contrast, patients with the nephrotic syndrome have a marked increase in serum LDL cholesterol but only a modest elevation of VLDL triglycerides. However, when their serum albumin falls below 2 g/dl, VLDL-triglyceride levels become more clearly abnormal. In these nephrotic patients, HDL cholesterol is either within the normal range or slightly subnormal and contributes to a low HDL/LDL ratio which has been associated with a tendency toward atherosclerosis. In epidemiological studies of subjects without kidney disease, there is a close association between an elevated LDL cholesterol and the development of atherosclerosis, and there is an inverse correlation between levels of HDL cholesterol and coronary artery disease. Regardless, at present, there is insufficient evidence to conclude that the lipid abnormalities of uremic subjects are causally related to the development of atherosclerosis.

The cause of hypertriglyceridemia in nonnephrotic uremic patients is multifactorial. Hyperinsulinemia with a resultant increase in triglyceride synthesis, the effects of various drugs, and the low levels of cofactors necessary for metabolism of free fatty acids have all been implicated. Most of the evidence suggests that hypertriglyceridemia is caused by decreased triglyceride clearance. Indeed, after an oral fat-loading test, peak postprandial triglyceride levels are higher and remain elevated longer in CRF patients than they do in hypertriglyceridemic, nonuremic subjects. This occurs despite a delay in fat absorption in most uremics. Normally, triglyceride clearance is largely accounted for by lipoprotein lipase. The activity of this enzyme as well as that of hepatic lipase is reduced in uremia. This may be due to diminished enzyme synthesis or to a change in levels of circulating activators or inhibitors of the enzymes. For example, it is known that apolipoprotein CII, a component of HDL and a cofactor for lipoprotein lipase activation, is reduced significantly in CRF. There also is evidence that triglyceride synthesis is increased in patients with CRF. Presumably, this is related to the hyperinsulinemia discussed previously.

Besides these abnormalities in triglyceride turnover, free fatty acids also may be increased in the plasma of uremic subjects. This has been linked to depletion of the quaternary amine, carnitine, from skeletal and cardiac muscle. Carnitine is necessary for the transport of fatty acids into mithochondria for oxidation. Indeed, plasma and tissue levels of carnitine are reduced in patients with CRF, probably because of diminished carnitine synthesis owing to reduced plasma levels of lysine, the precursor of carnitine. It remains to be established whether supplemental carnitine can normalize plasma lipids of uremic patients.

Knowledge of those factors affecting the pathogenesis of hyperlipidemia in CRF allows a more rational approach to dietary therapy. First, the distribution of calories can be changed so as to lower the contribution of excess carbohydrates in increasing triglyceride synthesis. When the proportion of carbohydrates contributing to the total calorie intake is lowered, plasma triglyceride levels will fall almost 35 percent over a period of several months. It is possible that this is related to lower plasma insulin levels. Second, plasma triglycerides can be lowered by raising the dietary polyunsaturated/saturated fat (P/S) ratio. For example, if the P/S ratio is raised above 4 while total daily cholesterol intake is kept at about 500 mg, serum triglyceride levels will fall by about 30 percent and the ratio of HDL cholesterol to total cholesterol will increase.

A very important aspect of conservative therapy of patients with CRF and especially those with lipid abnormalities is an exercise program. A careful study of the effects of a graded exercise program for hemodialysis patients during a 9-month period found that there was a 39 percent decrease in plasma triglycerides and a 23 percent increase in HDL cholesterol. These improvements tended to reverse when the exercise was stopped. Indeed, exercise seems to be a veritable panacea for many of the ills of the uremic patient in that it also was noted that exercise led to improved glucose tolerance, a decreased requirement for antihypertensive medications, and a reduction in the degree of anemia. Obviously, an exercise program also will benefit nondialysis patients.

Vitamins and trace minerals

Patients with renal insufficiency often require specific vitamins even when the diet is largely unrestricted. Supplemental water-soluble vitamins should be given both to predialysis and dialysis patients. However, this does not mean that a multivitamin preparation should be prescribed because supplemental vitamin A is not needed and additional vitamin D can cause hypercalcemia and increase the rate of loss of residual renal function. Its use should be restricted to patients with severe renal osteodystrophy (see Salomon and Mitch).

Water-soluble (B and C) vitamins are necessary because their intake is deficient when dietary protein is restricted. Unfortunately, the requirements for most water-soluble vitamins are not known, though requirements for vitamin C and B_6 (pyridoxine), 100 mg per day and 5 mg per day, respectively, exceed those of normal subjects. At least the minimum daily requirement for other water-soluble vitamins should be prescribed. In contrast, serum levels of vitamin A and its transport protein, retinol-binding protein, are increased in patients with CRF. Moreover, vitamin A stores are probably excessive. This is important because excess vitamin A has been correlated with the severity of renal osteodystrophy and the abnormalities of calcium metabolism in CRF. Consequently, vitamin A supplements should be avoided. The indications for administering vitamin D are complex and will be discussed in the section on management of the CRF patient.

The possibility that zinc is deficient in patients with renal failure has been studied extensively because zinc deficiency might cause both the impotence and decreased taste acuity of uremic patients as it does in zinc-deficient subjects with normal kidneys. However, the clinical course of patients treated with protein-restricted diets for long periods suggests that the development of serious zinc or other trace metal deficiencies is a rare complication of this therapy.

Salt intake

As CRF advances, the ability of the kidney to adapt to rapid changes in salt intake becomes progressively impaired. Nevertheless, the patient with CRF will remain in neutral salt balance (i.e., dietary salt equals salt losses) even with a creatinine clearance as low as 5 ml per minute. Indeed, it is unusual for nonnephrotic CRF patients on an unrestricted salt intake to develop edema despite the ongoing reduction in the number of functioning nephrons. This suggests that the compromised kidney is much more successful in eliminating salt and water than it is in clearing nitrogenous waste products. However, the inability of the kidney to adjust salt excretion rapidly in response to changes in salt intake must be considered when designing a diet for CRF patients or when unusual salt losses (e.g., diarrhea) occur.

When hypertension or excessive edema occur in CRF, moderate dietary salt restriction may be useful therapeutically, but every precaution must be taken to avoid a rapid loss of extracellular volume (ECV) as reflected in changes in body weight. Inappropriate salt restriction will lead to a negative salt balance, loss of ECV, and decreased renal perfusion. The consequences of restricting salt intake in patients with "salt-losing nephropathy" are well known and include rapid weight loss, a decline in renal blood flow, and eventually a decline in GFR. Although it has been demonstrated that patients with advanced CRF, even those with salt-losing nephropathy, can be safely salt-restricted if it is done slowly over a long period of time (months), this is of little practical use in managing most patients. However, a modest reduction in salt intake to 2 g of sodium per day may be very useful in the treatment of hypertension. For those patients without refractory hypertension, an optimal salt intake can be approximated by maintaining body weight at a level associated with "trace" ankle edema at the end of the day. Clearly, a daily weight record is indispensable in the long-term management of these patients. Any sudden change in weight reflects an important gain or loss of ECV signaling the need for appropriate adjustments in salt intake. Weight loss can be countered easily using high-sodium foods such as canned soup, while the cause of excessive weight loss is identified and eliminated. If weight is gained over a short period of time, salt, but not water, should be restricted unless hyponatremia is present. When sequential weights are unavailable, the presence or absence of edema or of postural hypotension will serve as clues to the adequacy of the ECV.

Certain diuretics can be used to manipulate the ECV or to treat hypertension. As in the case of too vigorous salt restriction, excessive diuresis can lead to precipitous falls in renal blood

TABLE 4
Nephrotoxic drugs

Drug category	Toxic effect and remarks
Antibiotics	
Aminoglycosides	Serum levels must be used to determine doses that will prevent nephro- and ototoxicity (high concentrations of penicillins can falsely reduce measured serum levels).
Vancomycin	Although less toxic than aminoglycosides, serum levels still are necessary to avoid toxicity.
Cephalosporins	May cause interstitial nephritis or vasculitis; cephaloridine should be avoided because of its direct nephrotoxicity.
Penicillins	Can cause interstitial nephritis or vasculitis.
Sulfonamides	Rarely causes interstitial nephritis.
Tetracycline	Outdated tetracycline may damage proximal tubules; demeclocycline may lower glomerular filtration rate (GFR).
Polymyxins	More nephrotoxic than aminoglycosides.
Amphotericin B	Tubular cell damage almost always occurs with effective doses.
Antiinflammatory drugs	
Prostaglandin inhibitors	All of these drugs may diminish GFR abruptly and increase azotemia, particularly in hypovolemic subjects and patients with renal disease. (These drugs also may cause interstitial nephritis.)
Penicillamine	Proteinuria occurs in as many as 20% of patients; progressive renal failure may occur also.
Gold	Proteinuria may occur but less frequently than with penicillamine.
Diuretics	In chronic renal failure, azotemia can increase with diuretic-induced hypovolemia.
Thiazides	Ineffective when creatinine clearance is less than 20 ml/min; may lower renal blood flow; can cause interstitial nephritis.
Furosemide	Rarely causes interstitial nephritis; may augment antibiotic-induced nephrotoxicity.

flow and GFR. The preferred diuretics for CRF patients are furosemide and ethacrynic acid, which are effective in increasing urinary salt loss even in individuals with advanced CRF. Larger doses than normal are usually necessary (e.g., 100 to 200 mg of furosemide) in order to ensure adequate drug delivery to its site of action in the kidney. The thiazide diuretics are generally avoided in CRF because they are ineffective when creatinine clearance is less than 20 ml per minute and they may reduce renal blood flow. If a long-acting diuretic is required, metolazone is preferable to the thiazides. When furosemide or ethacrynic acid is ineffective in controlling the ECV, diuresis may result from the combination of one of these drugs and metolazone. However, great care must be exercised to prevent too rapid

a contraction of the ECV and worsening of azotemia. Before using such a combination, the physician also should consider other reasons for diuretic resistance such as the concomitant administration of a prostaglandin inhibitor which often reduces the response to furosemide (Table 4).

THE PROGRESSIVE NATURE OF CRF

A remarkable fact about the clinical course of renal insufficiency is that the rate of loss of residual renal function in most patients is constant, suggesting that the disease is self-perpetuating. This has been recognized only recently because the clinical course of CRF traditionally has been

TABLE 4
Nephrotoxic drugs *(Cont.)*

Drug category	*Toxic effect and remarks*
Analgesics	Phenacetin alone or in combination with aspirin compounds can induce chronic renal failure.
Heavy metals	
Mercury compounds	Potent tubular toxins.
Platinum compounds	Dose-related nephrotoxicity can be minimized by adequate hydration.
Radiographic contrast dyes	Dehydration markedly augments their nephrotoxicity.
Cardiovascular drugs	
Captopril	Proteinuria is uncommon; GFR may decrease sharply in some patients with renovascular hypertension.
Hydralazine	Drug-induced lupus syndrome may involve the kidney. (Procainamide, isoniazid, and others also can cause a similar syndrome.)
Propranolol (and possibly other beta-adrenergic blocking agents)	Can reduce renal blood flow and GFR in patients with chronic renal failure; the exception may be nadoxolol.
Other drugs	
Lithium	Nephrogenic diabetes insipidus is common; chronic tubulointerstitial nephropathy is unusual.
Vitamin D	Potent analogues (1,25,di-hydroxycholecalciferol, 1α-hydroxycholecalciferol, dihydrotachysterol), although useful in selected patients with renal osteodystrophy, may worsen chronic renal failure particularly when serum phosphorus is high.
Drugs affecting serum creatinine	

Cephalosporins
   Cimetidine
   Trimethoprim
	Reduce tubular secretion of creatinine thereby raising serum creatinine.

L-dopa
   Methyldopa
   p-Aminohippuric acid (PAH)
   Acetoacetate/acetone
   Ascorbic acid
   Cefoxitin
	Can raise serum creatinine falsely.

estimated by studying groups of patients with the same or similar renal diseases because there was no simple method of estimating the rate of loss of renal function in an individual patient. For example, serial measurements of creatinine clearance are expensive, cumbersome, and difficult to perform accurately. Furthermore, the time course of the rise in serum creatinine in progressive renal failure is not easily analyzed. Figure 1 indicates that the rate of loss of creatinine clearance is indeed constant, and as creatinine clearance declines, serum creatinine rises at an increasingly rapid rate. If the reciprocal of the serum creatinine concentration with time is plotted for an individual patient, the relationship is quite linear (Fig. 3), permitting the rate of progression of renal insufficiency for an individual patient to be estimated easily and reliably. The slope of this relationship is representative of the rate of loss of creatinine clearance and can be used to estimate when a certain serum creatinine will be reached or whether a treatment has caused a significant change in the course of the disease. About seven determinations of serum creatinine over a period of 3 months usually are sufficient to establish the rate of decline in renal function, and a change in the slope of at least 15 percent usually signifies that a significant

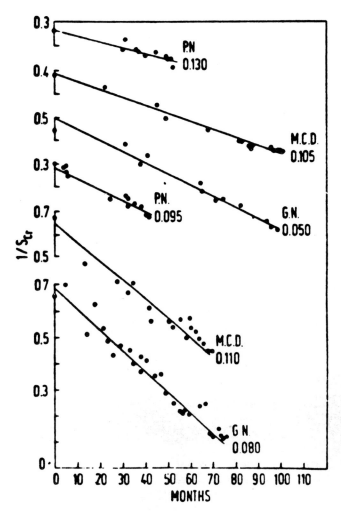

FIGURE 3

The large variation in rates of loss of residual renal function in patients with glomerulonephritis (GN), pyelonephritis (PN), or medullary cystic disease (MCD) is shown. The rates, estimated as changes in the reciprocal of serum creatinine concentration ($1/S_{Cr}$) with time, are displayed on the same plot by changing the unit divisions of the ordinate. The numbers refer to final measured value for $1/S_{Cr}$.

change in the progression of the disease has occurred.

This constancy of loss of renal function is inconsistent with episodic damage to the kidney as might occur with exogenous nephrotoxins. Moreover, few, if any, of the diseases that cause renal damage could explain the linear decline in renal function which would require that the pathological process be constantly active to the same degree.

The possibility that a change in diet could modify the constant loss of renal function was suggested decades ago. At least three mechanisms have been offered to explain how this might occur. The first is that accumulated waste products derived from dietary protein catabolism damage the kidney. Second, Addis suggested in the late 1940s that a high-protein diet increased

the workload of the kidney and that dietary protein restriction not only would reduce uremic symptoms but also might slow or reverse the progressive nature of CRF. Recently, this hypothesis has been reappraised by Brenner and his associates, and newer experimental evidence suggests that the hemodynamic adaptations including increased pressure and blood flow within the glomerular capillaries occur because of a high-protein diet (see Brenner et al.). This may contribute to the progressive loss of renal function. Third, hyperphosphatemia occurring as a consequence of the inability to excrete dietary phosphate leads to secondary hyperparathyroidism, causing calcium deposition in the kidney, which might reduce renal function. Lowering dietary protein always will lower dietary phosphates.

Nephrotoxicity of excess dietary protein

It was noted in 1922 that long-term feeding of normal rats with high-protein diets caused pathological damage to their kidneys and, subsequently, renal insufficiency. There are similar observations documenting the nephrotoxic effects of excess dietary protein in animals with experimentally reduced renal mass. In the same studies, it was shown that lowering dietary protein substantially reduces the histologic and functional damage caused by the experimental induction of CRF either by surgical or immunologic means..

Aside from a direct toxic effect, excess dietary protein may damage the kidney by inducing adaptive changes in renal hemodynamics. In this hypothesis, the increased single nephron glomerular filtration rate (SNGFR) and blood flow per residual nephron that follows renal damage in rats fed a high-protein diet leads to progressive glomerular damage and ultimately to sclerosis. The mesangial matrix of glomeruli expands and there are pathologic changes in glomerular endothelial cells. These pathological changes occur independently of any ongoing immune complex deposition or hypertension, and the pathology is ameliorated or eliminated by dietary protein restriction.

Calcium and phosphorus deposition in the kidney

When rats with CRF are fed a moderate amount of dietary protein (14 percent), calcium deposits develop within renal tubular basement membranes and there is glomerular sclerosis and a diffuse increase in the mesangial matrix in 80 to 95 percent of the remaining glomeruli. These calcium deposits often are associated with interstitial nephritis and suggest that abnormal mineral metabolism and secondary hyperparathyroidism may contribute to progressive renal damage. Since parathyroid hormone (PTH) administration to animals causes renal deposition of calcium and an interstitial nephritis, and since patients with primary hyperparathyroidism develop renal calcification and functional renal impairment, the potential nephrotoxicity of hyperparathyroidism has been suspected for years. In

fact, an association between secondary hyperparathyroidism induced by renal failure and subsequent progression of renal disease was suggested as early as 1937. It was noted that the renal calcium content of rats with CRF was proportional to the degree of parathyroid gland enlargement and that parathyroidectomy prevented further renal calcium deposition. Because of the association between a high serum phosphorus in CRF and the development of secondary hyperparathyroidism, it would seem logical to restrict dietary phosphate to prevent renal calcification. Indeed, when partially nephrectomized rats were fed a phosphate-restricted diet and given aluminum hydroxide to reduce phosphate absorption, they did not develop interstitial nephritis or the usual progressive increase in plasma urea nitrogen or creatinine concentrations. The contribution of hyperparathyroidism toward the progressive loss of renal function is still being debated; the effects of independently varying food and phosphorus intake on residual renal function of rats with CRF suggest that it is the lower food intake rather than simply a lower phosphorus intake that is more important in preserving renal function. Nevertheless, dietary phosphorus restriction clearly is beneficial in reducing the tendency toward renal osteodystrophy.

In humans, there also is evidence that abnormal mineral metabolism in CRF can contribute to progressive renal damage. For example, the rate of loss of residual renal function may accelerate when such patients are given vitamin D, particularly when they are hyperphosphatemic. For this reason, vitamin D or its analogues should be used cautiously in patients with renal insufficiency and must not be given if the serum phosphorus concentration is above the normal range.

CHANGES IN PROGRESSIVE RENAL INSUFFICIENCY IN HUMANS

Investigations of potential mechanisms underlying the constant loss of renal function in patients with CRF are understandably fewer than those carried out in animals. However, when the types of dietary intervention discussed above are used, the progression of renal insufficiency can be slowed, at least in some patients. On the other

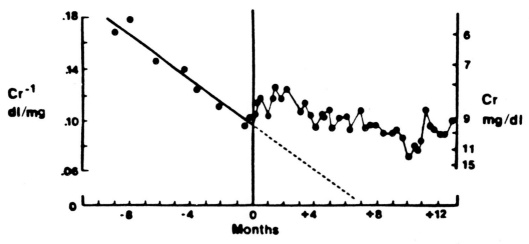

FIGURE 4

The clinical course of a patient with rapidly progressive glomerulonephritis before and after initiating nutritional therapy with a low-protein diet supplemented with ketoacids. The constant loss of renal function was interrupted for more than 1 year using this therapy.

hand (as detailed in Kelly and Mitch), when careful attention was not paid to restricting dietary protein, the average period of time before dialysis became necessary was about 3 months once the serum creatinine equaled 10 mg/dl.

Early attempts at nutritional therapy utilizing foods high in carbohydrates and in EAA (i.e., the "potato-egg" diet) produced results indicating that the prognosis could be improved; the average time before dialysis was extended to about 1 year. Such diets allow only a limited selection of foods thereby reducing their acceptance by patients, but recent studies using more palatable diets also have shown a beneficial effect of dietary protein restriction. For example, when a group of patients at the Mayo Clinic (Johnson et al.) who had an average serum creatinine of about 5 mg/dl were treated with dietary protein and phosphate restriction in an attempt to ameliorate secondary hyperparathyroidism, not only was the anticipated increase in PTH prevented, but also the average serum creatinine did not rise during 27 months. Although there was no control group treated simultaneously, it seems unlikely from historical controls that this could have been accomplished without dietary manipulation. In another study by Maschio and associates (Maschio et al.) dietary protein was limited to 0.6 g of protein per kilogram body weight per day, and it was found that the rise in serum creatinine was markedly slowed; the rate of rise was about one-twentieth that of patients whose diet was not regulated. It should be emphasized that this was a study of patients with early renal failure (serum creatinines 2 to 4 mg/dl). In our experience, a ketoacid-supplemented, low-protein diet combined with careful control of serum phosphorus, when compared with an unregulated diet, is more effective in slowing the rate of loss of residual renal function both in patients with early CRF and in patients with more advanced disease (Fig. 4).

In evaluating the effects of nutritional or other types of therapy on the course of CRF, it is important to remember that individual patients lose renal function at different rates. For this reason, the most convincing demonstration of a benefit from changing therapy is to observe a change in progression of CRF in the individual patient, easily estimated by plotting sequential values for the reciprocal of the serum creatinine against time. With this technique, each patient serves as his or her own control (Fig. 3) and the difficulties in finding a control subject of the same age, sex, and disease and with the same rate of progression are eliminated. This method has been used in the promising reports of relatively small numbers of patients studied in several different countries and, though not definitive, clearly raises the possibility that CRF need not always follow an inexorable course toward end-stage renal failure. If these early results are confirmed, the scope and importance of nutritional therapy of CRF will be increased markedly.

MANAGEMENT OF THE PATIENT WITH CRF

It should be emphasized that conservative management of CRF patients must include appropriate therapy for any reversible cause of kidney failure. Potentially treatable causes of CRF, such as active systemic vasculitis, or diabetes mellitus, should be given appropriate therapy. In addition, virtually any cause of acute renal failure may occur in the CRF patient with devastating results.

Obstruction to urinary flow at any point along the urinary tract can reduce renal function and thereby accelerate the course of CRF. Renal ultrasound provides a rapid, reliable procedure for evaluating possible urinary tract obstruction in CRF patients. Indeed, this technique has made the diagnostic intravenous pyelogram (IVP) virtually obsolete as a screening procedure for obstruction. The physician also must remember that chronic urinary tract infection often accompanies urinary obstruction. The diagnosis is made by urinalysis and appropriate antibiotic treatment should be based on the results of urine cultures. Antibiotic therapy alone may be successful unless the obstruction is relieved. Some drugs may be ineffective because they are insufficiently concentrated by the diseased kidney and do not achieve therapeutic levels in urine without reaching toxic levels in the plasma.

The risks of administering iodinated contrast material to the CRF patient must always be weighed against the potential benefits of the procedure because the dye may aggravate renal insufficiency. The risk appears to be greatest in those CRF patients with diabetes mellitus or multiple myeloma or in patients with any degree of dehydration. Thus, the usual practice of dehydrating patients before an IVP must be avoided. Because of the greater risk of inducing acute renal failure, the IVP should probably be avoided in advanced CRF in favor of newer diagnostic techniques such as the renal ultrasound or CT (computerized tomography) scan.

Inadequate renal perfusion is a common cause of worsening azotemia in the CRF patient. The first clue may be a rise in the SUN/creatinine ratio (normally 10). A decrease in renal perfusion and hence a decrease in GFR results in more avid salt and water reabsorption, consequently raising urea absorption and lowering urea clearance more than creatinine clearance. Besides an increase in the SUN/creatinine ratio, insidious loss of ECV (and decline in renal perfusion) may be detected by changes in weight. Therefore, it is critical that patients with CRF maintain a daily weight record and be instructed that weight loss of more than 2 lb can affect their kidney function adversely.

Many drugs adversely affect renal function. For a thorough discussion of drug use that is nephrotoxic (Table 4), the reader is referred to Schrier and Anderson. Clearly, any abrupt decline in renal function following administration of a newly prescribed drug should prompt consideration of the drug as the potential cause. In addition, drug interactions that are insignificant in the patient with normal renal function may become critically important in patients with CRF.

Some diseases which cause progressive loss of renal function may be reversed by appropriate therapy (e.g., Wegener's granulomatosis and lupus nephritis), but these usually require a renal biopsy for diagnosis. However, the risk of a percutaneous renal biopsy in a patient with CRF must be weighed carefully with any potential benefit of a definitive diagnosis.

The evidence presented indicates that nutritional therapy of CRF not only decreases the accumulation of unexcreted waste products without producing malnutrition, but also may have a very important impact on the course of the disease. We recommend that dietary protein restriction to 0.6 g/kg per day be initiated as soon as the SUN exceeds 60 mg/dl and possibly even earlier in order to preserve renal function. Since ketoanalogues of amino acids are not available commercially, dietary restriction to less than 0.6 g/kg per day will require an EAA supplement. This will require the assistance of a skilled dietician in order to design a diet similar to that shown in Table 3. During the initial months of the regimen, the patient should repeatedly review his or her protein-restricted diet with the dietician to ensure that calorie intake is adequate and that hidden sources of protein and phosphorus are not being consumed. The 24-h urea nitrogen excretion should be checked at least monthly during this initial period to monitor compliance with the diet. Generally, dietary habits are successfully altered within 3 to 6 months, after which the patient can be seen less frequently, though the urea nitrogen appearance rate should be monitored at least every 2 to 3 months in order to ensure continued compliance. The patient should maintain a daily weight record and feel at ease in calling both the dietician and the physician.

Long-term evaluation should include monthly measurements of SUN, calcium, phosphorus, and alkaline phosphatase. Serum albumin and transferrin concentrations should be measured at least every 2 months to ensure that protein nutrition is being maintained. Throughout, a graph of the reciprocal of serum creatinine concentration plotted against time (Fig. 3) should be maintained so that trends in the course of CRF can be detected easily.

Serum phosphorus concentration should be maintained below 4.3 mg/dl using dietary phosphorus restriction and aluminum-containing antacids. If constipation becomes a problem, sorbitol can be used. To overcome the decreased intestinal absorption of calcium, calcium intake should be about 1.5 g per day, which is difficult to achieve with a protein-restricted diet. However, if the serum phosphorus is normal, additional calcium can be given as calcium carbonate (or some other calcium salt) in order to raise calcium intake to 1.5 g per day and ensure neutral calcium balance.

Vitamin D should not be used in patients with hyperphosphatemia. Occasionally, in patients with renal osteodystrophy and persistent hypocalcemia, vitamin D may be useful. However, it is critical that serum calcium and renal function be monitored closely. If hypercalcemia or an accelerated loss of renal function occurs, vitamin D should be discontinued.

The decision as to when to begin dialysis therapy must be individualized and should not be made on the basis of a predetermined serum creatinine or creatinine clearance. Clearly, uncontrollable fluid retention and electrolyte abnormalities or pericarditis can force the initiation of chronic dialysis therapy. Likewise, the inability to control the symptoms of uremia with protein-restricted diets can preclude the use of nutritional therapy for patients with severe end-stage renal failure.

The principles of conservative therapy for the CRF patient that we have discussed, though somewhat difficult conceptually, are simple to implement in practice. Results from studies of experimental animals and patients indicate that dietary manipulation is effective in reducing the accumulation of waste products and thus uremic symptoms. These studies also suggest that nutritional therapy can slow the progressive loss of residual renal function. Thus, these principles for conservative management should be considered as an active alternative to more palliative therapeutic regimens that inevitably lead to dialysis.

Acknowledgments

Supported by an RCDA (AM 00750) from the National Institutes of Health. We thank P. Dolan for editorial assistance and C. Piper for design of the diets for patients with chronic renal failure.

References

BRENNER BM et al: Dietary protein intake and the progressive nature of kidney disease: The role of hemodynamically mediated glomerular injury in the pathogenesis of progressive glomerular sclerosis in aging, renal ablation, and intrinsic renal disease. N Engl J Med 307:652, 1982

JOHNSON MJ et al: The influence of maintaining normal serum phosphate and sodium on renal osteodystrophy, in *Vitamin D and Problems Related to Uremic Bone Disease*. Bern, Walter de Gruyter, 1975, pp 561–575

KELLY RA, MITCH WE: Creatinine, uric acid, and other nitrogenous waste products: Clinical implications of the imbalance between their production and elimination in uremia, in *Seminars in Nephrology* (in press)

————, ————: Nutrition in renal failure, in *The Systemic Consequences of Renal Failure*, G Eknoyan and JP Knochel (eds). New York, Grune & Stratton, (in press)

MASCHIO G et al: Effects of dietary protein and phosphorus restriction on the progression of early renal failure. Kidney Int 22:371, 1982

MITCH WE: The influence of the diet on progression of renal insufficiency. Ann Rev Med 35:249, 1984

MITCH WE et al: Long-term effects of a new ketoacid-amino acid supplement in patients with chronic renal failure. Kidney Int 22:48, 1982

———, WALSER M: A simple method of estimating progression of chronic renal failure. Lancet 2:1326, 1976

———, WILCOX CS: Disorders of body fluids, sodium and potassium in chronic renal failure. Am J Med 72:536, 1982

SALOMON DR, MITCH WE: Therapy of disordered divalent ion metabolism in chronic renal failure, in *Contemporary Issues in Nephrology,* BM Brenner and JH Stein (eds). New York, Churchill Livingstone, (in press)

SCHRIER RW, ANDERSON RJ (eds): *Clinical Use of Drugs in Patients with Kidney and Liver Disease.* Philadelphia, Saunders, 1981

WALSER M: Conservative management of the uremic patient, in *The Kidney,* 2d ed, BM Brenner and FC Rector (eds), Philadelphia, Saunders, 1981, pp 2383–2424

HIGH-FREQUENCY VENTILATION

THOMAS H. ROSSING, ARTHUR S. SLUTSKY, and JEFFREY M. DRAZEN

The conventional approach to mechanical ventilatory assistance is to use a breathing pattern similar to that found during spontaneous ventilation in normal humans. In the practice of adult medicine, this consists of delivering tidal volumes in the range of 8 to 15 ml per kilogram body weight at respiratory rates of 8 to 30 breaths per minute. This approach to mechanical ventilation has proved to be a very safe and effective method of achieving gas exchange in the majority of patients who require ventilatory support. However, in certain patients, conventional ventilatory techniques are associated with significant complications, mainly attributable to the high intrathoracic pressures that are sometimes required to maintain adequate ventilation. These large intrathoracic pressures are directly related to the large tidal volumes and the relatively noncompliant (stiff) lungs of many patients with pulmonary disease. As yet there is no solution to this problem, but a number of novel (although still experimental) approaches have been tried.

In this review we consider one such experimental approach, which consists of delivering small breaths at high frequencies. With this approach it is possible to achieve adequate alveolar ventilation using tidal volumes smaller than the anatomic dead space—a concept that is in direct conflict with conventional concepts of respiratory physiology. The success of this unconventional approach has stimulated investigation into the physical mechanisms that account for adequate gas exchange when the tidal volume is smaller than that required to bring fresh gas to the alveolar zone.

This new technique of mechanical ventilation is usually termed *high-frequency ventilation* (*HFV*). HFV has been applied in various ways using several different types of high-frequency ventilators and there is not yet a universally accepted definition of HFV. The purpose of this article is threefold: (1) to define HFV and HFV devices, (2) to describe some of the physical mechanisms thought to produce adequate gas exchange during HFV, and (3) to describe the proven clinical applications and the potential clinical pitfalls and benefits of HFV.

DEFINITION

As stated above, no precise definition of what constitutes HFV has yet been universally accepted. Definitions based on frequency alone are not adequate since the range of normal respiratory rates varies widely depending on age and species. Thus, a respiratory rate of 60 breaths per minute (1 Hz) would be considered high for a normal adult but normal for a neonate and low for certain animals (e.g., hummingbird). For the purpose of this discussion, we will define HFV as ventilation with frequencies greater than four times the normal resting value for the age and species (i.e., about 60 breaths per minute in adult humans).

TECHNIQUES OF HIGH-FREQUENCY VENTILATION

There are three basic techniques for delivering HFV (Table 1): (1) high-frequency positive-pressure ventilation, (2) high-frequency jet ventila-

TABLE 1
Comparison of techniques of mechanical ventilation

Type of ventilation	Rate, breaths per minute	Tidal volumes, ml	Expiration
Conventional mechanical ventilation	5–30	500	Passive
High-frequency positive-pressure ventilation	60–90	> 150	Passive
High-frequency jet ventilation	100–400	> 150	Passive
High-frequency oscillatory ventilation	100–1000	> 40	Active

tion, and (3) high-frequency oscillation. Even though there are similarities among these three approaches, each of them utilizes a distinct type of high-frequency ventilator. Further, although there have been attempts to use conventional ventilators to apply HFV, most investigators have used specially designed high-frequency ventilators for the following reasons. (1) The pressures required to generate flow at high respiratory rates are so large that gas compression in the conventional ventilator and tubing make use of these devices tenuous. As a result, most high-frequency ventilators are designed to have a very small compressible volume. (2) Moreover, most conventional ventilators cannot operate at frequencies greater than about 100 breaths per minute, and even this value may be too low for certain clinical applications.

FIGURE 1
Schematic diagram of gas flow during high-frequency positive-pressure ventilation.

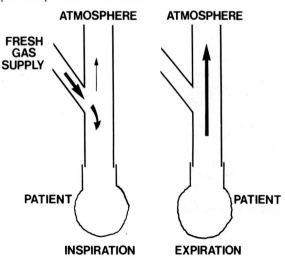

ATMOSPHERE ATMOSPHERE

FRESH GAS SUPPLY

PATIENT PATIENT

INSPIRATION EXPIRATION

High-frequency positive-pressure ventilation (HFPPV)

This mode of ventilation was originally developed by Sjostrand and his colleagues in the late 1960s. With this system, the ventilator delivers positive-pressure breaths to the patient via a sidearm port in such a way that most of the gas enters the patient while the small amount of the gas which is expelled via an exit port prevents entrainment of ambient air (Fig. 1). Exhalation is passive and the pressure within the airways is determined by the specific choice of frequency and delivered tidal volume and by the mechanical characteristics of the patient's respiratory system. Ventilatory rates used in HFPPV have ranged from 60 to 90 breaths per minute, with inspiratory/expiratory (I/E) ratios of about 1:4 to 1:5. The tidal volumes delivered by this ventilator are difficult to measure but are thought to be greater than the dead space. The main advantage of HFPPV is the ease with which it can be applied, especially during operative procedures; one disadvantage is that airway pressure cannot be independently controlled.

High-frequency jet ventilation (HFJV)

The technique of jet ventilation was originally introduced by Sanders in 1967 as a means of supporting gas exchange during bronchoscopy. Klain and Smith modified the technique for use at high frequencies, and were able to maintain normal blood gases in dogs at respiratory rates as high as 400 breaths per minute. As shown in Fig. 2, during HFJV a pulse of gas is injected rapidly into the airway via a narrow lumen catheter (14 to 16 gauge). In accordance with the

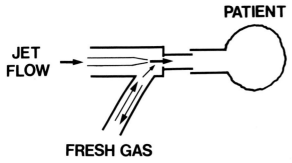

FIGURE 2
Schematic diagram of gas flow during high-frequency jet ventilation.

Venturi principle, the pressure immediately surrounding the injector catheter falls, and additional gas is entrained. As a result, the tidal volume delivered to the patient is greater than the volume leaving the catheter. The high-frequency jet can be produced by a number of different methods, depending on the valving technique (e.g., solenoid, fluidic, or pneumatic valves). The flow delivered by the jet is determined by the driving pressure of the ventilator (up to 50 lb/in^2) as well as the characteristics of the catheter system. Because the actual volume delivered to the subject includes the entrained volume, which is difficult to measure, the actual tidal volume is not known with certainty. As in HFPPV, exhalation is passive and the airway pressure is again determined by the flow characteristics of the jet and the respiratory mechanics of the patient. Because of its simplicity and reliability, HFJV has been widely used. Rates have usually ranged from 100 to 400 ventilator breaths per minute with I/E ratios of about 1:4 to 1:6. Tidal volumes are thought to be greater than the anatomic dead space.

High-frequency oscillatory ventilation (HFOV)

HFOV is a technique that differs in several respects from both HFPPV and HFJV. First, during HFOV both the inspiratory and expiratory phases are actively controlled by the ventilator—the ventilator creates a positive pressure to push the gas into the lungs and creates a negative pressure to "pull" the gas out of the lungs. This is in direct contrast to HFPPV and HFJV where exhalation is passive. Second, the flow waveform during HFOV is usually sinusoidal with an I/E ratio of 1:1 as opposed to the pulse or jet waveform observed with the other forms of HFV. Third, the oscillatory pump is usually a sealed unit and does not by itself deliver fresh gas to the subject. Rather, nonrespired gas is delivered by either (1) having the oscillations traverse a "fresh gas bias flow" (Fig. 3) which effectively removes CO_2 and replenishes the O_2 consumed by the subject or (2) removing CO_2 via a CO_2 absorber circuit with oxygen added at a rate equal to the O_2 consumed. To date HFOV has been used primarily as a research tool, since it allows precise control of tidal volume and airway pressure—variables which are of great importance in studying the mechanisms of gas transport during HFV. Tidal volumes employed may be as low as 40 ml, and frequencies may exceed 1000 ventilator breaths per minute.

PHYSIOLOGY OF HFV

One of the most interesting aspects of HFV is that tidal volumes can be less than the dead space volume. Classical respiratory physiology considers the airways as a dead space volume in series with an alveolar volume (Fig. 4A). In this model, it is necessary to inspire a volume greater than that occupied by the dead space volume in order to ventilate the alveolar zone. This model may be formulated according to the following equation:

FIGURE 3
Schematic diagram of gas flow during high-frequency oscillatory ventilation.

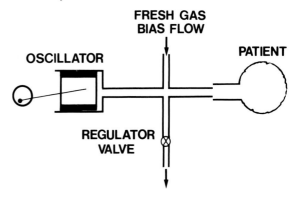

A)

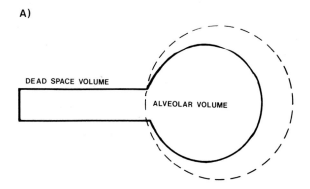

B)

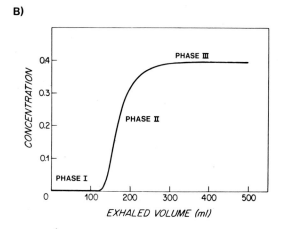

FIGURE 4

A. Classical model of ventilation. Gas must traverse the dead space volume to reach the alveoli. B. Single-breath nitrogen washout curve. Nitrogen washout following single breaths of 100% O_2 consists of initial phase with no nitrogen followed by mixing of gas from the alveoli during phase 2.

$$V_A = f (V_T - V_D)$$

where V_A = alveolar minute ventilation
    f = respiratory frequency
    V_T = tidal volume
    V_D = dead space volume

Clearly, if V_D is greater than V_T no alveolar ventilation should occur. There is a substantial amount of clinical experience and physiologic data to support the validity of the dead space model.

For example, in the classic studies of Fowler, subjects breathing air inspired a single breath of 100 percent oxygen, and from the beginning to the end of the subsequent expiration the concentration of nitrogen in the expired gas was measured. At least three distinct phases were seen (Fig. 4B). In phase 1 the expired gas contained no nitrogen and consisted predominantly of dead space gas. In phase 2 the concentration of nitrogen in the expired gas rose rapidly from zero to a certain concentration at which it reached a plateau (phase 3). Fowler hypothesized that phase 1 represented gas which was not in contact with the blood. That is, phase 1 consisted entirely of dead space gas, while phase 2 consisted of gas from various parts of the alveolar zones as they mixed at or near the airway opening. Phase 3 represented gas coming from the alveolar zones.

Despite the data supporting the dead space model of ventilation, there are many studies both in animals and in humans demonstrating that small tidal volumes (less than the dead space) can be used to provide adequate alveolar gas exchange. To explain these observations, the physical mechanisms that mediate gas transport during HFV must be examined. Physiologists have proposed a number of physical models which can be grouped into three categories: (1) augmented dispersion, (2) convective transport, and (3) a mixture of these two categories. Models of augmented dispersion describe gas transport based on ideas which are similar to those of Fick's law of molecular diffusion:

$$\text{Tracer flux} = D_{mol} \cdot \text{area} \cdot \text{concentration gradient}$$

This formulation states that the rate of diffusion of a substance depends on three factors: the diffusion coefficient D_{mol} (molecular diffusivity, which is a physical property of the gas being transported and the medium in which it is being transported), the area, and the concentration gradient over this area. In other words, the equation predicts that the rate at which material will be transported by molecular diffusion increases as the concentration gradient, the area, or the molecular diffusivity increases. Examining a process where this mode of material transport dominates (such as is the case for oxygen transport in the tissues) makes it easy to appreciate that the amount of material transported in a given setting could be increased by increasing the concentration gradient for the material or the area over which this concentration gradient is established. Molecular diffusivity is a physical constant and cannot be altered.

The concept of augmented dispersion as a mechanism for gas transport is based on the idea that, in a given setting, material transport can be described by an equation similar to the equation for molecular diffusion. However, rather than being based on molecular diffusivity, the constant of proportionality, termed *effective diffusivity* in the new equation, results from the combined effects of axial convection and radial transport. A simple example may help clarify how these two processes can enhance gas transport.

Suppose a drop of blue ink is placed in a glass of clear water. Over time, the ink will diffuse into the water and the entire liquid turns light blue. Viewed in the context of material transport, the ink was transported from the drop to the remainder of the water in the glass at a given rate which would be analogous to the material flux in Fick's law. If the same experiment is repeated except that, rather than putting the ink in the water when the water is still, the ink and water are stirred, the process of convection inherent in the stirring gives rise to rapid and enhanced mixing. By observing how long it takes for the water to turn blue, a flux for the amount of ink transported due to the stirring can be computed. This effective diffusivity would be much greater than the molecular diffusivity of ink in still water. Engineers and physical scientists have analyzed situations analogous to the lung and have provided very specific mathematical descriptions of the gas transport which can be effected by small-volume oscillations when combined with radial mixing. These equations can be applied to the lung by using these mathematical descriptions along with known airway size and branching patterns in order to compute gas exchange rates.

Although the details of this transport are beyond the scope of this discussion, these analyses predict that the major factor influencing the rate of gas transport by small-volume oscillations will be the flow rate, rather than the specific frequency or tidal volume used to achieve that flow. This is, to some extent, a simplification; it can be shown that for the product of a given fre-

quency and tidal volume, a larger tidal volume will produce slightly more efficient gas transport than a smaller one.

There are two models which fall into the category of convective dispersion. These are (1) the ventilation of nearby air spaces and (2) the asynchronous ventilation theory. In the nearby air space model, the lung is viewed as a collection of air spaces, each of which has a separate dead space volume. Analysis of the lungs of humans and experimental animals has suggested that the volume between the carina tracheae and the various alveolar air spaces can vary substantially. That is, some alveoli have a very small dead space volume while other alveoli have a very large dead space volume. Thus, if the tidal volume is smaller than the overall total dead space but larger than the dead space of some individual airway units, it may be possible to ventilate some "nearby alveoli" and produce adequate pulmonary ventilation. In contrast to the predictions made by the augmented dispersion model cited above, models based on airway geometries suggest that there will be a very strong dependence of gas transport on tidal volume at a given frequency over a range of tidal volumes which encompass the smallest dead space pathway to the largest dead space pathway. The augmented dispersion model predicted a relatively weaker dependence of tidal volume over such a range.

The second convective model is based on the asynchronous ventilation theory. This model is based on the concept that at "normal" respiratory frequencies (10 to 20 breaths per minute) the distribution of tidal volume depends almost entirely on local parenchymal compliance. However, as the respiratory frequency increases, airway resistance and gas inertance will also influence the distribution of tidal ventilation. Because the airways branch in an asymmetric fashion and contribute the bulk of airway resistance and gas inertance, changes in lung volume based on these properties will probably be nonuniform. Not only will the initial distribution of tidal volume be nonuniform, but computations based on realistic airway models have shown that during the course of a single respiratory cycle at high respiratory frequencies (such as may be encountered during HFV) gas may actually go from one alveolar zone to another before leaving the respiratory system. This asynchrony of ventilation could serve to make gas within the overall alveolar region quite homogeneous. This homogeneity could lead to enhancement of gas transport by reducing total dead space to that of the common dead space. For example, if such a mechanism applies to the lung, then only the common dead space (i.e., the tracheal dead space) could influence gas exchange. In contrast to the two previously mentioned models, no mathematical formulation has been made of this particular model and no specific predictions can be made which allow separation from the other models.

The third category of models is mixed models which incorporate the concepts of augmented dispersion and of convection. As yet no formal analysis based on a combination of these mechanisms has emerged. However, as the physics of gas exchange under the circumstances of HFV becomes better developed, more comprehensive models based on combinations of mechanisms may emerge.

In summary, explanations of the gas exchange which occurs with tidal volumes substantially less than the anatomic dead space have been offered, although at present no comprehensive theory exists.

Animal studies

The stimulus for the development of the HFV technique was the need for a method to support pulmonary gas exchange while studying the carotid sinus reflex in dogs. In such studies HFV produced several other interesting effects. For example, HFV appeared to reflexly inhibit spontaneous breathing, regardless of arterial oxygen and carbon dioxide tensions. It was also observed that airway pressures were low during HFV, suggesting that the risk of barotrauma might be reduced by this new approach. These observations stimulated further animal studies designed to determine the physiologic and physical mechanisms underlying this new type of ventilation. An important observation in this respect was that carbon dioxide transport observed in normal dogs undergoing HFV is largely determined by the total gas flow in the airways, which is directly related to the product of the tidal volume and the ventilation frequency even at rates of over 1000 ventilator breaths per minute. This

result is in accord with the theoretical predictions mentioned above.

Perhaps the observation that eucapnia could be produced by HFV in healthy dogs should not have been surprising, since the normal canine pattern of breathing consists of rapid shallow panting that is similar to HFV. However, the successful use of HFV in normal animals could not predict similar success in diseased lungs, so studies of HFV in animal models of disease were necessary before attempting to use this technique clinically.

Animal models of airway constriction, pulmonary edema, surfactant deficiency, and airway injury have now been studied. Several techniques have been employed to produce airway constriction, including intravenous histamine infusion and inhalation of methacholine aerosol. Eucapnic gas exchange can usually be produced by HFV in the setting of histamine-induced small airway constriction; however, short-term ventilatory effectiveness in dogs reaches a maximum at a frequency of about 500 breaths per minute most likely because of the dynamic airway collapse observed in this setting. Above this frequency, ventilation either remains at a plateau value or even declines slightly as frequency is increased.

Lung injury, atelectasis, and airway closure are other conditions that could have major impacts on the efficiency of gas transport during HFV. Oleic acid infusion has been used to produce pulmonary edema in both dogs and rabbits that were then ventilated at rapid rates. Adequate carbon dioxide exchange under these circumstances could be produced by HFV, and arterial oxygen tensions during HFV were equal to or greater than those observed during conventional mechanical ventilation using large tidal volumes and slow ventilator rates.

In other studies hypoxemia was induced in rabbits by saline lung lavage, which is thought to remove surfactant and destabilize the small air spaces. The utility of this animal model is that it produces atelectasis and reduced compliance similar to that noted in the respiratory distress syndrome of the newborn. In these animals HFV has been shown to be remarkably more effective than conventional techniques in maintaining an adequate arterial oxygen tension and decreasing the incidence of barotrauma.

Animal models also have been used to investigate new methods for delivering HFV. For example, externally applied, small-volume oscillations have been successfully utilized to produce gas exchange in tracheotomized cats. Another approach used in dogs has been to deliver the rapid breaths via a small catheter inserted percutaneously into the trachea. This transtracheal approach permits spontaneous breathing by the animal during the delivery of up to 200 ventilator breaths per minute. Several other experiments have shown that HFV may be of value in animals with major airway disruption, such as bronchopleural fistula. In this case, although a portion of each breath is lost through the fistula, the gas flow patterns in the airways suffice to produce gas transport. Thus, these animal studies suggest that HFV may eventually have clinical potential in the areas of emergency resuscitation and airway surgery.

Clinical experiments

Early success in using HFV to support ventilation in normal animals led to the clinical use of this technique in patients without major parenchymal lung disease. Among the first clinical uses for HFV was supporting gas exchange during rigid bronchoscopy and laryngoscopy. These studies indicated that the distribution of inspired gas may be more homogeneous during HFV than during conventional mechanical ventilation. This technique resulted in a reduction in the arterial-alveolar oxygen gradient, probably due to improved matching of ventilation to perfusion. A major advantage was that the small tidal volumes used during HFV resulted in less movement of the airways, which is an obvious advantage during bronchoscopy and laryngoscopy.

Despite the successful clinical use of HFV in these settings, little systematic information is available about the physiologic basis for successful HFV in humans. One study in nonintubated normal human subjects showed that spontaneous ventilation fell and breath-holding time rose during external chest vibration applied at 100 breaths per minute, but information about gas exchange was not reported. In other studies, CO_2 elimination at rates equal to or greater than metabolic CO_2 production and prolonged breath-holding have been demonstrated in normal hu-

man subjects who suppressed their own respirations while rapid, small ventilator breaths were delivered via a mouthpiece or an endotracheal tube. More recently, the effectiveness of HFV has also been demonstrated in intubated postoperative patients and in patients requiring prolonged mechanical ventilation because of respiratory muscle paralysis. From these experiments it has been determined that tidal volumes smaller than the dead space can be used to transport CO_2 from the human lung, and the effectiveness of such ventilation improves as the breathing frequency rises to about 250 breaths per minute. Above this frequency the effectivenss of HFV rises no further, reaching a plateau similar to that seen in dogs with bronchoconstriction. It is likely that the collapsible characteristics of the tracheobronchial tree may give rise to this plateau effect by absorbing a fraction of the tidal volume delivered at the trachea and preventing its delivery to the alveolar zone. Not only will absorption of a fraction of the tidal volume decrease the efficiency of HFV, it can also lead to repetitive airway collapse and expansion which itself may induce cough. However, ventilation at frequencies below the plateau in HFV efficiency (less than 250 breaths per minute) is tolerated well by patients.

While surprisingly few systematic studies of HFV have been undertaken in humans with normal lungs, there is now increasing anecdotal experience to support using HFV in patients with acute disease of the lung or airways. For example, an encouraging finding in some postoperative patients is that the calculated pulmonary shunt appeared to fall significantly during HFV, as compared to conventional mechanical ventilation. However, such case reports and small uncontrolled series do not permit any well-founded conclusions about the ultimate clinical role of HFV. They do point out promising areas for future human and animal research.

Airway disruption

Perhaps the most promising clinical research application at this point is the use of HFV in patients with airway disruption, such as bronchopleural fistula. Conventional ventilation is limited in this circumstance by convective loss of tidal volume to the pleural space and the atmosphere. At low frequencies, gas is distributed on the basis of local compliance; since a fistula is an infinite compliance, most tidal volume is lost to the fistula, preventing the usual inflation and deflation of the lung. However, in HFV gas flow patterns are dictated by the airways, not the parenchyma, and the mixing of gas produced by the small rapid breaths suffices to provide adequate gas transport to the alveolar zone. By changing the physical mechanisms which influence the distribution of airflow within the airways, HFV can support gas exchange even while the fistula is patent. However, at this point it is only possible to state that while HFV appears to be a promising, alternative ventilatory technique which merits further investigation, there are no comparative data demonstrating any better clinical outcomes for patients treated with HFV.

HFV has been used as a method of intraoperative ventilatory support in Sweden and in some centers in the United States. For example, during laryngeal or tracheal surgery there is often competition between the surgeon and the anesthetist for the airway. This competition can be minimized by delivering HFV through a small endotracheal cannula occupying only a fraction of the space required by a standard endotracheal tube. The use of small tidal volumes also has advantages where the motion generated during ventilation with large tidal volumes is an impediment to the surgeon, as in thoracic surgery or neurosurgery. This type of ventilation remains only one of the options which can be selected for operative ventilation. Questions need to be answered concerning the safety, expense, moment-to-moment physiologic monitoring, and operative time and outcome before the ultimate clinical role of HFV in the operating room is known.

DIFFUSE LUNG DISEASE

Although airway disruption and airway surgery are potential uses for HFV, conventional ventilation techniques are usually adequate in patients with these problems. This is not always the case in patients with respiratory failure due to advanced chronic obstructive lung disease or to the respiratory distress syndromes of the infant or adult. In these disease states ventilatory support is often difficult using standard respirators. Therefore, it is in these conditions that a new means of ventilatory support is needed most.

The major impediment to adequate ventilation differs for these two types of respiratory failure. In advanced emphysema or bronchitis, the most common problems are deranged matching of ventilation to perfusion, usually due to abnormal airway resistances and obstruction to airflow during expiration. The few studies that have attempted to use HFV in this population have found a reduction in the amount of blood perfusing poorly ventilated alveoli, and a resultant rise in arterial oxygen tension. Theoretically, this occurs because HFV may distribute gas more uniformly throughout the lung than conventional ventilators. However, air trapping due to airflow obstruction during expiration also may be more diffuse (see "Risks") and this complication may be more significant than the improvement in oxygenation.

In contrast, patients with hyaline membrane disease or the adult respiratory distress syndrome (ARDS) have reduced lung compliance. Despite high pressures in the trachea, the lung gas volume may be reduced. Treatment includes the use of high airway pressures to prevent airway closure and to distend the stiff lungs. Such high airway pressures may cause cardiovascular problems (i.e., decreased cardiac output) and barotrauma, such as pneumothorax or pulmonary interstitial emphysema. It is possible that the incidence of such problems would decrease if patients could be adequately ventilated at lower pressures.

Initial studies of HFV in the infant respiratory distress syndrome have been as promising as the animal model described above. Compared to conventional types of ventilation, HFV provided higher arterial oxygen tensions and permitted a reduction in the inspired oxygen concentration. Further, arterial carbon dioxide tension was lower during HFV, and the infants did not attempt to breathe in competition with the ventilator. In one series, five infants who developed severe pulmonary interstitial emphysema during conventional mechanical ventilation showed dramatic clinical improvement with the institution of HFV, as well as resolution of their interstitial emphysema. While these results are encouraging, the effect of HFV on clinical outcome, including the incidence of pneumothorax and survival, has not yet been compared to conventional techniques.

Results of trials of HFV in ARDS have been less encouraging. In part this may derive from the nature of the patient population. For example, ARDS may occur as a result of severe disease outside of the lung, such as sepsis or trauma. Therefore, survival depends not only on the adequacy of ventilatory support, but also on the successful treatment of the underlying disease. As a result, the natural history of ARDS is quite variable, which complicates assessment of different ventilation strategies. Although there are theoretical reasons to believe that HFV might be beneficial in this group of patients, and while there are anecdotal reports of survival in patients supported by HFV, these presumed benefits are not yet established. Until more careful, randomized trials show that HFV is associated with better survival or a lower incidence of barotrauma, it is possible only to state that HFV is an experimental and unproven clinical tool which merits further study before it is widely employed.

RISKS

At present an adequate assessment of the risks and benefits of HFV is lacking, and the expense of purchasing new HFV ventilators is not justified. Future research must attempt to identify patients who are likely to benefit from HFV and evaluate the risks of applying this new technology.

Since clinical use has been limited, it is difficult to know how frequently complications of HFV will occur. Among the potential problems are several related to mucociliary clearance. The rapid flow of gas in the airways during HFV may affect mucus production in several ways. First, the rapid flow of gas may be an irritant if it produces turbulence or excessive motion in the airways. Second, the rapid flow of gas during HFV may produce excessive drying of the airways if the gas is not adequately humidified. This drying effect may also change the character of airway secretions and indirectly impede mucociliary transport. Finally, the rapid reversals of flow during HFV may directly impede the motion of the cilia, or may transfer mucus away from

the central airways, which could enhance the risk of infection.

Other potential problems which require further investigation involve progressive trapping of liquid or gas within the lung. To understand the potential problems of fluid trapping, it is necessary to allude to the mechanisms underlying lymph transport. As is true in other organ systems, transport of lymph is not an active process in the same sense that the circulation of the blood is directly due to active pumping of the heart. Rather, the flow of lymph is mediated by the motion of the tissues surrounding the lymph vessels. Thus, inflation and deflation of the lungs may play an important role in producing the transport of excess water from the pleural space and lung interstitium.

Similarly, the potential problem of air trapping in the lung must be explained in terms of the time sequence of inspiration and expiration. During normal, unassisted breathing, contraction of the inspiratory muscles produces active inspiration of gas during only a small part of each breath. The remainder of each breath consists of a longer period during which gas flows passively out of the lung as a result of the elastic recoil of the lung and chest wall. A similar ratio of inspiration and expiration is utilized during most types of mechanical ventilatory assistance. If insufficient time is allotted to expiration, expiration may be incomplete when the next inspiration occurs. Repetitive failure to complete expiration would result in the net accumulation of gas within the alveoli. If this process occurs predominantly in certain locations, some portions of the lung would become overdistended, leading to abnormal matching of ventilation to perfusion, and possibly to pneumothorax. If gas trapping occurs diffusely, the entire lung would become hyperinflated, leading to probable cardiovascular compromise. Since gas-trapping is commonly observed in patients with airway obstruction during conventional mechanical ventilation, it seems likely that if this problem also occurs during HFV, it will probably occur in this same group of patients with airway obstruction.

The final group of potential problems involve the reaction of the airways to the pressures and flows generated during HFV. Although the tidal volumes used are small, the rate at which gas flows into and out of the airways is very rapid.

TABLE 2
Possible advantages of high-frequency ventilation (HFV)

Clinical setting	Problems with conventional mechanical ventilation	Possible benefits of HFV
Ventilatory failure arterial $PCO_2 > 50$ mmHg	High pressures with risk of pneumothorax and reduced cardiac output	Lower pressures and reduced risk
Bronchopleural fistula	Loss of tidal volume through persistent fistula	More effective ventilation; more rapid healing
Hypoxemia	Mismatching of ventilation and perfusion; risk of barotrauma with high levels of positive end expiratory pressure	Improved matching of ventilation and perfusion
Surgical procedures	Large endotracheal tube; movement of lungs and chest	Less airway interference and less motion of surgical fields

Such rapid flows within the airways might produce shearing forces and tracheal motion that could damage the airway epithelium. Similarly, although the airway pressures during HFV should be lower than during conventional ventilation, the actual flow of gas into the trachea during HFV may be quite high. If the exit for this gas becomes occluded, airway pressures would rise quickly, posing life-threatening problems due to barotrauma or cardiovascular compromise. Until safety considerations, such as alarms or pressure-limiting systems, are adequately assured, HFV must be considered to pose an unknown risk to patient safety.

CONCLUSIONS

The field of high-frequency ventilation has opened exciting new opportunities for the respiratory physiologist, the anesthesiologist, and the intensive care specialist (see Table 2). It is likely that some type of HFV may become a valuable tool for maintaining adequate gas exchange during tracheal surgery, thoracic surgery, and perhaps neurosurgery. It is also probable that this mode of ventilatory support may be useful in the treatment of bronchopleural fistula. However, the role of this new technique in the areas of emergency resuscitation, obstructive airway disease, and the respiratory distress syndromes of the adult or infant remains to be defined. Further basic and clinical research into the physiology and safety of HFV must be undertaken before this new ventilatory technique assumes an important role in clinical medicine.

References

BOHN DJ et al: Ventilation by high frequency oscillation. J Appl Physiol 48:710, 1980

BUTLER et al: Ventilation by high-frequency oscillations in humans. Anesth Analg (Cleve) 59:577, 1980

CARLON GC et al: High frequency jet ventilation: Theoretical considerations and clinical observations. Chest 81:350, 1982

DEDERIAN et al: High frequency positive pressure jet ventilation in bilateral bronchopleural fistulae. Crit Care Med 10:119, 1982

FREDBERG JJ: Augmented diffusion in the airways can support pulmonary gas exchange. J Appl Physiol 49:232, 1980

GALLAGHER TJ et al: Present status of high frequency ventilation. Crit Care Med 10:613, 1982

GILLESPIE DJ: High frequency ventilation: A new concept in mechanical ventilation. Mayo Clin Proc 58:187, 1983

GOLDSTEIN D et al: CO_2 elimination by high frequency ventilation (4 to 10 Hz) in normal subjects. Am Rev Respir Dis 123:251, 1981

HASELTON FR, SCHERER PW: Bronchial bifurcations and respiratory mass transport. Science 208:69, 1980

KLAIN M, SMITH RB: High frequency percutaneous transtracheal jet ventilation. Crit Care Med 5:280, 1977

ROSSING TH et al: Tidal volume and frequency dependence of carbon dioxide elimination by high-frequency ventilation. N Engl J Med 305:1375, 1981

SCHMID ER et al: Intrapulmonary gas transport and perfusion during high-frequency oscillation. J Appl Physiol 51:1507, 1981

SJOSTRAND U: High-frequency positive-pressure ventilation (HFPPV): A review. Crit Care Med 8:345, 1980

SJOSTRAND UH, ERIKSSON IA: High rates and low volumes in mechanical ventilation: Not just a matter of ventilatory frequency. Anesth Analg (Cleve) 59:567, 1980

SLUTSKY AS et al: Effects of frequency, tidal volume, and lung volume on CO_2 elimination in dogs by high frequency (2–30 Hz), low tidal volume ventilation. J Clin Invest 68:1475, 1981

SMITH RB: Ventilation at high respiratory frequencies. Anaesthesia 37:1011, 1982

TURNBULL AD et al: High frequency jet ventilation in major airway or pulmonary disruption. Ann Thorac Surg 32:468, 1981

ALTERATIONS IN THYROID FUNCTION TESTS IN NONTHYROIDAL DISEASE

P. REED LARSEN

Changes in thyroid physiology during acute and chronic medical illnesses may influence the assessment of thyroid status by conventional biochemical tests. Understanding such changes in thyroid function is important because the symptoms of the primary disease may confound the clinical presentation of any coexisting disorders of the thyroid gland itself and because it may be impossible to obtain an adequate history from the seriously ill patient, making interpretation of the biochemical tests critical for establishing the diagnosis. The fact that hyper- or hypothyroidism occurs in about 4 percent of the female population emphasizes the importance of separating this group from those in whom changes in thyroid function are secondary.

The changes that occur in thyroid physiology during acute illnesses are summarized in Table 1. Particularly prominent is the reduced extrathyroidal conversion of thyroxine (T_4) to triiodothyronine (T_3), a process termed *iodothyronine 5' deiodination*. Since this reaction is also involved in the degradation of much of the reverse

TABLE 1
Changes in thyroid physiology during acute medical illnesses

1. Reduced extrathyroidal T_4 to T_3 conversion in the liver and kidney usually associated with impaired degradation of T_3.
2. Inhibition of thyroid-stimulating hormone secretion probably in proportion to the severity of the illness.
3. Decrease in T_4 binding to plasma proteins due to an inhibitor released into the circulation during the illness. T_3 binding is less affected.
4. Reduction in serum thyroid-hormone-binding proteins due to a decrease in hepatic protein synthesis.

triiodothyronine (rT_3), blood rT_3 concentrations are usually increased. Despite the decrease in serum T_3, secretion of thyroid-stimulating hormone (TSH) does not usually rise and may even be suppressed in sick patients. Alteration in the normal relation between serum T_4 and T_3 and the binding proteins is common, and the concentrations of the binding proteins may be reduced. Taken together, these changes complicate the interpretation of the state of thyroid function. To understand the pathophysiology of these alterations, it is necessary to review briefly some of the underlying normal physiology, particularly in reference to extrathyroidal T_4 to T_3 conversion and the regulation of TSH secretion.

THE PHYSIOLOGY OF EXTRATHYROIDAL T_4 to T_3 CONVERSION

The structures of T_4 and of the products of its deiodination are presented in Fig. 1. About 80 percent of T_4 is successively monodeiodinated in either the 5' or 5 positions to the various iodothyronines. Approximately one-third of the T_4 secreted each day is first metabolized via 5' deiodination, giving rise to most of the T_3 produced each day in humans. This conversion occurs primarily in the liver and kidney, and the T_3 that is formed is released into the plasma. Since virtually all of the metabolic activity of T_4 can be accounted for by the T_3 produced from it, T_4 acts as a prohormone at physiological concentrations. Accordingly, alteration of T_4 to T_3 conversion can have important acute effects on the thyroid status, independent of the hypothalamic-pituitary feedback system.

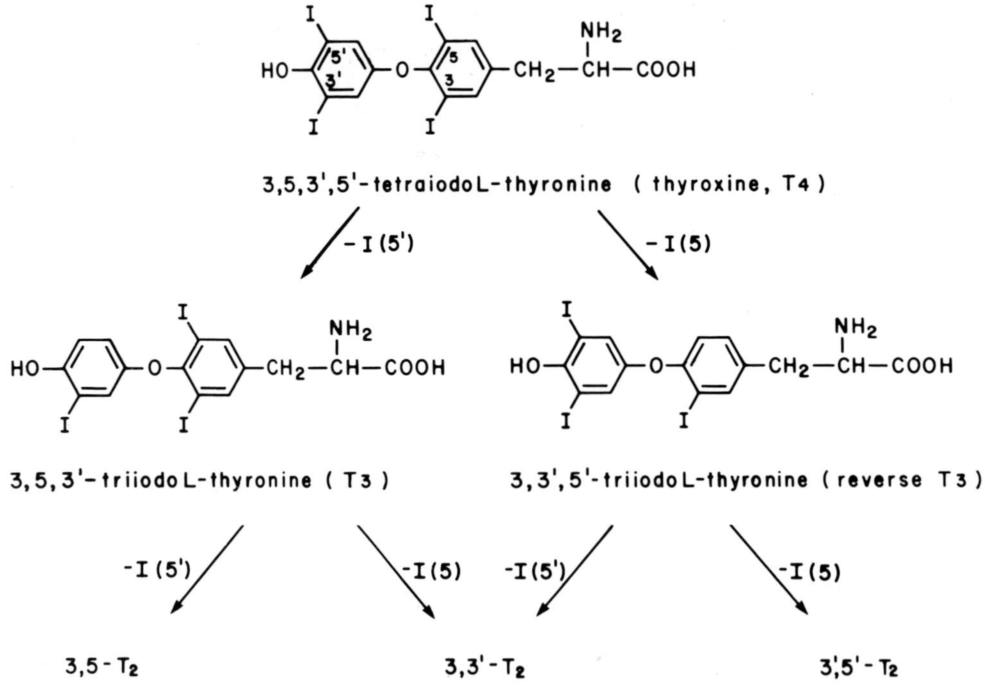

FIGURE 1

Formulas of the biologically important iodothyronines and their deiodination products. Arrows labeled 5' and 5 refer to iodothyronine 5'- and 5-monodeiodination reactions.

Another 30 to 40 percent of T_4 metabolized each day is deiodinated in the inner ring to produce the rT_3, which has no metabolic effects and is thought to be an inactive degradation product of T_4. Since a major fraction of rT_3 is deiodinated in the outer ring to 3,3'-diiodothyronine by the same liver and kidney iodothyronine 5'-deiodinase that causes the transformation of T_4 to T_3, inhibition of this enzyme causes an elevation in serum rT_3 (due to the slowing of its clearance), as well as a decrease in serum T_3. Thus, the typical pattern to be expected from inhibition of iodothyronine 5' deiodination is a fall in T_3 and an increase in serum rT_3. This phenomenon occurs in a variety of physiological conditions, including nonthyroidal illness, and can be caused by a number of pharmacological agents (Table 2). The exception to this general pattern occurs in renal disease, where serum T_3 falls but serum rT_3 does not increase.

While the deiodination of T_4 to T_3 in liver and kidney appears to be a simple chemical modifi-

cation, the responsible enzyme has yet to be isolated. The reaction requires the presence of a cofactor in the cytosol which participates in the regeneration of a sulfhydryl group in the active center of the enzyme. A characteristic aspect of the reaction in the liver and kidney is its inhibition by propylthiouracil, which is thought to form a stable mixed disulfide with the enzyme-iodide intermediate produced during the deiodination reaction. The propylthiouracil-enzyme complex is relatively resistant to reactivation by the tissue cofactor, and the reaction slows. The concentration of the cytosolic cofactor somehow

TABLE 2

Common causes of inhibition of T_4 to T_3 conversion

1. Severe illness or surgery
2. Fasting (carbohydrate deprivation)
3. Significant hepatic or renal disease
4. Normal human fetus
5. Pharmacological inhibitors
   a Propylthiouracil [not methimazole (Tapazole)]
   b Iopanoic acid (Telepaque) and sodium ipodate (Oragrafin-Sodium)
   c Amiodarone
   d Propranolol
   e Glucocorticoids in pharmacological dosage

depends on glucose uptake by the cell since fasting, particularly carbohydrate deprivation, causes a decrease in T_4 to T_3 conversion. The cofactor has not been identified, but it may be a nonprotein sulfhydryl. The inhibitory effect of illness or surgical stress on T_4 to T_3 conversion is thought to be a consequence of depletion of this critical tissue cofactor. Since T_3 is the metabolically active thyroid hormone, decrease in T_4 to T_3 conversion may be a protective adaptation in situations in which conservation of protein is desirable.

T_3 is produced from T_4 in brain, pituitary, and brown adipose tissue in the rodent by another enzymatic process that is kinetically different from that occurring in liver and kidney. While the reaction is stimulated by sulfhydryl-containing cofactors, it is not inhibited by propylthiouracil. This enzyme has been designated propylthiouracil-insensitive, or type II iodothyronine 5'-deiodinase, to differentiate it from the type I enzyme in the liver and kidney. One important aspect of this deiodination reaction is that it supplies one-half or more of the intracellular T_3 to the cerebral cortex and the pituitary gland. In the euthyroid rat, type II deiodinase may contribute one-fifth of the serum T_3. In hypothyroidism the activity of this enzyme increases so as to buffer the intracellular T_3 concentration in these tissues against the consequences of a decrease in serum T_4. Circulating T_4 provides direct feedback inhibition of TSH secretion via this mechanism. The effect of a competitive inhibitor of T_4 to T_3 conversion, such as iopanoic acid, is to cause an increase in TSH secretion not only due to the fall in circulating T_3 as a consequence of inhibition of the type I deiodinase but also due to a decrease in local T_3 production from T_4 in the pituitary gland. In contrast, the activity of the type II 5'-deiodinase in rats is not greatly reduced by starvation.

CHANGES IN THYROID PHYSIOLOGY OCCURRING DURING MEDICAL ILLNESS IN HUMANS

The most common change in thyroid physiology in the sick patient is a decrease in T_4 to T_3 conversion (Table 1). The result is a fall in the serum T_3, elevation in serum rT_3, and no change in

serum T_4. Since both serum T_3 and T_4 feed back on the pituitary to regulate TSH secretion, one would expect that the decrease in serum T_3 would cause an increase in TSH release with a consequent increase in serum T_4. This increased TSH secretion does not usually occur in sick patients for reasons which are not understood. TSH secretion is increased after administration of pharmacological inhibitors of T_4 to T_3 conversion such as propylthiouracil or the oral cholecystographic dyes, suggesting that a suppression of TSH release is a feature of severe illness. In general, the sicker the patient, the more impaired TSH secretion and the lower the serum T_4. In the acutely ill patient, TSH release after the administrations of thyrotropin-releasing hormone (TRH) may also be reduced, suggesting a decrease in pituitary responsiveness to TRH. This could be due to decrease in endogenous TRH secretion, to release of hypothalamic suppressors of TSH release such as dopamine or somatostatin, or to illness-related changes in the cells that secrete TSH. It has not been possible to determine which, if any, of these is the major cause of the decreased TSH response, but a similar reduction in TSH secretion occurs during fasting in the rat. The tendency for TSH secretion to be inappropriately low for the ambient thyroid hormone levels may be further exacerbated when dopamine is administered for maintenance of blood pressure. In experimental animals the release of TSH is suppressed by this monoamine, and in humans it can even suppress the elevated plasma TSH levels in patients with primary hypothyroidism into the normal range. Thus, in a patient with a reduced serum T_4 who is receiving dopamine, a normal serum TSH concentration cannot be interpreted as unequivocal evidence that primary hypothyroidism is not present.

An exception to the general rule that reductions in T_4 to T_3 conversion due to stress or disease do not give rise to elevations in serum TSH occurs in some patients with liver disease. In such patients, the failure of hepatic conversion of T_4 to T_3 is presumably not associated with systemic manifestations severe enough to result in suppression of TSH secretion. This situation may be analogous to that which occurs in the experimental animal given propylthiouracil.

In some sick people the binding of T_4, and to

some extent of T_3, to the circulating plasma proteins may be decreased due to an interfering protein released into the serum. This substance may also inhibit the uptake of T_4 into cells and the uptake to nonspecific adsorbing surfaces such as charcoal. The fact that T_3 binding to serum proteins is not as greatly affected as is that of T_4 leads to difficulties in the interpretation of tests which depend on tracer T_3 for assessing the free fraction of thyroid hormones. When the serum concentration of thyroxine-binding globulin (TBG) is altered, changes in T_3 binding parallel those in the binding of T_4. In the presence of the putative T_4-binding inhibitor of illness, the increase in the free fraction of T_4 is not reflected in a proportional increase in the T_3 resin or charcoal uptake. Therefore, the free T_4 index[1] is lower than is the free T_4. In fact, free T_4 concentrations measured by dialysis are more often elevated than reduced in patients with acute medical illnesses even though estimates of the free T_4 index suggest otherwise.

Sick patients, particularly those with chronic illnesses, may have reductions in serum TBG, albumin, or thyroxine-binding prealbumin (TBPA). In acute illness, the concentration of serum TBPA falls most rapidly of the three though this has only a modest effect on the total serum T_4 or T_3. In patients with hepatic cirrhosis, there may be a decrease in albumin and TBPA but an increase in TBG due to an increase in the serum estrogen/testosterone ratio characteristic of that abnormality. On the other hand, in severe hepatic failure the synthesis of all proteins is reduced, and both serum total T_4 and T_3 decrease as a result of the TBG deficiency.

Finally, there occasionally may be a rise in the serum total T_4 concentration in the severely ill patient. If euthyroid, such patients tend to have marked decreases in serum T_3, and this pattern is possibly caused by a marked inhibition of T_4 deiodination with persistent TSH secretion. Alternatively, a similar pattern can occur in sick patients with underlying autonomous thyroid function such as may be present in multinodular goiter or in euthyroid Graves' disease. The same

biochemical pattern can also be seen in patients with typical hyperthyroidism who become ill with a consequent decrease in T_4 to T_3 conversion. Methods for making the proper diagnosis in such patients are discussed below.

PREVALENCE OF ABNORMALITIES IN PATIENTS WITH ACUTE MEDICAL ILLNESSES

Many reports of abnormal thyroid function tests in patients with nonthyroidal illness are highly selective and do not reflect the typical patterns to be expected in the sick population in general. While the study of patients with extreme abnormalities is important for understanding of the pathophysiology, it is also necessary to appreciate the usual pattern that is to be anticipated. Results from one such study are shown in Fig. 2 in which 98 unselected patients admitted to a medical service through the emergency room had serum thyroid function tests. Two had primary thyroid disease, one was hyperthyroid, and the other hypothyroid; the remainder were euthyroid. Total serum T_4 concentrations were normal in 82 percent of the group. To obtain an indirect estimate of the free T_4, the free T_4 index was calculated using a normalized T_3 charcoal uptake. In 8 of the 17 individuals with a reduced total serum T_4, the free T_4 index was normal, indicating that a reduced TBG was the cause of the abnormality. Two patients with a normal total T_4 had a low free T_4 index. Of the eleven patients with a low free T_4 index, five were receiving phenytoin, a drug known to compete with T_4 for TBG-binding sites and to cause a reduction in the serum free T_4. If the five patients receiving phenytoin and the two patients with recognized thyroid disorders are eliminated, over 90 percent of the euthyroid patients were biochemically, as well as clinically, euthyroid on the basis of this screening test.

To examine the relationship between the free T_4 index and the free T_4 in ill patients, equilibrium dialysis was performed. Twenty-one percent of the patients had an elevated free T_4. The discrepancy between the free T_4 index and the free T_4 is presumably due to the presence in the serum of the T_4-binding inhibitor described above. More detailed characterization of the patients with normal and high free T_4 values is

---

[1] *The free T_4 index is the product of the total serum T_4 ($\mu g/dl$) and the ratio of the serum T_3 charcoal (or resin) uptake divided by the charcoal uptake of the standard serum for that day. Thus, the normal T_4 index is 0.8 to 1.2 times the serum T_4.*

TABLE 3
Thyroid hormone and binding protein concentrations in acutely ill euthyroid subjects with normal or elevated free thyroxine

	N	Free T_4,* ng/dl	T_4, μg/dl	Free T_4 index†	T_3, ng/dl	rT_3, ng/dl	Thyroxine-binding globulin, mg/l	Thyroxine-binding prealbumin, mg/dl
Normal range	38	0.98–2.30	5.0–10.7	4.7–10.6	75–222	13–32	15–30	21–48
Patients with normal free T_4								
Mean	67	1.74	6.7	6.3	87	32	23	25†
SEM		0.04	0.2	0.1	5	2	1	1
Patients with high free T_4								
Mean	19	2.69	8.1*	8.0*	65	50	22	16†
SEM		0.06	0.3	6	6	1	2	
p Value, high free T_4 group vs. normal free T_4 group				< 0.01	< 0.05	0.005	N.S.‡	< 0.05

* As determined by equilibrium dialysis.
† The product of the total T_4 (μg/dl) and the ratio of the T_3 charcoal (or resin) uptake divided by the uptake of the standard serum for that day (normal range is 0.8 to 1.2).
‡ N.S. = not significant.
SOURCE: *Kaplan et al.*

provided in Table 3. The concentrations of serum T_4, rT_3, and thyroid-hormone-binding proteins are typical of those reported in unselected patients with acute illness. The serum T_3 is reduced in both groups, although it is reduced to a greater extent in the high free T_4 group than in the individuals with a normal free T_4. In addition, the rT_3 concentration is higher in patients with an elevated free T_4. This could be a result of the higher serum T_4 (the substrate from which rT_3 is

derived) or of more complete inhibition of the type I deiodinase in these patients. The latter explanation is consistent with the lower serum T_3 concentration in this group. The serum TBG values were not different in the two groups, but the serum TBPA, a marker for the severity of acute illness, was lower in the group with the high free T_4. Serum TSH concentrations were normal in both groups. These results do not allow a conclusion as to the cause of the high

FIGURE 2
Relationships of serum total T_4, free T_4 index (FT4I), and free T_4 measurements in acutely ill patients. Free T_4 measurements could not be performed in five patients. To calculate percent values, the number of patients for whom the indicated measurement was performed was used as the denominator. (From Kaplan et al.)

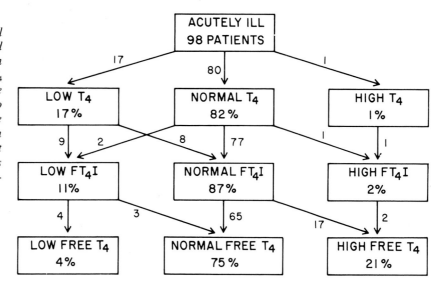

serum free T_4 in patients with serious illnesses. At least two possibilities are suggested. Patients with high free T_4 values may be sicker than those with a normal free T_4 and therefore have a greater release of the T_4-binding inhibitor into the circulation. The lower serum T_3 and higher serum rT_3 could be explained on that basis. Alternatively, the high free T_4 may be a compensatory response of the pituitary gland to the more severe reduction in serum T_3 in these individuals.

THE DIAGNOSTIC APPROACH TO THE PATIENT WITH NONTHYROIDAL ILLNESS

Given this information, how do we approach the patient with nonthyroidal illness in whom an assessment of thyroid hormone status is required? The diagnostic strategy in these patients is not greatly different from that ordinarily used when thyroid dysfunction is suspected. Alterations in the serum T_4 due to altered serum TBG concentrations must be separated from abnormalities caused by disturbances in thyroid hormone secretion rate. This basic distinction is made by calculation of the free T_4 index or by measurement of free T_4 using one of the many kits which are now commercially available. It should be mentioned that none of these kits quantitate the free T_4 per se but calculate it based on the kinetics of interactions between labeled T_4 (or T_4 analogues) and the serum-binding proteins. Measurement of free T_4 by equilibrium dialysis is not practical on a routine basis. If the free T_4 index is normal, it is safe to assume that the patient is not hypothyroid. The question of mild hyperthyroidism cannot be eliminated by this initial assessment, but it is unlikely that significant hyperthyroidism is present when serum T_4 is normal.

Since the most common abnormality in the sick patient is a reduced serum free T_4 index, a suitable diagnostic approach to this situation is outlined in Fig. 3. Administration of T_3, salicylates, or phenytoin can cause a reduction in the free T_4 index. If ingestion of these three drugs can be eliminated by history or by appropriate serum assays, then the differential diagnosis includes hypothyroidism, either primary or secondary, or an illness-associated abnormality in T_4 binding. The serum TSH concentration should

be measured; an elevation indicates primary hypothyroidism. If the serum TSH is normal (or low) then the decision is whether the patient has secondary hypothyroidism or an illness-associated abnormality in T_4 binding or secretion. If the patient is receiving dopamine, the possibility of an underlying primary hypothyroidism still remains. If the free T_4 index is very low (<2 units), then it is wise to measure serum cortisol, which is often greater than 20 μg/dl in the stressed patient with normal adrenal function. If the serum cortisol is below 20 μg/dl, the possibility of hypothalamic-pituitary abnormality must be considered. Depending on the clinical situation, such patients may require temporary treatment with appropriate amounts of glucocorticoid and thyroid hormone until a more definitive endocrinological workup can be performed. If serum cortisol levels are appropriate (>20 μg/dl) but serum T_4 is reduced, it is likely that the patient is euthyroid and has a severe illness-induced abnormality in thyroid physiology.

Patients with a reduced serum T_4 due solely to acute illness generally have an elevation in serum rT_3 concentrations. However, it is not always possible to separate acutely ill euthyroid from acutely ill hypothyroid patients with this assay. The serum TSH is a better discriminator since over 95 percent of hypothyroid patients have primary hypothyroidism. In the rare situation where the possibility of secondary hypothyroidism vs. illness-induced hypothyroxinemia is being considered, measurement of serum rT_3 may provide helpful information. If the level is elevated (more than two times the upper normal limit) then the diagnosis is likely to be illness-induced hypothyroxinemia. However, if the serum rT_3 is closer to the normal range, then it is not helpful in differentiating these two causes of hypothyroxinemia.

At this point, a decision as to whether or not to treat the patient with T_4 depends on the individual clinical circumstances. If there is a significant possibility of thyroid disease, the author prefers to give L-thyroxine, 2.25 μg per kilogram body weight orally or 1.2 μg per kilogram body weight intravenously as a single bolus once daily. Such treatment is not often necessary but does not adversely affect euthyroid individuals and will be beneficial to the patients with true hypothyroidism.

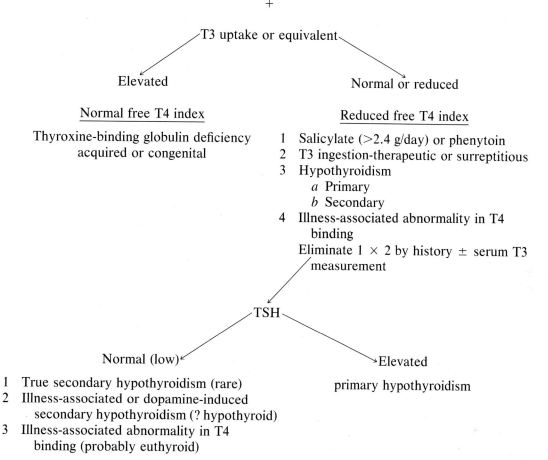

Reduced serum T4 in a severely ill patient

+

T3 uptake or equivalent

Elevated   Normal or reduced

Normal free T4 index   Reduced free T4 index

Thyroxine-binding globulin deficiency   1 Salicylate (>2.4 g/day) or phenytoin
acquired or congenital   2 T3 ingestion-therapeutic or surreptitious
                                        3 Hypothyroidism
                                             a Primary
                                             b Secondary
                                        4 Illness-associated abnormality in T4
                                             binding
                                        Eliminate 1 × 2 by history ± serum T3
                                        measurement

                                        TSH

Normal (low)   Elevated

1 True secondary hypothyroidism (rare)   primary hypothyroidism
2 Illness-associated or dopamine-induced
     secondary hypothyroidism (? hypothyroid)
3 Illness-associated abnormality in T4
     binding (probably euthyroid)

FIGURE 3
Evaluation of a reduced serum T₄ in a severely ill patient.

EVALUATION OF AN INCREASED SERUM T₄ OR FREE T₄ INDEX IN SICK PATIENTS

The diagnoses to be considered in these patients are shown in Table 4. In the case of an elevated total T_4, the first step is to eliminate an elevation in serum TBG as the cause. Such patients have reduced T_3 uptakes and normal free T_4 indexes. If the free T_4 index is elevated, then one should consider a number of situations including the acute illness as an explanation for this abnormality. It should be emphasized that a high free T_4 index is rarely due to illness per se, appearing in only one of the 98 patients surveyed (Fig. 2). Exceptions to this general rule include patients with acute psychosis and those with hyperemesis gravidarum in whom an elevation in the free T_4 index may occur during the acute illness, usually associated with a normal serum T_3 concentration. These abnormalities disappear with time, with or without antithyroid drug treatment. One very confusing aspect of such patients is that the TSH response to TRH may be abnormal or "flat" (see below) even though true hyperthyroidism is not present. Depending on the clinical circumstances, it may be necessary to institute antithyroid therapy in such patients until the acute situation has resolved.

TABLE 4
Causes of elevation in the serum thyroxine (T$_4$) concentration

1 Increased serum thyroxine-binding globulin
2 Hyperthyroidism
3 Acute psychotic illness
4 Hyperemesis gravidarum
5 Familial hyperthyroxinemia due to a circulating albumin or prealbumin molecule with abnormally high affinity for T$_4$ (but not T$_3$)
6 Drug-induced blockade of T$_4$ to T$_3$ conversion with compensatory increase in thyroid-stimulating hormone secretion
  a Oral cholecystographic agents
  b Amiodarone
  c High-dose propranolol
7 Illness-induced blockade of T$_4$ to T$_3$ conversion (Such subjects may have underlying autonomous thyroid function.)
8 Thyroid hormone resistance
  a All tissues (patient euthyroid or hypothyroid)
  b Pituitary resistance only (patient hyperthyroid)
9 Endogenous anti-T$_4$ antibodies

In general, measuring the serum T$_3$ concentration provides useful information in acutely ill patients with an elevated free T$_4$ index (see Fig. 3). If the total serum T$_3$ is greater than 160 ng/dl (assuming serum TBG is normal) hyperthyroidism is usually present. Even in the hyperthyroid patient, sickness may reduce the serum T$_3$ to the normal range as a result of impairment of peripheral T$_4$ to T$_3$ conversion. Therefore, a normal serum T$_3$ concentration does not exclude the diagnosis of hyperthyroidism. If typical hyperthyroidism is present, treatment should be instituted immediately with a combination of propylthiouracil and iodide.

If the serum T$_3$ is normal or low, then it is usually not possible to make an unequivocal diagnosis. A rare cause of this biochemical pattern is familial hyperthyroxinemia in which an abnormal albumin (or rarely prealbumin) with a high affinity for T$_4$ but not for T$_3$ is formed. The albumin acts as a TBG-like protein that binds T$_4$ but not T$_3$. Therefore, such patients have an elevated total T$_4$, but the serum T$_3$ and T$_3$ resin or charcoal uptake tests are usually normal.

Drug-induced blockade of T$_4$ to T$_3$ conversion may also occur, the principle offending drugs being iopanoic acid (Telepaque), sodium ipodate (Oragrafin-Sodium), amiodarone, or, rarely, high doses of propranolol (greater than 120 mg per day). These drugs block T$_4$ to T$_3$ conversion suf-

ficiently that compensatory TSH secretion is initiated. The oral cholecystographic agents and amiodarone can impair hepatic, renal, pituitary, and cerebral conversion of T$_4$ to T$_3$. Propranolol interacts predominantly with cell membranes in the liver and kidney to inhibit T$_4$ to T$_3$ conversion. This property is not shared by β-adrenergic blocking agents that do not have this membrane-stabilizing effect and is not a function of β-adrenergic blockade itself.

Thyroid hormone resistance is a rare disorder, usually familial, in which levels of serum T$_4$ and T$_3$ and TSH are elevated. Subjects may be euthyroid or hypothyroid depending on the severity of the defect and whether all tissues are equally affected. If only the pituitary or hypothalamus is resistant, then the subject has elevated serum TSH concentration and may even be hyperthyroid in other tissues.

The possibility that endogenous anti-T$_4$ antibodies are present must be kept in mind although such instances are rare. Whether or not endogenous T$_4$ antibodies cause an increase or decrease in the estimated serum T$_4$ depends on the method used for the T$_4$ assay. In those methods in which immobilized antibody or rabbit first antibody precipitation is employed to separate T$_4$, "bound" and "free" serum containing T$_4$ antibody produces a falsely elevated serum T$_4$. In those assays in which charcoal or resin is used to separate bound and free hormone, the value is usually artifactually reduced.

When greater assurance is required that the patient is not hyperthyroid, a TRH test should be performed. This test requires measurement of the baseline serum TSH, administration of 200 to 500 μg of TRH intravenously, and measurement of TSH 20 to 30 min later. Any increase in TSH after TRH administration indicates that hyperthyroidism is not present except for the rare form of hyperthyroidism caused by excess TSH secretion. An absent response to TRH is consistent with hyperthyroidism but does not establish this diagnosis. Increasing age in humans is associated with attenuation of the normal TSH response to TRH, and acute illness or dopamine infusion may also blunt the TSH response to TRH. In patients with hyperthyroxinemia on the basis of abnormal circulating proteins, type I or II deiodinase blocking agents, or endogenous T$_4$ antibodies, the TRH test is normal. If there is no

TSH reponse to TRH, it is necessary to determine appropriate therapy on an individual basis. If there is a strong clinical suggestion of hyperthyroidism, then it is the author's practice to treat with propylthiouracil and iodide as though the patient had thyrotoxicosis, allowing the resolution of the acute illness before obtaining a precise diagnosis as to the thyroid status. Fortunately, the institution of short-term ($\simeq 1$ week) antithyroid drug therapy with propylthiouracil and iodide does not cause major abnormalities in the euthyroid state. Such treatment of the hyperthyroid patient with other illnesses may prevent development of thyroid storm or other lethal complications of the disease and thus may be lifesaving.

Any patient who shows an elevated free T_4 index as a consequence of acute illness should be evaluated for underlying autonomous thyroid function after recovery from the primary illness. A number of such patients prove to be hyperthyroid.

SUMMARY

Acute medical or surgical illnesses can cause a variety of abnormalities in thyroid function tests. In general, the serum T_4 is normal or low, and serum T_3 is almost invariably reduced. The differential diagnosis of the causes of these abnormalities is similar to that for less severely ill subjects, but the effects of the illness may confuse the laboratory findings. In particular, patients with hyperthyroidism may have only an elevation in serum T_4 and not T_3 as a consequence of inhibition of peripheral T_4 to T_3 conversion. Alternatively, the serum free T_4 index may be low in patients with severe illness even though the estimates of free T_4 by more precise means are normal or increased. Such individuals often have evidence of circulating inhibitors of T_4 binding to serum proteins. If a serum TSH is normal in patients with a reduced free T_4 index and the patient has not received salicylates, phenytoin, or exogenous T_3, then the explanation is likely to be the illness itself. On occasion it is impossible to eliminate the diagnosis of underlying hypothyroidism, particularly that due to hypothalamic or pituitary dysfunction, and temporary replacement therapy with thyroid hormone must be provided until the acute episode

has resolved. In such patients, the serum cortisol should be evaluated as well and replacement therapy with glucocorticoid should be considered because of the possibility of combined deficits.

There are many causes of an elevated serum free T_4 index. Acute illness per se is not a common cause of this biochemical abnormality, and therefore the diagnosis of hyperthyroidism must be considered in such patients. If this diagnosis cannot be excluded, then treatment with propylthiouracil and iodide should be given until the acute illness has resolved and the usual evaluation performed. The importance of informed clinical judgment in deciding whether to institute therapy for thyroid disease in an acutely ill patient cannot be overemphasized.

References

BACCI V et al: The relationship between serum triiodothyronine and thyrotropin during systemic illness. J Clin Endocrinol Metab 54:1229, 1982

BERMUDEZ F et al: High incidence of decreased serum triiodothyronine concentration in patients with nonthyroidal disease. J Clin Endocrinol Metab 41:27, 1975

BOUILLON R et al: Thyroid function in patients with hyperemesis gravidarum. Am J Obstet Gynecol 143:922, 1982

CHOPRA IJ et al: Misleadingly low free thyroxine index and usefulness of reverse triiodothyronine measurement in nonthyroidal illnesses. Ann Intern Med 90:905, 1979

——— et al: An inhibitor of the binding of thyroid hormones to serum proteins is present in extrathyroidal tissues. Science 215:407, 1982

DOCTER R et al: Inherited thyroxine excess: A serum abnormality due to an increased affinity for modified albumin. Clin Endocrinol 15:363, 1981

GARDNER DF et al: Effect of triiodothyronine replacement on the metabolic and pituitary responses to starvation. N Engl J Med 300:579, 1979

GAVIN LA et al: The diagnostic dilemma of isolated hyperthyroxinemia in acute illness. JAMA 242:251, 1979

GOOCH BR et al: Abnormalities in thyroid function tests in patients admitted to a medical service. Arch Intern Med 142:1801, 1982

KAPLAN MM et al: Prevalence of abnormal thyroid function test results in patients with acute medical illnesses. Am J Med 72:9, 1982

LARSEN PR: Thyroid-pituitary interaction: Feedback regulation of thyrotropin secretion by thyroid hormones. N Engl J Med 306:23, 1982

———— et al: Relationships between circulating and intracellular thyroid hormones: Physiological and clinical implications. Endocr Rev 2:87, 1981

LEVY RP et al: Serum thyroid hormone abnormalities in psychiatric disease. Metabolism 30:1060, 1981

LIM VS et al: Thyroid dysfunction in chronic renal failure: A study of the pituitary-thyroid axis and peripheral turnover kinetics of thyroxine and triiodothyronine. J Clin Invest 60:522, 1977

MATURLO SJ et al: Variable thyrotropin response to thyrotropin-releasing hormone after small decreases in plasma free thyroid hormone concentrations in patients with nonthyroidal diseases. J Clin Invest 66:451, 1980

MELMED S et al: A comparison of methods for assessing thyroid function in nonthyroidal illness. J Clin Endocrinol Metab 54:300, 1982

OPPENHEIMER JH et al: Evidence for a factor in the sera of patients with nonthyroidal disease which inhibits iodothyronine binding by solid matrices, serum proteins, and rat hepatocytes. J Clin Endocrinol Metab 54:757, 1982

SCHUSSLER GC et al: Increased serum thyroid hormone binding and decreased free hormone in chronic active liver disease. N Engl. J Med 299:510, 1978

SILVA JE et al: Evidence for two tissue-specific pathways for in vivo thyroxine 5′-deiodination in the rat. J Clin Invest 69:1176, 1982

SLAG MF et al: Hypothyroxinemia in critically ill patients as a predictor of high mortality. JAMA 245:43, 1981

SPRATT DI et al: Hyperthyroxinemia in patients with acute psychiatric disorders. Am J Med 73:41, 1982

VISSER TJ et al: Evidence for two pathways of iodothyronine 5′-deiodination in rat pituitary that differ in kinetics, propylthiouracil sensitivity, and response to hypothyroidism. J Clin Invest 71:992, 1983

CLINICAL USE OF ASSAYS FOR SOMATOMEDIN AND INSULIN-LIKE GROWTH FACTORS

RAYMOND L. HINTZ

The somatomedins and insulin-like growth factors are a group of insulin-like peptides that have anabolic actions on a number of tissues (Van Wyk et al.). Over the past two decades, a large amount of information has accrued to link some of these hormonal peptides to the action of growth hormone. In addition, these substances may play a role in modulating the action of insulin. Three different lines of evidence (see below) have provided insight into the role of these substances.

Salmon and Daughaday, while exploring the potential in vitro actions of growth hormones on cartilage, discovered that growth hormone did not act directly on cartilage tissue but acted through a growth hormone–dependent intermediary that appeared in plasma when hypophysectomized rats were treated with growth hormone (Fig. 1). This plasma factor was provisionally named *sulfation factor,* and it was recognized

FIGURE 1
The original concept of sulfation factor. GH is growth hormone.

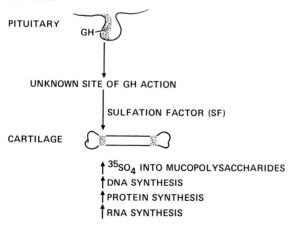

that an understanding of the role of sulfation factor was important in understanding growth hormone action. Subsequently, bioassays for sulfation factor were utilized as a clinical tool for diagnosing deficiency or excess of growth hormone. However, the bioassays for sulfation factor were tedious and had relatively poor reproducibility, and when radioimmunoassay techniques were developed for measurement of growth hormone, use of bioassays for sulfation factor as a diagnostic tool quickly waned.

A second line of evidence arose from the observation by Froesch et al. that more insulin-like activity is measurable in serum by bioassay than can be accounted for by immunoreactive insulin. This bioactivity in excess of insulin activity was termed nonsuppressible insulin-like activity (NSILA), since the insulin-like bioactivity was not suppressible by large amounts of anti-insulin antiserum (Fig. 2). The biological relevance of this nonsuppressible insulin-like activity was uncertain, the majority of workers feeling that immunoassayable insulin is the biologically relevant measurement. As a result, interest in NSILA waned during the mid-1960s (Burgi et al.).

A third route of evidence arose from the observations of Temin that a large proportion of the growth-stimulating activities of fetal calf serum on cells in tissue culture is due to an insulin-like peptide that he named *multiplication-stimulating activity* (MSA) (see Dulak and Temin).

It then became clear that sulfation factor has insulin-like as well as multiplication-stimulating activities. A unifying hypothesis was proposed that these three types of activities are in fact due to an interrelated group of insulin-like peptides under growth hormone control (Daughaday et

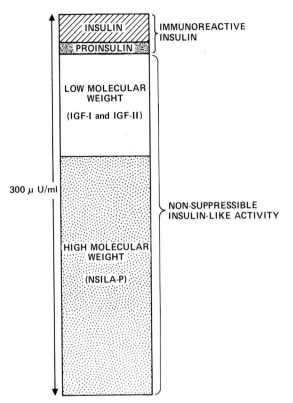

FIGURE 2

Schematic diagram of the different forms of insulin-like activity in plasma. IGF-I and IGF-II are the two insulin-like growth factors; NSILA-P is nonsuppressible insulin-like activity in plasma.

al., 1972), and the term *somatomedin* (SM) was proposed for these hormonal peptides. This intuition proved correct when a Swiss team working on the purification of NSILA isolated and sequenced not one but two peptides of the somatomedin group (Rinderknecht and Humbel, 1978a and 1978b). Both peptides possess a striking structural relationship to human proinsulin, thus explaining the insulin-like biological actions. These workers proposed a new nomenclature and termed these substances insulin-like growth factors I and II (IGF-I and IGF-II).

The multiple terminologies applied to these substances made it difficult to evaluate contributions from different laboratories. However, it is now established that the somatomedin peptides in human plasma are relatively small in number and that some of the terminologies are merely different names for identical substances. SM-C, described by Van Wyk, and IGF-I, se-

quenced by Rinderknecht and Humbel, are the same peptide. IGF-II is chemically and structurally distinct; MSA is now believed to be the homologue of IGF-I in the rat. SM-A is probably a mixture of SM-C–IGF-I and IGF-II peptides, although the final proof is not yet available. SM-B is not a member of the somatomedin group either structurally or biologically (Haldin et al.). Thus, it seems likely that there are in fact only two somatomedin peptides circulating in human plasma, the SM-C–IGF-I and IGF-II peptides. This dual system of somatomedin peptides is also present in other species (Hintz and Liu, 1982).

THE SOMATOMEDIN PEPTIDES

The somatomedins share a common general structure (Fig. 3). Like proinsulin, they have A and B regions with two connecting disulfide bonds and one intrachain disulfide bond. In these A and B regions there is greater than 50 percent homology with human insulin. Furthermore, 19 of the 21 amino acid positions that are constant in insulin molecules from a wide variety of species are also constant in the SM-IGF peptides. Also similar to proinsulin, the somatomedins contain a C-peptide region that is analogous to but shorter than the C peptide of proinsulin (8- and 12-amino acids long as compared to 31 in human proinsulin). In addition, the SM-C–peptide region does not possess Arg-Arg or Arg-Lys amino acid pairs to delineate it for proteolytic removal, also unlike the situation with proinsulin-insulin. The SM-IGF peptides are believed to remain as single-chain amino acid peptides. Also unlike insulin and proinsulin, both IGF-I and IGF-II have C-terminal extensions called the *D region*. The three-dimensional structures of the somatomedins have not yet been determined, but computer modeling studies using the known three-dimensional structure of insulin and the amino acid sequence of the insulin-like growth factors suggest that there is also a large degree of three-dimensional homology between the somatomedins and insulin (Blundell et al.). Differences in the putative receptor-binding regions of insulin and the somatomedins could explain the incomplete cross reactions of these related peptides with their receptors. Differences in the structures of the B-chain regions, which are the most antigenic regions in the molecules, may

IGF-I   NH$_2$ - Gly - Pro - Glu - Thr - Leu - Cys - Gly - Ala - Glu - Leu - Val - Asp - Ala - Leu - Gln - Phe - Val - Cys - Gly - Asp - Arg - Gly - Phe - Tyr - Phe - Asn - Lys - Pro - Thr -
IGF-II NH$_2$ - Ala - Tyr - Arg - Pro - Ser - Glu - Thr - Leu - Cys - Gly - Gly - Glu - Leu - Val - Asp - Thr - Leu - Gln - Phe - Val - Cys - Gly - Asp - Arg - Gly - Phe - Tyr - Phe - Ser - Arg - Pro -
HPI   NH$_2$ - Phe - Val - Asn - Gln - His - Leu - Cys - Gly - Ser - His - Leu - Val - Glu - Ala - Leu - Tyr - Leu - Val - Cys - Gly - Glu - Arg - Gly - Phe - Phe - Tyr - Thr - Pro - Lys - Thr -
} B region

IGF-I   - Gly - Tyr - Gly - Ser - Ser - Ser - Arg - Arg - Ala - Pro - Gln - Thr -
IGF-II - Ser - Arg - Val - Ser - Arg - Arg - Ser - Arg -
HPI   - Arg - Arg - Glu - Ala - Glu - Asp - Leu - Gln - Val - Gly - Gln - Val - Glu - Leu - Gly - Gly - Gly - Pro - Gly - Ala - Gly - Ser - Leu - Gln - Pro - Leu - Ala - Leu - Glu - Gly - Ser - Leu - Gln - Lys - Arg -
} C region

IGF-I   - Gly - Ile - Val - Asp - Glu - Cys - Cys - Phe - Arg - Ser - Cys - Asp - Leu - Arg - Arg - Leu - Glu - Met - Tyr - Cys - Ala -
IGF-II - Gly - Ile - Val - Glu - Glu - Cys - Cys - Phe - Arg - Ser - Cys - Asp - Leu - Ala - Leu - Leu - Glu - Thr - Tyr - Cys - Ala -
HPI   - Gly - Ile - Val - Glu - Gln - Cys - Cys - Thr - Ser - Ile - Cys - Ser - Leu - Tyr - Gln - Leu - Glu - Asn - Tyr - Cys - Asn - COOH
} A region

IGF-I   - Pro - Leu - Lys - Pro - Ala - Lys - Ser - Ala - COOH
IGF-II - Thr - Pro - Ala - Lys - Ser - Glu - COOH
HPI
} D region

FIGURE 3

Homologies between the sequences of somatomedin-C-insulin-like growth factor I. (SM-C-IGF-I), insulin-like growth factor II (IGF-II), and human proinsulin (HPI) peptides. Dashed lines enclose the amino acids that are the same.

explain the lack of cross reaction between most antisera against insulin and the insulin-like growth factors.

The insulin-like growth factors also differ from insulin and proinsulin in regard to their transport in plasma. Insulin and proinsulin circulate free in plasma, whereas the SM-IGF peptides in the plasma are tightly bound in two complex forms of approximately 150,000 and 50,000 mol. The 150,000-mol wt complex is usually predominant and appears to consist of three subunits: the somatomedin peptide, a second subunit of approximately 40,000 mol wt that contains the ability to bind to the somatomedin peptide, and a third subunit that is acid labile (Fig. 4). The smaller complex is apparently composed of the binding-protein subunits and the somatomedin peptides (Hintz and Liu, 1979; Furlanetto). The physiologic role of these complexes is not established, but somatomedins have half-lives of up to 18 h, much longer than that of other peptide hormones (Kaufmann et al., Cohen and Nislet). The proportion of unbound or free somatomedin peptides in plasma is less than 1 percent of the total amount (Daughaday et al., 1982). Whether only the free somatomedin is active or whether the complex forms are also active is unclear (Hintz and Liu, 1980). Because the bulk of somatomedins in plasma are in the complex forms and because there is an excess of unsaturated binding protein(s) in plasma, the measurement of somatomedin activity in plasma is complicated.

PHYSIOLOGY OF THE SOMATOMEDIN PEPTIDES

The general outlines of somatomedin pathophysiology appear clear. The level of SM-C–IGF-I peptide is under tight growth hormone control. Concentrations are high in states where growth hormone secretion is increased, and are decreased in situations where growth hormone secretion is decreased. Thus, the concentration of SM-C-IGF-I can serve as a useful index of growth hormone secretion. Because of the long half-life of SM-C-IGF-I in plasma, measurement of the level at a single time point is a potential index of the integrated growth hormone secretion over a 24-h period, thus making unnecessary the use of the stimulation tests that are usually required for assessments of growth hormone it-

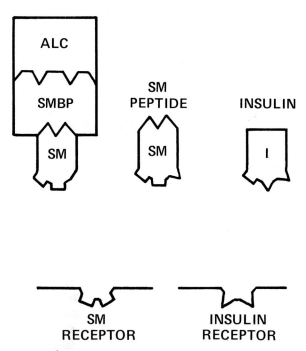

FIGURE 4

Model of the somatomedin (SM) complexes in plasma. I, insulin; SM, somatomedin; SMBP, somatomedin-binding peptide; ALC, acid labile component.

self. The long half-life also obviates the necessity of measurements in multiple samples for an accurate assessment of average SM-C levels. SM-C-IGF-I is believed to be the major mediator by which growth hormone promotes growth, since SM-C-IGF-I alone is sufficient to promote somatic growth in the absence of growth hormone (Schoenle et al.). Thus, measurement of somatomedin levels may be particularly useful in circumstances in which growth hormone is uncoupled from somatomedin secretion.

Less is known about the pathophysiology of IGF-II levels in human plasma, but it correlates less well than SM-C-IGF-I with growth hormone secretion. While IGF-II levels are low in hypopituitary states, the proportional decrease is less than that of SM-C-IGF-I. At the other end of the spectrum, subjects with growth hormone excess and acromegaly do not have increased IGF-II.

Since in normal plasma there is a threefold higher concentration of IGF-II than of IGF-I, the specificity of any assay for IGF-I must be clearly defined. Relatively small changes in IGF-II can easily mask changes in SM-C-IGF-I if the assay is not completely specific. The question of specificity applies both to some bioassays and some radioreceptor assays. Thus, a knowledge of the various assays for somatomedin and their specificities is necessary before deciding which should be used and how to interpret the results.

ASSAYS FOR THE SOMATOMEDINS

As is true for other hormones, the first assays for the somatomedin peptides were bioassays, and much of the present knowledge of somatomedin pathophysiology was elucidated with these bioassays. However, the reproducibility of such bioassays is poor compared to that of radioligand assay methods. Furthermore, bioassays are tedious, expensive, and complex to perform and have not received widespread use in clinical medicine. The receptor assays represented a great advance in reproducibility, but it was not until the development of the radioimmunoassays for the somatomedins that the measurement of these peptides became applicable for clinical medicine.

SM-C-IGF-I

The features of several radioimmunoassays for SM-C-IGF-I are summarized in Table 1. The first, developed by Furlanetto et al. using a rabbit antisera against purified SM-C conjugated to bovine albumin, is commercially available in the United States. This antisera has a high specificity for SM-C-IGF-I, with a 50:1 ratio of detection of SM-C-IGF-I compared to IGF-II. In addition, half-maximum displacement is achieved with less than 1ng/ml of pure SM-C-IGF-I. The problems caused by the existence of free SM-binding protein sites in plasma and by the complex forms of somatomedin are circumvented by using a nonequilibrium method of incubation, in which the linearity of plasma curves is similar to that of purified peptide standard. The levels of somatomedin measured in plasma by this method appear to be less than the total content of SM-C-IGF-I. Furthermore, the assay is affected by a variety of factors such as anticoagulants, ionic environment, and types of glassware. Modifications of this radioimmunoassay using either acid chromatography or acid ethanol extraction for partially removing somatomedin peptides from plasma before assay have been proposed by both Daughaday et al. and the Stanford group (Kemp et al.). These modifications remove the binding protein and allow the assay of the total amount of SM-C-IGF-I peptide present, but the modifications also make the assay more complicated. Another antisera against purified IGF-I was developed by Zapf and colleagues in Switzerland. This immunoassay appears to be somewhat less specific and less sensitive for IGF-I than the antisera of Furlanetto et al. The latter assay utilized chromatography to separate the SM-IGF peptides from binding protein prior to assay. Similar immunoassays against SM-C-IGF-I have also been developed by Bala and Bhaumick, Baxter et al., and Liu et al. An immunoassay developed against SM-C by Hall et al. appears to be specific mainly for SM-C-IGF-I.

Another approach to developing antisera has been developed by Hintz and coworkers. Using a synthetic C-peptide fragment of IGF-I conjugated to thyroglobulin, they showed that some

TABLE 1
Radioimmunoassays for somatomedin-C-insulin-like growth factor I (SM-C-IGF-I) peptide

Assay	Sensitivity, B/BO = 0.5	Specificity, IGF-I/IGF-II
Furlanetto	0.6 ng/ml	50
Zapf	2.2	27
Hall	1.2	100
Bala	0.8	10
Hintz		
C peptide	60.0	>1000
Carboxyterminal	8.0	200
Baxter		
Polyclonal	2.0	?
Monoclonal	4.0	9

antisera against the conjugated peptide cross react successfully with the intact SM-C-IGF-I in plasma. This antisera has the advantage of extreme specificity with less than 1 part in 1000 cross reaction to IGF-II or other somatomedin peptides. While the sensitivity is not as great as that of some of the other antisera, the relatively large amount of SM-C-IGF-I in plasma makes the assay usable for clinical determinations. As in the Zapf assay, the latter assay prevents interference by the free SM-binding protein sites in plasma by acid stripping each sample before assay. This immunoassay is also now commercially available in the United States. Baxter et al. have recently described a monoclonal antibody against IGF-I which appears to be both sensitive and specific. Such monoclonal antibodies may eventually make the clinical assay of somatomedin peptides more widespread and available.

IGF-II

Radioimmunoassays for IGF-II are less well developed, but two such assays have been described. Zapf and coworkers have developed a radioimmunoassay utilizing an antisera against purified IGF-II, which has been utilized for studies of the physiology of IGF-II and IGF-I. Another assay for IGF-II was developed by Hintz et al. and utilizes as the antigen the synthetic C-peptide region of IGF-II cross-linked to thyroglobulin. The antisera not only cross react with intact IGF-II but also allow the use of iodinated, tyrosylated C-peptide region of IGF-II as the radioligand. The published data from these two IGF-II immunoassays are similar. In both cases the average plasma level of IGF-II in normal adults is about 600 ng/ml, and the levels are lower in subjects with hypopituitarism. However, the proportional difference in IGF-II levels between hypopituitary subjects and normal controls is less than that of SM-C-IGF-I. A striking feature of both immunoassays is that acromegalic patients with high levels of IGF-II nevertheless have normal levels of IGF-II. Thus, a small amount of growth hormone may be sufficient to ensure maximal synthesis of IGF-II, and additional growth hormone may not increase the rate of synthesis. Alternatively, the amount of binding protein available may limit the amount of IGF-II in plasma.

CLINICAL CORRELATES

The two commercially available immunoassays for SM-C-IGF-I have reasonable specificity. What clinically important uses can be made of this determination? Because it is transported in plasma in a complex form and consequently has a long half-life, SM-C-IGF-I exhibits little diurnal variation. Thus, assay of a single specimen drawn at any time during the day can serve as a reasonable estimate of average somatomedin levels throughout a 24-h period, and consequently SM-C levels can be used as a simple assessment of the rate of growth hormone secretion.

SM-C-IGF-I has been studied extensively as a screening test for the two major abnormalities of growth hormone secretion: hypopituitarism and acromegaly. A single sample of SM-C-IGF-I can serve as a reasonable screen for growth hormone deficiency. The finding that the SM-C–IGF-I level is normal for age in a child above age 5 or in an adult essentially rules out the possibility of growth hormone deficiency.

However, there are other causes of low somatomedins summarized in Table 2. Newborns and children of less than 5 years of age have low levels of SM-C when compared to older children and adults. Because of this, the lower limits of normal for age overlap with the values found in subjects with growth hormone deficiency, and many infants and children have somatomedin levels that do not distinguish between the low, but normal for age, levels of SM-C-IGF-I and the abnormally low values (Hintz et al.). In rare syndromes of growth hormone resistance (i.e., Laron dwarfism and its variants), growth hormone levels are usually high and appear to be biologically active. However, these individuals resemble growth hormone–deficient patients and have low levels of SM-C-IGF-I. This disorder appears to be due to an inherited failure to respond to growth hormone and enhance the production of SM-C-IGF-I. At the other end of the age spectrum, a significant percentage of otherwise normal elderly individuals have low levels of SM-C-IGF-I in association with disordered growth hormone secretion (Rudman et al., 1981). It is not known whether these low levels of somatomedin and growth hormone levels are clinically important to the aging process. Malnutrition is another cause of low somatomedin levels, and many malnourished subjects have high levels of

TABLE 2

Causes of low somatomedin-C-insulin-like growth factor I (SM-C-IGF-I) levels in plasma

Growth hormone deficiency
Growth hormone resistance syndrome (Laron dwarfism and its variants)
Ineffective growth hormone syndrome
Newborn and < 5 years old
Aging
Malnutrition
Cirrhosis and hepatic failure
Hypothyroidism
Severe acute illness

growth hormone, suggesting that malnutrition causes an acquired form of growth hormone resistance (Hintz et al., 1978). In addition, hypothyroidism, cirrhosis, hepatic failure, and many forms of acute severe illness are associated with low somatomedin levels. Thus, the finding of low somatomedin level is a cause for further diagnostic tests to determine whether the low SM-C–IGF-I level is due to growth hormone deficiency or has another cause.

Rudman et al. (1980) have reported that some patients with constitutional growth failure have normal response of plasma growth hormone to provocative tests but low somatomedin levels, and that the group with low somatomedin levels responded to therapy with growth hormone. Consequently, Rudman et al. proposed that the finding of low somatomedin level associated with normal responses of growth hormone to provocative tests may be an indication for treating children with growth hormone. In other studies of children with constitutional growth failure associated with low somatomedin levels for age, there was no correlation between growth response and somatomedin levels (Gertner et al.; Van Vliet et al.). Thus, the role of somatomedin levels in predicting the response of this important group of patients to therapy remains unsettled. Growth failure of this type may result from an ineffective growth hormone due to some structural abnormality of the molecule or, alternatively, some subtle defect in the neural control of growth hormone secretion. Carefully controlled trials of growth hormone therapy must be performed to determine which of these patients will respond favorably to growth hormone treatment.

SM-C-IGF-I levels are also useful in diagnosing cases of growth hormone excess, particularly in the diagnosis and follow-up of acromegaly (Clemmons et al.) and pituitary gigantism. Most patients with acromegaly, irrespective of plasma levels of growth hormone, have elevations of plasma levels of SM-C-IGF-I. Thus, the assay can serve as a useful screening procedure for acromegaly in subjects with clinical signs suggestive of the diagnosis. Clemmons et al. have also reported that measurement of SM-C-IGF-I is the single most useful chemical assessment of the activity of acromegaly after treatment. While this finding has been disputed, the measurement of SM-C-IGF-I is undoubtedly a useful aid in both diagnosis and follow-up of patients with acromegaly. Analogous to the situation with low somatomedin levels, several clinical situations may lead to increased plasma SM-C–IGF-I levels (Table 3). The diagnosis of pituitary gigantism is complicated by the fact that levels of SM-C–IGF-I normally increase during adolescence (Bala et al.); indeed, during the rapid-growth phase of adolescence, levels of SM-C-IGF-I in normal children may be within the range diagnostic of acromegaly in adults. Relatively high levels of the hormone have also been reported in subjects with obesity, renal failure, and hypercortisolism. In addition, there are technical problems that may result in falsely elevated levels if plasma is not handled correctly (Chatelain et al.). This phenomenon appears to be due to a dissociation of the bound form of the molecule into the smaller units, which are more accessible to the antibody, and does not occur in the immunoassays utilizing acid-treated or acid-chromographed plasma. In summary, a single elevated somatomedin value is not diagnostic of growth hormone excess and must be interpreted in relation to the information available on the patient. It must be kept in mind that occasional patients with growth failure have

TABLE 3
Causes of high somatomedin-C–insulin-like growth factor I

Acromegaly
Pituitary gigantism
Adolescence
Somatomedin resistance syndrome

been reported to have elevated levels of SM-C-IGF-I. In theory these individuals may have a block in somatomedin action leading to growth failure accompanied by a failure of suppression of growth hormone levels due to defective somatomedin feedback on the pituitary or hypothalamus.

Less is known about the pathophysiology of IGF-II; it appears that measurement of IGF-II will be of less value than of SM-C-IGF-I for the screening of hypopituitarism. An exception to this may be in children of very young age. IGF-II values are remarkably constant in normal individuals from 1 year of age to adulthood (Zapf et al.), and the measurement of IGF-II levels may be useful as a screen for growth hormone deficiency in children under age 5. Since the values of IGF-II are not elevated in situations of growth hormone excess, the measurement will be of no use in acromegaly. One situation where elevated IGF-II values would be predicted to be elevated is in the plasma of subjects with hypoglycemia associated with tumors that do not produce insulin. However, the work of Zapf et al. suggests that the levels of immunoassayable IGF-II are not routinely increased in such cases. Thus, the clinical usefulness of an IGF-II radioimmunoassay has not been established.

CONCLUSIONS

The somatomedins are a group of peptides under the control of growth hormone and other hormonal or nonhormonal factors. Two distinct somatomedins circulate in human plasma, SM-C-IGF-I and IGF-II. These hormonal peptides have insulin-like and growth-promoting actions in vitro. In addition, SM-C-IGF-I causes growth in the absence of growth hormone and appears to play a role in the feedback control of growth hormone secretion. The somatomedin peptides have strong homologies and presumably share a common evolutionary ancestor with proinsulin. Radioimmunoassays for SM-C-IGF-I are now

reasonably well developed and are available for clinical use. Because the somatomedin peptides have a long half-life and, therefore, show little variation during the day, the measurement of SM-C-IGF-I is a useful means of assessing growth hormone–secretion rates and of screening for growth hormone deficiency and growth hormone excess in both adults and children. As is true for other radioimmunoassays, there are a variety of clinical situations that lead to falsely elevated or falsely low SM-C-IGF-I levels. In addition, sM-C-IGF-I levels change strikingly with age, and a single value cannot be interpreted without careful consideration of the overall clinical setting. It is uncertain whether the measurement of IGF-II will be of clinical importance. Whether the somatomedin peptides are the sole mediators of growth hormone action also remains to be determined. However, these peptides occupy a unique niche between classical hormones and tissue-growth factors, and elucidation of their exact role in normal and pathological states will almost certainly provide major insight into the normal growth process.

References

BALA RM, BHAUMICK B: Radioimmunoassay of a basic somatomedin: Comparison of various assay techniques and somatomedin levels in various sera. J Clin Endocrinol Metab 49:770, 1979

——— et al: Serum immunoreactive somatomedin levels in normal adults, pregnant women at term, children at various ages, and children with constitutionally delayed growth. J Clin Endocrinol Metab 52:508, 1981

BAXTER RC et al: Radioimmunoassay for somatomedin-C: Comparison with radioreceptor assay in patients with growth-hormone disorders, hypothyroidism, and renal failure. Clin Chem 28:488, 1982

——— et al: Monoclonal antibody against human somatomedin-C–insulin-like growth factor-I. J Clin Endocrinol Metab 54:474, 1982

BLUNDELL TL et al: Insulin-like growth factor: A model for tertiary structure accounting for immunoreactivity and receptor binding. Proc Natl Acad Sci USA 75:180, 1978

BURGI H et al: Nonsuppressible insulin-like activity of human serum: I. Physicochemical properties, extraction and partial purification. Biochim Biophys Acta 121:349, 1966

CHATELAIN PG et al: Effect of in vitro action of serum proteases or exposure to acid on measurable immunoreactive somatomedin-C in serum. J Clin Endocrinol Metab 56:376, 1982

CLEMMONS DR et al: Evaluation of acromegaly by radioimmunoassay of somatomedin-C. N Engl J Med 301:1138, 1979

COHEN KL, NISSLET SP: The serum half-life of somatomedin activity: Evidence for growth hormone dependence. Acta Endocrinol (Copenh) 83:243, 1976

DAUGHADAY WH et al: Characterization of somatomedin binding in human serum by ultracentrifugation and gel filtration. J Clin Endocrinol Metab 55:916, 1982

—— et al: Inhibition of access of bound somatomedin to membrane receptor and immunobinding sites: A comparison of radioreceptor and radioimmunoassay of somatomedin in native and acid ethanol extracted serum. J Clin Endocrinol Metab 51:781, 1980

—— et al: Somatomedin: Proposed designation for sulfation factor. Nature 235:197, 1972

DULAK NC, TEMIN HM: A partially purified polypeptide fraction from rat liver cell conditioned medium with multiplication-stimulating activity for embryo fibroblasts. J Cell Physiol 81:153, 1973

FROESCH ER et al: Antibody-suppressible and non-suppressible insulin-like activities in serum and their physiologic significance. J Clin Invest 42:1816, 1963

FURLANETTO RW: The somatomedin C binding protein: Evidence for a heterologous subunit structure. J Clin Endocrinol Metab 51:12, 1980

—— et al: Estimation of somatomedin C levels in normals and patient with pituitary disease by RIA. J Clin Invest 60:648, 1977

GERTNER J et al: Insulin-like growth factor-I levels do not predict response to growth hormone in hormonally normal short children. Pediatr Res 17:457A, 1983

HALDIN C-H et al: Somatomedin B: Mitogenic activity derived from contaminant epidermal growth factor. Science 213:1122, 1981

HALL K et al: Immunoreactive somatomedin A in human serum. J Clin Endocrinol Metab 48:271, 1979

HINTZ RL et al: Characterization of an insulin-like growth factor-I/somatomedin-C radioimmunoassay specific for the C-peptide region. J Clin Endocrinol Metab 55:927, 1982

—— et al: Interaction of somatomedin-C with an antibody directed against the synthetic C-peptide region of insulin-like growth factor-I. J Clin Endocrinol Metab 50:405, 1980

—— et al: Plasma somatomedin and growth hormone values in children with protein calorie malnutrition. J Pediat 92:153, 1978

HINTZ RL, LIU F: A radioimmunoassay for insulin-like growth factor II specific for the C-peptide region. J Clin Endocrinol Metab 54:442, 1982

——, ——: Somatomedin plasma binding proteins, in *Growth Hormone and Other Biologically Active Peptides,* A. Pecile and E. Muller (eds). Amsterdam, Excerpta Medica, 1980, p 133

——, ——: Human somatomedin plasma binding proteins, in *Somatomedin and Related Peptides,* G. Giordano (ed). Amsterdam, Excerpta Medica, 1979, p 143

KAUFMANN U et al: Demonstration of a specific serum carrier protein of nonsuppressible insulin-like activity in vivo. J Clin Endocrinol Metab 44:169, 1977

KEMP SF et al: Acute somatomedin response to growth hormone: Radioreceptor assay versus radioimmunoassay. J Clin Endocrinol Metab 52:616, 1981

KLAPPER DG et al: Sequence analysis of somatomedin-C: Confirmation of identity with insulin-like growth factor I. Endocrinology 112:2215, 1983

LARON Z: Syndrome of familial dwarfism and high plasma immunoreactive growth hormone. Isr J Med Sci 10:1247, 1974

LIU F et al: An improved RIA for insulin-like growth factor-I using synthetic radioligand and standard. Clin Res 31:124A, 1983

RINDERKNECHT E, HUMBEL RE: The amino acid sequence of human insulin-like growth factor I and its structural homology with proinsulin. J Biol Chem 253:2769, 1978a

——, ——: Primary structure of human insulin-like growth factor II. FEBS Lett 89:283, 1978b

RUDMAN D et al: Impaired GH secretion in the adult population. J Clin Invest 67:1361, 1981

—— et al: Further observations on four subgroups of normal variant short stature. J Clin Endocrinol Metab 51:1378, 1980

SALMON WD JR, DAUGHADAY WN: A hormonally controlled serum factor which stimulates sulfate incorporation by cartilage in vitro. J Lab Clin Med 49:825, 1957

SCHOENLE E et al: Insulin-like growth factor I stimulates growth in hypophysectomized rats. Nature 296:252, 1982

VAN VLIET G et al: HGH therapy can increase height velocity in short children with normal serum somatomedin-C and GH by RIA. Clin Res 31:125A, 1983

VAN WYK JJ et al: The somatomedins: A family of insulin-like hormones under growth hormone control. Recent Prog Horm Res 30:259, 1974

ZAPF J et al: Radioimmunological determination of insulin-like growth factors I and II in normal subjects and in patients with growth disorder and extrapancreatic tumor hypoglycemia. J Clin Invest 68:1321, 1981

—— et al: Serum levels of insulin-like growth factor and its carrier protein in various metabolic disorders. Acta Endocrinol (Copenh) 95:505, 1980

RECENT ADVANCES IN NEUROIMMUNOLOGY

HOWARD L. WEINER and STEPHEN L. HAUSER

The science of neuroimmunology can be divided into two broad areas of investigation. The first consists of the study of immunologic mechanisms responsible for human disorders and the application of that understanding to the development of specific immunotherapies. The second involves the use of immunologic methods in order to study the basic structure, development, and function of the nervous system.

Jerne was first to suggest that the immune and nervous systems share certain essential characteristics, including the property of memory, the ability to respond in a precise way to a large number of external influences, and the formation of a self-modulating excitability and inhibitory network. In addition, several functionally important surface structures and chemical signals are known to be shared between the immune and nervous systems. On the most practical level, some of the major diseases affecting the nervous system are likely due to an aberration of immune function.

This article will begin by reviewing basic concepts of immunology which are essential to an understanding of this area. Following this, current research findings in a number of nervous system diseases of known or suspected immunologic origin will be summarized. Finally, an update will be presented on the use of immunologic probes in neurobiology in order to provide the reader with a basic foundation with which to understand future developments in this rapidly expanding field.

THE CLONAL NATURE OF THE IMMUNE SYSTEM

The clonal nature of the immune system implies that each lymphocyte and its progeny stem from individual ancestors and bear unique membrane receptors capable of binding a specific physical determinant or antigen. When a lymphocyte is exposed to that antigenic determinant, whether it be a virus or foreign-tissue transplant, the lymphocyte divides, or undergoes clonal expansion. The expanded clone (consisting of as many as 10^7 cells) then carries out its appropriate immune function. Thus, the specificity and diversity of the mammalian immune system (i.e., one's immunologic repertoire) comprises an estimated 10^5 to 10^8 different clones of lymphocytes, each with a unique specificity. These lymphocytes are created during ontogeny, are present before antigen stimulation, and increase in number afterward. It is likely that some self-reactive clones are deleted early in development, while others are present in the mature animal but are not operational because of regulatory influences. With the breakdown of regulatory mechanisms and the expansion of autoreactive clones, "autoimmunity" may result.

Monoclonal antibodies

Monoclonal antibodies are extraordinarily powerful biologic tools which are playing a major role in almost all areas of biologic research because of their ability to define single antigenic determinants. Monoclonal antibodies differ from conventional antibodies because they have a single, unique, specificity. For example, the serum from an animal immunized with a virus contains hundreds of antibodies directed at different determinants on the virus. A monoclonal antibody reacts with only one determinant on the virus. Monoclonal antibodies are produced by injecting a mouse or rat with the antigen against which the monoclonals are to be made (e.g., a virus) and fusing the spleen of the injected animal with myeloma cells. The fusion results in the immor-

251

talization of a single immunoglobulin-producing B lymphocyte as a hybridoma clone of cells that can be carried in a cell culture. Each hybridoma serves as a cellular factory which produces an individual antibody of unique specificity. In immunology, monoclonal antibodies have been used to define different subsets of lymphocytes and to identify antigens unique to neurons, astrocytes, and oligodendroglia (discussed later in this review). Theoretically, they can be used therapeutically. For example, if a brain tumor has a unique surface protein that does not exist on other cells, and monoclonal antibodies could be made against that protein, the monoclonal antibody could be "tagged" with a toxin and used specifically to destroy tumor cells.

Regulation of the immune response

A balance between a complex series of inducer and suppressor signals is required for the maintenance of immune homeostasis, and abnormalities in this system of regulation may result in clinical disease syndromes. Advances in the understanding of immunoregulation have occurred both in murine models and in human disease states. In general, the basic immunologic principles established in murine models have found their counterpart in humans, although by necessity at a simpler level. Although it is not necessary to review this entire area, three major concepts which have become central to an understanding of immunoregulation will now be defined: immunoregulatory T cells, idiotype-antiidiotype networks, and immune-response genes.

Immunoregulatory T cells   *T cells,* or *thymus-derived lymphocytes* (so named because they mature to immunocompetent T cells within the environment of the thymus), are the fundamental immunoregulatory cells of the immune system. The regulatory nature of T cells has been demonstrated by their ability to modulate the immune response both in vivo (in the mouse) and in vitro. Different subsets of regulatory T cells have been identified on the basis of surface glycoproteins which serve as phenotypic markers for the functional properties of the cell. The development of monoclonal antibodies which se-

lectively identify distinct T-cell subpopulations has, within the past 5 years, resulted in important new insights into the function of these cells in health and disease.

Regulatory T cells consist of suppressor and helper (or inducer) cells. These cells regulate both humoral immunity (B-cell production of antibody) and cellular immune responses (e.g., graft rejection, delayed-type hypersensitivity, and cytotoxic responses against virally infected cells). In addition, other effector cells including macrophages, polymorphonuclear leukocytes, and mast cells are under the influence of immunoregulatory T cells and their products.

In human peripheral blood, 65 percent of lymphocytes are T cells; the remainder are B cells (immunoglobulin-bearing cells), monocytes, or cells without T- or B-cell markers (null cells). The T3 monoclonal antibody identifies all T cells in the peripheral blood, T4 identifies the inducer (or helper) population (60 percent of T cells), and T5 or T8 identifies the suppressor-cell and the cytotoxic-cell population (30 percent of T cells). The T suppressor cell and T cytotoxic cell, although functionally distinct, cannot currently be distinguished with monoclonal antibody markers. Thus, the cell that is identified by the T5 or T8 marker is often referred to as a suppressor-cytotoxic cell. These subsets are analogous to the Lyt1 + (inducer or helper cell) and Lyt2,3 + (suppressor-cytotoxic) T-cell subsets in mice. The T4 subset has been further subdivided based on reactivity with serum from patients with juvenile rheumatoid arthritis (JRA). T4 + JRA + cells induce T5/8 suppressor-cell activation while T4 + JRA − cells induce help for B-cell differentiation and immunoglobulin production and for cytotoxic T-cell effector function (see Fig. 1). The T4 + JRA + subset has a similar counterpart in the Lyt1 + Qal + murine subpopulation. The human T4 + subset can also be divided into cells which do or do not express Ia antigen on their surface following activation. The present scheme of immunoregulatory T-cell function will undergo multiple changes as it is further dissected and as new monoclonal antibody markers are developed.

The study of a variety of human diseases using both these markers plus in vitro studies of T-cell function has provided major insights into mechanisms of altered immunoregulation (see Table 1

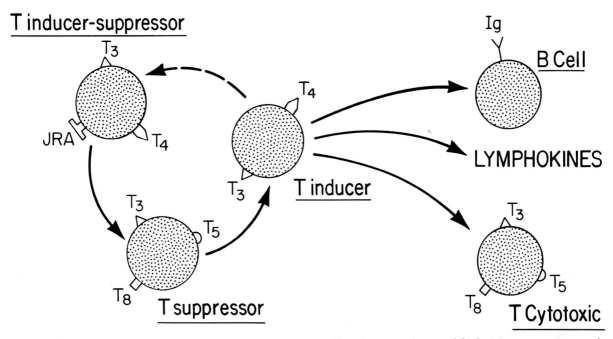

FIGURE 1

Immunoregulatory T-cell network in humans. Interacting networks of T cells regulate the immune response and can be identified on the basis of surface glycoproteins which serve as phenotypic markers for the functional properties of the cell. For example, T inducer cells (which bear T4 and T3 markers) induce B cells (which have immunoglobulin or Ig on their surface) to produce immunoglobulin. B cells without T inducer cells will not produce Ig when stimulated. If sufficient T suppressor cells (which bear T3, T5, and T8 markers) are added to B cells and T inducer cells, the production of antibody by B cells is shut off. T inducer cells also produce lymphokines which are sol-

uble substances that amplify the immune response and induce T cytotoxic cells. Although T suppressor and T cytotoxic cells have different functional properties, surface markers have yet to be found that distinguish these cells. A subgroup of T inducer cells possess the JRA marker (a surface structure reactive with serum from patients with juvenile rheumatoid arthritis). These cells are believed to be inducers of suppressor cells. Based on murine studies, a cell that induces the inducer-suppressor cell (represented by the dotted line) may exist, though it has yet to be described in humans. In summary, all T cells possess the T3 marker, inducer cells possess the T4 marker, and suppressor-cytotoxic cells possess the T5 and T8 markers.

for summary). For example, some patients with acquired agammaglobulinemia are unable to trigger B-cell synthesis of immunoglobulin because of an absent or defective T4+ population, while other patients with agammaglobulinemia have normal T cells but possess B-cell abnormalities. In terms of neurologic disease, a loss of T5/8 suppressor-cytotoxic cells occurs during acute attacks of multiple sclerosis with reconstitution of these cells during recovery (discussed below).

Idiotypes and the network hypothesis The *network hypothesis* refers to communication between lymphocytes by a series of reactions against their own cell-surface antigen receptors or idiotypes. *Idiotype* refers to the site on the

lymphocyte receptor that combines with antigen, and a clone of lymphocytes shares a common idiotype. For the B cell, the antigen-specific receptor is immunoglobulin and the idiotypic site on the immunoglobulin molecule consists of both heavy chain and light chain determinants. Similarly, antigen-specific idiotypes are also present on most T cells. The network hypothesis states that these idiotypes themselves are immunogenic, and during the course of the immune response, clones of cells are expanded that make antiidiotypic or antiantigen receptor antibodies. In an analogous way, a third-order cell may be generated (anti-antiidiotypic), which may bear a receptor similar or identical to the original idiotype. This network of receptor-antireceptor in-

TABLE 1
Abnormalities of immunoregulatory T cells in human disease states

Disorders characterized by
  decreased suppression
    Active multiple sclerosis
    Lupus erythematosus
    Acute graft-vs.-host disease
    Hemolytic anemia
    Hyper-IgE syndrome
    Renal graft rejection
    Juvenile rheumatoid arthritis (decreased
      inducer-suppressor subset)
Disorders characterized by
  increased suppression
    Epstein-Barr virus infection
    Chronic graft-vs.-host disease
    Acquired agammaglobulinemia (type 1)
    Cytomegalovirus infection
    Lepromatous leprosy (specific suppression to
      lepromin antigen)
    Sarcoid
    Acquired immunodeficiency
Disorders characterized by
  defective help
    Acquired agammaglobulinemia (type 2)

teractions ultimately results in a modulating or regulatory influence on the immune response. The experimental study of the network hypothesis is currently a major focus of immunologic investigation.

To give an example of how the network hypothesis might function during the course of the normal immune response to a virus, assume that a virus has one antigenic determinant. That determinant will bind specifically to lymphocytes that have the appropriate receptor or idiotype on their surface, resulting in an expansion of those clones. That expansion ultimately involves antibody production, which is the result of collaboration between a T inducer cell and a B cell, both with the same idiotypic receptor on their surface. (The viral antigen is presented to the cells by a macrophage or antigen-presenting cell and communication between the T and B cell is mediated by a variety of soluble factors.) The antiviral antibodies produced by the B cell bear idiotypic determinants that can bind the virus. In addition, the determinants are themselves immunogenic and serve as antigens, so that antiidiotypic antibodies are made. These antiidiotypic antibodies do not bind virus, but bind to the cell surface receptor that originally bound the virus. This last step makes it possible for anti-antiidiotypic an-

tibodies to be produced. Ultimately, this cascade results in the generation of a suppressive influence that turns off the immune response. Current theories of the T-cell regulation in the mouse involve the generation of a hierarchy of the T suppressor cells bearing idiotypic and antiidiotypic determinants (see Fig. 2). These networks are continuously being redefined as more experimental data accumulate.

A wide variety of experimental murine systems are currently being used to study idiotype-antiidiotype interactions, and this approach has been applied to human illness as well. For example, antiidiotypic antibodies against oligoclonal IgG from the cerebrospinal fluid of multiple sclerosis patients have been made in an attempt to determine the antigenic specificity of the immunoglobulin. Antiidiotypic antibodies have been used to inhibit immunoglobulin production in vitro by B cells from patients with malignant gammopathies. It is theoretically possible that exquisite manipulation of the immune response by antiidiotypic antibodies directed at specific clones of immunoreactive cells might one day occur. One neurologic disease where this may have application is myasthenia gravis where it would be theoretically possible to inactivate specific clones of lymphocytes that react with the acetylcholine receptor. In fact, idiotypic restriction for myasthenia gravis autoantibodies has been reported, suggesting that there may be restricted clones of B cells that produce autoantibodies in the disease.

Immune-response genes As discussed above, most antigens elicit a complex network of functionally distinct T cells that regulate B cells and each other. Idiotypic-antiidiotypic relationships act within this network. A third level of immune regulation involves *immune-response genes,* genes which code for antigens within the major histocompatibility complex (MHC). In a manner not clearly understood, these antigens have a profound effect on the immune response. In the mouse, there is evidence that these gene products act in part by determining the way in which macrophages present antigens to T cells, thus influencing whether or not T cells will respond and whether the responding cells will be helper or suppressor. In addition, the gene products coded for in the MHC may function by

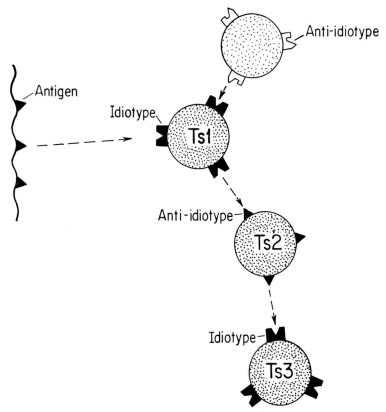

FIGURE 2
Activation of a suppressor-cell network in the mouse. Antigen binds to specific receptors (idiotypes) on the surface of some T cells. These cells, the first-order cells of the suppressor network, are termed Ts1. Ts1 products then react with a second population of cells, Ts2, that possess complementary (antiidiotypic), receptors, or receptors which bind the idiotype. This population in turn reacts with a third subset of cells, Ts3, with anti-antiidiotypic (or idiotypic) receptors. Ts3 appears to represent the active cell which mediates suppression. Note that, while the antiidiotype may be antigenically similar to the initial antigen, this is not always the case.

determining the ultimate T-cell repertoire during the course of T-cell maturation in the thymus. Thus, in certain instances, susceptibility to autoimmunity is strongly influenced by immune-response genes. In animals, for example, the development of experimental allergic encephalomyelitis is linked to certain histocompatibility antigens.

Immune-response genes are associated with the MHC, and the MHC is divided into different loci or alleles. These loci have been studied both in humans and in the mouse using antisera (or cell surface reactivity) which identify cell surface markers unique for each loci, much in the same way that different surface antigens identify blood types, though the MHC is more complex. The MHC is designated HLA in humans and H-2 in the mouse. The human MHC contains four major loci termed HLA-A, B, C, and D. Within each loci there are various alleles, HLA-A3, HLA-A5, HLA-A8, and so on. The susceptibility to a variety of diseases is associated with particular haplotypes, with the strongest association

between HLA-B27 and ankylosing spondylitis and Reiter's disease. The largest category of HLA-associated diseases is linked to alleles of the HLA-D locus and includes celiac disease, thyrotoxicosis, juvenile-onset diabetes, rheumatoid arthritis, systemic lupus erythematosus, chronic active hepatitis, and Sjögren's syndrome. Two neurologic diseases associated with alleles in the MHC are multiple sclerosis, which is associated with HLA-DR2, and myasthenia gravis, which is associated with HLA-B8. Of note is that the D locus may be involved in the regulation of suppressor and helper T-cell networks. The murine counterpart of the D locus is subdivided into several regions that determine the structure of antigens on B cells, macrophages, and T cells. The identification of analogous antigens in the human may make it possible to identify more precisely those people at risk for a particular disease. In humans, most diseases thus far linked to particular HLA loci have a definite or suspected autoimmune pathogenesis.

AUTOIMMUNITY AND THE NERVOUS SYSTEM

Autoimmunity, or a loss of immunologic tolerance (unreactivity) to "self" antigens, may be due to a failure of immune regulation, to a failure to delete self-reactive clones during development, or to a change in the structure of an antigen following viral infection or other environmental exposure. In some situations, more than one mechanism may be necessary for autoimmunity to result. Many important human disease states are currently thought to be autoimmune in origin, including a number of nervous system diseases (see Table 3). For each disease, the development of specific and effective treatment may ultimately depend upon an understanding of the pathophysiologic basis of the symptoms and signs and upon the application of that understanding to each clinical situation. Three central questions must be answered in each of these diseases:

1 Against what *antigen(s)* of the nervous system is the autoimmune response directed?

2 What is the *mechanism* of immune damage?

3 What initiates or *triggers* the autoimmune response?

The three major diseases of the nervous system which appear to be autoimmune in nature are myasthenia gravis, multiple sclerosis, and acute inflammatory polyneuropathy (Guillain-Barré syndrome); these diseases will be discussed using a framework of the three central questions outlined above. Of the three questions, it will become clear that two can be readily answered for myasthenia gravis, one for acute inflammatory polyneuropathy, and none for multiple sclerosis. The immunologic basis of other neurologic diseases will be discussed later in the article on cross-reacting antigens of the nervous system.

Myasthenia gravis

What is the antigen? The antigen against which the autoimmune response is directed in myasthenia is the acetylcholine receptor (AChR). Anti-AChR antibody is present in the serum of approximately 90 percent of myasthenic patients, the titer of which correlates, albeit imperfectly, with disease activity. By using monoclonal antibodies which identify different determinants on the AChR, it is clear that autoantibodies in myasthenia are present against multiple determinants on the receptor, and all of them are not related to disease activity.

What is the mechanism of immune damage? Immune damage is the result of antibody-mediated dysfunction of the AChR at the postsynaptic junction. The most provocative natural experiment which suggested that myasthenia was an antibody-mediated disease was the finding of neonatal myasthenia in children of myasthenic mothers. Direct experimental evidence came

TABLE 2
Analysis of T-cell subsets in neurologic disease

	Percent reactivity with monoclonal antibodies*			T4:T5/8 ratio†	
Patient group	*T3*	*T4*	*T5/8*	*4*	*4*
Normals‡, § N = 40	67 + 3	41 + 2	20 + 5	40	0
Active multiple sclerosis, N = 15	38 + 4	27 + 3	5 + 2	4	11
Inactive multiple sclerosis, N = 18	46 + 4	31 + 3	14 + 2	17	1
Acute Guillain-Barré syndrome, N = 12	64 + 4	47 + 4	20 + 2	12	0
Acute myasthenia gravis, N = 12	50 + 5	35 + 5	19 + 2	11	1
Other neurologic diseases, N = 26¶	53 + 4	34 + 2	17 + 2	26	0

* *Results are expressed as mean + S.E.M.*
† *The T4:T5/8 ratio reflects the relative numbers of helper to suppressor T cells in the peripheral blood. In normal individuals, the T4:T5/8 ratio is less than 4.*
‡ *p = 0.05 between patient and normal control groups.*
§ *p = 0.00001 (Fisher's exact test).*
¶ *Includes vascular, inflammatory, infectious, degenerative, and malignant diseases.*

with the transfer of disease from myasthenics to animals using the IgG fraction of myasthenic serum. Only antibodies against certain determinants on the AChR cause myasthenia, just as some, but not all, monoclonal antibodies directed at different specificities of the AChR cause disease when injected into mice.

There is more than one mechanism of dysfunction of the AChR that is induced by anti-AChR antibody. Mechanisms include complement-dependent damage to the postsynaptic membrane, increased AChR degradation caused by cross-linking of AChR by divalent antibody, and direct block of AChR function by binding of antibody to the binding site of AChR and α-bungarotoxin. Antibodies can also modify rather than block AChR function.

Cellular immune mechanisms may also play a role in myasthenia (especially in certain disease subcategories), as cell-mediated immunity against the AChR has been demonstrated in myasthenics.

What triggers the autoimmune response? The major clue in this area is the association of myasthenia with abnormalities of the thymus gland. In addition, myasthenics have an increase of certain HLA types, which must in some way predispose them to the development of autoimmunity and which distinguish different clinical categories (young females with thymic hyperplasia have an increased prevalence of HLA-B8, while this allele is uncommon in older males and patients with thymomas). Consistent abnormalities of immunoregulatory cells have not been found in myasthenia (see Table 2).

The linkage of thymic abnormalities to an autoimmune attack against the AChR may be through shared antigens between these two structures. It has been reported that thymic lymphocytes have a surface antigen which cross reacts with the AChR, and cultured thymic epithelial cells can display musclelike antigens including AChR. In addition, nicotinic receptors on peripheral-blood lymphocytes have been reported. It is possible that AChR-specific helper cells are generated in the thymus and migrate to the periphery where they promote anti-AChR antibody synthesis or that there is a deficiency of specific clonally restricted suppressor T cells in myasthenics. No present evidence indicates

that a virus triggers myasthenia. One speculation concerning the pathogenesis of myasthenia is that all people have low levels of anti-AChR antibodies, but because of an as yet undefined dysfunction of immunoregulation, myasthenia develops in some individuals. In this regard, it is known that myasthenics have an increased incidence of other "autoimmune diseases" such as thyroiditis, hyperthyroidism, red cell aplasia, and lupus erythematosus. Of note is that this clustering of other autoimmune diseases is not generally seen in multiple sclerosis or acute inflammatory polyneuropathy.

Multiple sclerosis

What is the antigen? It is assumed that a component of white matter must be the antigen against which an autoimmune response is directed. A great deal of interest has centered on myelin basic protein (MBP), as it has been shown to be the encephalitogenic determinant for producing experimental allergic encephalomyelitis in animals (see Table 3 and below). Reactivity of cerebrospinal fluid lymphocytes against MBP exists, MBP components can be identified in the cerebrospinal fluid by radioimmunoassay, some patients have cerebrospinal fluid antibodies to MBP, investigators have shown cell-mediated immunity against MBP in multiple sclerosis (MS) (though this is controversial), and sera from MS patients affect myelin in a variety of in vitro assays. It is possible that these reactions against myelin are secondary to myelin breakdown, or that if myelin is the target antigen an appropriate assay has yet to be developed. Of note is that in a recent trial of treatment of MS with MBP, some patients developed a "primary take" to MBP as demonstrated by skin testing. These results suggest that they had not been previously sensitized to MBP antigen (i.e., that immunoreactive cells sensitized to MBP did not exist prior to the skin testing and thus were not responsible for the demyelinating process).

A structure on the surface of the oligodendrocyte such as galactocerebroside could be the antigen. This would explain the specificity of MS for the central nervous system and the early loss of oligodendrocytes from the evolving MS plaque. Early reports of antioligodendrocyte an-

TABLE 3
Autoimmune diseases of the nervous system

	Site	*Antigen*	*Mechanism*	*Trigger*
Definite				
Myasthenia gravis	Postsynaptic neuromuscular junction	Acetylcholine receptor (also in experimental allergic myasthenia gravis)	Antibody and complement	? Thymic abnormalities
Suspected				
Multiple sclerosis	Central nervous system (CNS) white matter	Unknown [myelin basic protein (MBP) in experimental allergic encephalomyelitis (EAE)]	Unknown (Lyt1+ cells in EAE)	? Loss of suppression ? Virus
Acute inflammatory polyneuritis (Guillain-Barré syndrome)	Peripheral nervous system (PNS) white matter	Unknown (P2 protein in experimental allergic neuritis)	Macrophage stripping of PNS myelin	Viral infection
Neuropathy-associated with IgM paraproteinemia	PNS white matter	Myelin-associated glycoprotein (MAG)	Antibody	Unknown
Acute disseminated encephalomyelitis	CNS white matter	? MBP	Unknown	Viral infection
Sydenham's chorea	? Caudate and/or subthalamic neurons	Unknown	Antibody	Streptococcal infection; ? shared antigen with caudate and/ or subthalamic neurons
Myasthenic (Eaton-Lambert) syndrome)	Presynaptic neuromuscular junction	Unknown	Antibody	Tumor in some patients; ? shared antigen
Paraneoplastic cerebellar degeneration	Cerebellar cortex	Unknown	? Antibody	Tumor; ? shared same antigen
Systemic lupus erythematosus	? CNS neurons	Unknown	? Antibody	? Loss of suppression; ? Virus
Polymyositis	Muscle	Unknown	Unknown	? Loss of suppression; ? Virus

tibodies in the serum of patients with MS have not been confirmed, and the binding appears to have been an artifact of nonspecific binding of antibody by the Fc portion of the immunoglobulin molecule. Several investigators are attempting to define specific antigens on the surface of the oligodendrocyte which could be tested as the inciting antigen.

The elevated immunoglobulin in the cerebrospinal fluid of MS patients has never been shown to react with white matter or other central nervous system structures, and its specificity remains an enigma. Although cerebrospinal fluid IgG is locally produced within the central nervous system, clonally restricted B cells and oligoclonal IgG can be demonstrated in the peripheral blood of MS patients. In addition, the number of immunoglobulin-bearing cells in the peripheral blood appears to correlate with cerebrospinal fluid IgG levels in MS patients. Some investigators believe that the IgG in the cerebrospinal fluid is produced by B-cell clones that migrate to the central nervous system during the course of an attack and are trapped there, producing IgG against an unrelated antigen to which the cell was exposed in the periphery.

Other potential targets of an autoimmune reaction (either humoral or cellular) against central nervous system white matter include myelin-associated glycoprotein and myelin gangliosides.

What is the mechanism of immune damage in MS?   Immune injury can occur via the following mechanisms: antibody plus complement, cytotoxic T cells, immune-complex injury, and antibody-dependent cellular cytotoxicity. Although there are multiple studies of these mechanisms in MS, none has been shown to be clearly linked to the disease, and the line of investigation has been hampered by lack of a specific antigen. Nonetheless, several investigators working independently with different systems have recently shown that marked perturbations of immunoregulatory cells (viz., the loss of suppressor cells) occur in the peripheral blood of MS patients during disease activity. This was first shown using a functional assay for suppressor-cell activity and, most recently, using monoclonal antibodies that identify T-cell subsets. Cells bearing the T5/8

marker are reduced, or even absent from the blood during acute attacks of MS and reappear when the attack is over. In a serial study of patients with relapsing, remitting MS where T-cell phenotypes were measured weekly, there was a close correlation in most patients between clinical activity and the frequency of increases in the T4/T8 (helper/suppressor) ratio. In some instances, a drop in suppressor cells occurred as early as 1 week prior to an attack, at a time when the patient was clinically stable. Changes in suppressor-cytotoxic cells have also been found in childhood MS. These changes in immunoregulatory T cells are the first immune aberration in MS so clearly linked to disease activity. The aberration can be measured in the peripheral blood and may ultimately provide an insight into the pathogenesis of the disease.

Reduced numbers of circulating suppressor-cytotoxic cells are not seen in a variety of neurologic diseases (malignant, infectious, vascular) and thus far have not been found in two other autoimmune diseases of the nervous system, myasthenia gravis and acute inflammatory polyneuropathy (Guillain-Barré syndrome) (see Table 2). Similar changes are seen, however, in systemic lupus erythematosus, graft-vs.-host disease, acute renal graft rejection, and hemolytic anemia, demonstrating that these changes are common to a number of autoimmune diseases which do not affect the nervous system.

The loss of suppressor-cytotoxic cells with disease activity in MS cannot by itself explain the specificity of white matter injury. An entire subset of regulatory T cells is decreased, representing thousands of clones, each with a unique idiotype and clonally restricted specificity. If T-cell subset changes play a primary role in the pathogenesis of MS (something as yet unproved), one possible explanation for the specificity of injury is that the loss of a suppressor influence on the immune system allows previously primed cells which have specificity for central nervous system white matter to escape immune regulation, migrate to the central nervous system, and cause injury. The specific immune mechanisms which are then activated may be determined by a combination of prior environmental exposure and an individual's immune-response genes. This may explain why a loss of

TABLE 4
Animal models of autoimmune nervous system diseases

	Experimental allergic myasthenia gravis (EAMG)	*Experimental allergic encephalitis (EAE)*	*Experimental allergic neuritis (EAN)*
Human disease counterpart	Myasthenia gravis	Multiple sclerosis (MS)	Acute inflammatory polyneuropathy (AIP)
Antigen	Acetylcholine receptor	Myelin basic protein (in some models, proteolipid protein or galactocerebroside)	P2 protein
Mechanism	Antibody and complement	Lyt1 + cells; ? antibody in some models	Sensitized cells; ? antibody in some models
Passive transfer	Serum	Lyt1 + cells	Cells
Analogy to human disease	Excellent	Unknown; acute EAE resembles acute disseminated encephalomyelitis more than it does MS; chronic relapsing EAE may be a closer model of MS	Unknown; pathology of EAN and AIP are similar

suppresssor-cytotoxic cells might result in MS in some people and lupus in others.

Where do these cells go and what does their loss mean? One possibility is that they are destroyed. In lupus, autoantibodies exist which react with the T5/8 subset, and one postulate is that the loss of T5/8 cells from the blood of MS patients is secondary to an antibody which recognizes a determinant present both on the T5/8 cell and central nervous system white matter. Lymphocytotoxic antibodies have been reported as well, though their significance is not clear. We have been unable to find antibodies in MS sera that react with isolated T-cell subsets in vitro and currently believe that autoantibodies against T5/8 cells do not play a pathophysiologic role in the loss of T5/8 cells from the peripheral blood of MS patients. A second possibility is that T5/8 cells migrate to the central nervous system where they are effector (cytotoxic) cells for the autoimmune response. In this regard, identification of lymphocyte subpopulations present in the cerebrospinal fluid of patients with active MS has failed to show large numbers of T5/8 cells. More recently, direct characterization of T-cell subsets from brain has revealed that T8 cells are overrepresented in central nervous system perivascular infiltrates in MS compared with peripheral blood, suggesting the possibility that T8 cells may be migrating to the central nervous system in MS.

The mechanism by which immunoregulatory cells change in the peripheral blood of patients with certain inflammatory diseases and their role in the pathogenesis of these diseases remain major biologic questions. It is probable that these changes are secondary phenomena in some diseases and are primarily linked to the genesis of the autoimmune response in others.

What triggers the autoimmune response? It is clear that something triggers a perturbation in circulating immunoregulatory T cells when MS is active. It does not appear to be a virus. Certain viral infections such as infectious mononucleosis result in an increase, rather than a decrease, in T5/8 cells and we have observed no changes in T-cell subsets in normal individuals or in MS patients with simple viral illnesses. In addition, previous investigators have been unable to correlate viral infections with attacks of MS, although some patients may report worsening of their disease following viral infection. Clinically, MS attacks usually occur without clearly inciting events. Thus, either the event occurred too far prior to the attack to be identified or the event(s) that triggers the attacks is(are) yet to be discovered. It does appear, however, that the MS patient is primed; epidemiologic evidence suggests that this priming may involve a prior viral exposure. As discussed above, this priming occurs predominantly in individuals with certain immune-response genes.

Acute inflammatory polyneuropathy (Guillain-Barré syndrome)

What is the antigen?   In acute inflammatory polyneuropathy (AIP), the antigen appears to be a component of peripheral nerve. Three proteins, P0, P1, and P2, account for approximately 70 percent of peripheral nervous system myelin. P0 is restricted to the peripheral nervous system, P1 is probably identical to central nervous system MBP, and P2 is the antigen which in animals elicits experimental allergic neuritis, a disease virtually identical to AIP (see below). Cell-mediated immunity against peripheral nerve extracts has been demonstrated in AIP by a variety of investigators, but not against the P2 protein. Other investigators have produced EAN in rabbits by injecting galactocerebroside, suggesting that it might be the antigen. Thus, the antigen against which the autoimmune attack is directed in AIP is unknown.

What is the mechanism of immune damage? In AIP, the pathologic mechanism of damage can be visualized under the electron microscope (viz., macrophages penetrate the basement membrane around nerve fibers and strip what appears to be normal myelin from the body of the Schwann cell). Why the macrophages do this and whereby they obtain their specificity is not known. Of note is that macrophage stripping of central nervous system myelin has not been consistently observed in MS, although phagocytic cells may be involved in myelin breakdown.

A number of experiments have shown that cell-mediated immunity against an as yet undetermined component of peripheral nerve exists in AIP. Recently there has been interest in the participation of humoral factors (e.g., antibody, immune complexes) in AIP, as it has been possible to induce demyelination of mouse peripheral nerve by injecting serum from patients with AIP. It is likely that both cellular and humoral components contribute.

What triggers the autoimmune response?
A viral infection in some way must trigger the autoimmune response in the majority (50 to 70 percent) of patients with AIP. Many studies have shown an increased incidence of antecedent respiratory infections and gastrointestinal illnesses in patients with AIP and have suggested an association with cytomegalovirus, Epstein-Barr virus, Coxsackie, echo, influenza, varicella, measles, and mumps viruses. Following A/New Jersey influenza vaccinations in 1976 and 1977, there was an increased incidence of AIP, although this has not occurred with other influenza vaccination programs.

Antecedent surgery and Hodgkin's disease have been reported to be associated with AIP, as has mycoplasma infection. Marek's disease, a disease of chickens associated with a herpes virus, is similar pathologically to AIP, but the mechanism of injury has yet to be elucidated.

It is remarkable that a wide variety of infectious agents (RNA viruses, DNA viruses, enveloped viruses, nonenveloped viruses) can provoke an identical, specific, autoimmune attack against the peripheral nervous system. It must be assumed that these agents act via a final common pathway and either trigger some underlying mechanism (a second agent or a common response against a viral infection such as interferon production) or share a common antigenic structure with the peripheral nervous system.

A potential insight into autoimmunity is contained in the difference between AIP and chronic inflammatory polyneuropathy. There is no HLA linkage in the acute syndrome, whereas there is in the chronic form. This may imply that the development of a relapsing autoimmune reaction against the nervous system (? MS) requires an initial insult (perhaps in association with a viral infection or following trauma), and in people with certain immune-response genes, this insult in turn leads to an abnormal immunoregulatory cycle and recurrent attacks. Of note is that patients with AIP have normal ratios of circulating regulatory T cells (Table 2). In this regard, T-cell subset analysis in patients with chronic inflammatory polyneuropathy will be of interest.

EXPERIMENTAL MODELS OF AUTOIMMUNE NEUROLOGIC DISEASE

Animal models of autoimmune neurologic disease

Animal models of autoallergy to nervous system antigens have been of major importance to the study of immune-mediated nervous system diseases. As shown in Table 4, each of the three diseases discussed in the previous sections has laboratory equivalents which serve as putative diseases models for the human condition. These experimental diseases are induced (or triggered) by injection of the appropriate antigen (or tissue) with an immunostimulator, usually Freund's adjuvant. Thus, experimental allergic myasthenia gravis (EAMG) serves as a model for myasthenia gravis, experimental allergic encephalomyelitis (EAE) for multiple sclerosis, and experimental allergic neuritis (EAN) for acute inflammatory polyneuritis.

EAMG is produced by the inoculation of AChR in adjuvant and is manifested by weakness with fatigability, reduced miniature end-plate potentials, decreased amplitude of the muscle action potential to repetitive stimulation, and clinical response to physostigmine. Antibody and complement can be visualized by electron microscopy at the postsynaptic portion of the neuromuscular junction. In all of these respects, EAMG appears to be an excellent disease model for human myasthenia gravis. Certain forms of EAMG appear to be mediated by antibody, and animal-to-animal transfer of disease can be accomplished using serum from affected animals. Analysis of AChR-specific autoantibodies in EAMG using monoclonal antibodies has revealed that antibodies are produced against multiple portions of the receptor molecule, and that some antibodies are more important than others in the production of signs of disease.

EAE, first described in 1932, is an inflammatory central nervous system demyelinating disease. Two recent advances in EAE methodology have resulted in the development of a closer human disease model and have permitted new insights into the immunologic basis of EAE. In the first, spontaneously relapsing and remitting models of EAE have now been described which closely resemble MS both clinically and pathologically. In the second, the recent development of a reliable method of EAE induction in mice now permits the study of EAE using the tools of murine immunology. Thus, it has recently been demonstrated that Lyt1+2− inducer T-cells play a critical role in the induction of acute EAE in the mouse, suggesting that the immunologic mechanism of EAE is that of a delayed-type hypersensitivity response.

MBP is known to be an effective antigen for the induction of EAE in most species. Sensitivity to MBP has been very difficult to demonstrate in patients with MS. The recent findings that other nervous system antigens, alone or in combination with MBP, are important in the induction of relapsing EAE may have major importance for the study of MS.

The clinical course and pathology of nerve lesions in EAN closely resemble that found in AIP. The antigen responsible for EAN appears to be a basic protein of peripheral nerve myelin termed *P2 protein*. Animal-to-animal transfer of EAN requires sensitized cells, although humoral factors recently have also been implicated in EAN. As previously noted, sensitivity to P2 protein has *not* been found in patients with AIP.

IMMUNOTHERAPY IN AUTOIMMUNE DISEASE

The ultimate goal in these disorders is to devise effective therapy. As knowledge of immunoregulation increases and when both the antigen involved and the mechanism of damage in these diseases are known, appropriate immunotherapy should be forthcoming.

Current immunotherapy involves gross manipulation of the immune response which in some instances is quite effective. Myasthenia gravis is helped by removing the thymus, by steroid therapy, and, in acute situations, by removing autoantibodies with plasmapheresis. In MS, studies have demonstrated that ACTH or intensive immunosuppressive regimens are of benefit; in addition, studies are in progress to assess the efficacy of plasmapheresis in MS, even though an offending autoantibody has not been identified. Similarly, the effectiveness of plasmapheresis in AIP is currently being evaluated, and steroids are of benefit in chronic inflammatory polyneuritis.

More sophisticated forms of therapy than those described above are theoretically possible. For example, if the underlying immune abnormality in MS is indeed the loss of a balance between subclasses of immunoregulatory T cells, then monoclonal antibodies (either human or murine) directed at classes of immunoregulatory cells might be used to modulate the immune response. Drugs which may have selective effects on immunoregulation could also be used. An even more specific immunotherapeutic approach would be the removal or inactivation of idiotype-specific immunoreactive cells that are directing the autoimmune attack. This approach is feasible in experimental myasthenia gravis by the administration of monoclonal antiidiotypic antibodies directed against the idiotype (anti-AChR antibody) which causes the disease. This experiment has already been performed but did not prevent disease, perhaps because the antiidiotypic antibody was too specific (i.e., it did not recognize a broad enough number of reacting clones that were responsible for the disease). Although the efficacy of the above modes of therapy remain hypothetical at present, it is likely that these or other specific forms of immunotherapy will ultimately be employed in clinical situations as the pathophysiologic mechanisms of clinical immunoregulatory abnormalities are better understood.

ANTIGENIC SPECIFICITY OF THE NERVOUS SYSTEM

The generation and specificity of an immune response are determined by the reaction of the immune system to a specific antigen with which it is presented (e.g., the development of specific antiviral antibodies following a viral infection). In addition, the immune system itself is subdivided into various functional classes of cells which can be identified by unique structures on their surface. In an analogous way, "antigenic specificity" of the nervous system exists and is determined by unique cell surface (and in some instances intracellular) structures which are immunogenic and which are present on different classes of cells in the nervous system. These structures are of paramount importance for the study of nervous system tissue in vitro as they allow the unequivocal identification of functional classes and subclasses of neural cells. Furthermore, probes which recognize specific cell surface structures provide a tool by which different cell types may be isolated and studied in vitro. Some of these structures serve as receptors for neurotransmitters and drugs. In addition, specific cell surface structures may serve as targets against which autoimmune responses are directed and function as receptors by which viruses infect the nervous system. Thus, at the most basic level, *neuroimmunology* is the characterization of surface structures on cells of the nervous system and the study of their relationship to cell type, cell function, and cell vulnerability to injury (Fig. 3).

Methods of identifying specific nervous system antigens

Until recently, the primary method of identifying nervous system antigens has relied either on conventional antibodies (heteroantisera) prepared by injecting nervous system tissue into animals or on the binding properties of certain natural toxins for neural cells. For example, heteroantisera against isolated fractions of neurons, oligodendroglia, or tumor-cell lines have been prepared by injecting these preparations into rabbits, and neural specificity has been achieved by removing antibodies against irrelevant tissue via absorption techniques. Some antigens are present on tissue other than nervous system tissue, and investigators have utilized this natural cross reaction to study the nervous system. For example, the Thy 1 antigen is present on the surface of both murine T lymphocytes and central nervous system tissue. Thus, anti-Thy 1 antiserum not only reacts with murine T cells, but with central nervous system tissue as well. Tetanus toxin, which probably binds to specific gangliosides, preferentially reacts with neurons in tissue culture and thus is used as a standard neuronal marker.

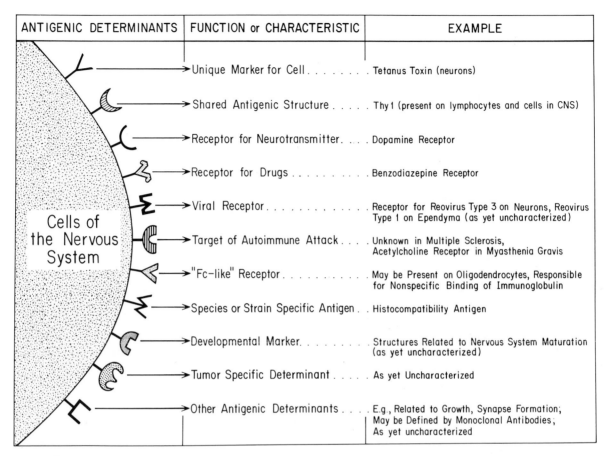

ANTIGENIC DETERMINANTS	FUNCTION or CHARACTERISTIC	EXAMPLE
	Unique Marker for Cell	Tetanus Toxin (neurons)
	Shared Antigenic Structure	Thy1 (present on lymphocytes and cells in CNS)
	Receptor for Neurotransmitter	Dopamine Receptor
	Receptor for Drugs	Benzodiazepine Receptor
	Viral Receptor	Receptor for Reovirus Type 3 on Neurons, Reovirus Type 1 on Ependyma (as yet uncharacterized)
Cells of the Nervous System	Target of Autoimmune Attack	Unknown in Multiple Sclerosis, Acetylcholine Receptor in Myasthenia Gravis
	"Fc-like" Receptor	May be Present on Oligodendrocytes, Responsible for Nonspecific Binding of Immunoglobulin
	Species or Strain Specific Antigen	Histocompatibility Antigen
	Developmental Marker	Structures Related to Nervous System Maturation (as yet uncharacterized)
	Tumor Specific Determinant	As yet Uncharacterized
	Other Antigenic Determinants	E.g., Related to Growth, Synapse Formation; May be Defined by Monoclonal Antibodies; As yet uncharacterized

FIGURE 3

Schematic representation of antigenic specificity of the nervous system. Note that a single determinant may serve more than one function. For example, the acetylcholine receptor not only serves as a neurotransmitter receptor, but is the target of an autoimmune attack in myasthenia gravis and has been reported to be viral receptor for rabies virus. Many of the antigenic determinants on nervous system tissue have yet to be characterized. (This schematic representation is not intended to be all-inclusive.)

With the advent of hybridoma technology and the ability to make monoclonal antibodies against nervous tissue, a new level of sophistication for the immunologic definition of nervous system antigens has become possible. Two recent experiments will be described to illustrate the fine specificity that can be obtained with monoclonal antibody probes of nervous tissue antigens. In the first, Barnstable raised monoclonals which recognize different cell types in the rat retina. This was accomplished by injecting mice with crude membrane pellets prepared from rat retinas, fusing the spleen cells from the injected animals with myeloma cells, and then screening antibody-producing clones. Screening was first performed by simple binding of antibody to retinal membrane preparations and then by specific immunofluorescence. Barnstable described seven monoclonal antibodies, three of which react with specific regions of the rat photoreceptor cell surface. In the second experiment, Zipser and McKay reported even more dramatic specificity and antigenic diversity in neurons by preparing monoclonal antibodies against leech neurons. In their experiment, mice were immunized with the entire isolated nervous system of the leech, spleens from the immunized animals were fused with myeloma cells, and 475 hybridomas obtained from the fusions were screened on intact ganglia. Of the 475, 300 bound the leech nervous system and 41 of these labeled specific subsets of neurons. For example, one monoclonal antibody only stained a bilateral set of five cell bodies in the supraesophageal ganglion. This experiment with monoclonal antibodies demonstrates that it is possible to identify antigens which are restricted to small groups of neurons and implies that a tremendous degree of antigenic diversity within the nervous system can be identified using this technique. These studies also raise major theoretical questions related to organization of the nervous system: As defined by surface (or intracellular) markers, how many unique neuronal subpopulations are there? Could each neuron have its own antigenic marker? More importantly, what is the role of the structures identified by monoclonal antibodies in nervous system function and development?

An enormous advantage of hybridoma technology for the study of the nervous system is that one does not need cell populations of morphologic or biochemical purity to produce monospecific antibodies. Yet, although monoclonal antibodies are easily generated, a large amount of work is then required to fully characterize the reactivity of each individual monoclonal antibody. Complete characterization ultimately entails biochemical identification of the antigen with which the monoclonal antibody reacts. Some monoclonal antibodies may be ''too specific'' for practical use in biologic investigation. For example, they may identify such a restricted portion of the antigen being studied that there is significant cross reaction with other antigens. This has created difficulties in the development of monoclonal antibodies against neurotransmitters.

Over the next few years, a large number of monoclonal antibodies will be described which not only will recognize the entire variety of cell types in the central and peripheral nervous system but will create new subdivisions and subsets of cells within the current categories. Since a secreting hybridoma line can produce unlimited quantities of the same monospecific antibody, ultimately a catalogue of standard reagents will be available to investigators.

Utilization of nervous system cell surface markers in biologic investigation

One of the major uses of cell surface markers is for the positive identification of the various nervous system cell types in tissue culture. It is not always possible to identify neural elements solely on the basis of light-microscopic morphology (e.g., neurons from glia in early cell culture or mixed neuronal and glial elements in heterogeneous cultures), and for many investigations it is impractical to use electrical properties for the definition of neurons. Using an analogy to immunology, virtually all lymphocytes look identical when viewed under the microscope. The identification of surface markers which are specific for functional lymphocyte subclasses (e.g., which identify T-cell subsets) has been of major importance in immunologic investigation. Similarly, nervous system markers which distinguish neurons and the major classes of glial cells in culture have fulfilled an important function in neurobiologic investigation.

In addition to identifying neural classes, antibodies to unique neural cell surface structures can be used to positively or negatively enrich for cell populations. For example, it is possible that a particular class of neurons could be labeled by a monoclonal antibody that recognizes a unique surface structure on those neurons. That antibody could then be labeled with a fluoresceinated tag and the cells purified on an automated fluorescence-activated cell sorter in an analogous way that lymphocyte subsets are purified. In another approach, it is possible to enrich for certain neural cell classes by binding antibody specific for those neuronal cells to plates, overlaying a mixed population of cells, and harvesting only those cells which bind to the plates. Furthermore, ''negative selection'' with antibody can be utilized specifically to lyse a cell poulation. For example, fibroblasts that may make up 10 to 20 percent of a Schwann cell preparation can be eliminated by treating the cell population with anti-Thy 1 antibody (which binds to fibroblasts but not Schwann cells) and then adding complement to lyse the fibroblasts.

In addition, antibodies which recognize unique antigenic structures on the surface of neural cells can be used in a variety of ways for investigating the biology of both normal and abnormal nervous system function, as described in the following examples. (1) Monoclonal antibodies to cell surface components may alter cell shape, cell-recognition patterns, and cellular differentiation or may block more complex functions such as synaptogenesis. Thus, they can be used to define which determinants on the cell surface are required for neural function and/or differentiation. (2) Monoclonal antibodies can be used to define the unique nervous system structures which are targets of autoimmune injury. Thus, in the experimental model of myasthenia gravis, monoclonal antibodies against certain determinants on the AChR cause muscle weakness when injected into animals, whereas monoclonal antibodies against other determinants on the AChR have no effect. (3) Although at this time theoretical, monoclonal antibodies against specific nervous system structures might have profound effects on nervous system function when administered in vivo.

Cell types of the nervous system and their antigens

It is beyond the scope of the present review to describe in detail the currently defined neural antigens and their markers. In many instances markers recognize determinants which are present on more than one cell type in the nervous system and there are differences in the species specificity of these markers depending on the antibody being used. In addition, with the advent of monoclonal antibody technology, there is an exponentially increasing number of reagents being generated that may be identifying new antigenic determinants. Thus, for the purpose of this review, the major subclasses and standard antigenic determinants are presented in Fig. 4; a more detailed partial listing of antigenic determinants is presented in Table 5. For a more complete listing, the reader is referred to the references at the end of this review.

Neurons The standard marker for neurons in culture is tetanus toxin. Monoclonal antibodies have been described which distinguish neurons in the central and peripheral nervous system, and a variety of antibodies have been described which identify antigens on neuronal cell lines such as neuroblastoma and pheochromocytoma. Another approach for the investigation of unique neuronal populations has been the generation of antisera which identify neurotransmitters or the enzymes responsible for neurotransmitter synthesis or their degradation. Thus, antisera to 5-hydroxytryptamine, glutamic acid decarboxylase (GABAergic neurons), and choline acetyltransferase (acetylcholine-containing neurons) have been used to identify populations of neurons

within the central nervous system. Peptidergic pathways in the brain have also been mapped using heteroantisera, and the neuroanatomic localization of more than two-dozen peptides has been characterized. Recently, a monoclonal antibody specific for substance P has been produced as has one for choline acetyltransferase. Thus, immunologic probes made against classical neurotransmitters or neuropeptides may be used to selectively identify restricted populations of neurons.

Oligodendrocytes The standard marker for oligodendrocytes is galactocerebroside which is easily labeled with antigalactocerebroside antibody. Monoclonal antibodies which recognize oligodendrocytes have been described, as have monoclonal antibodies against galactocerebroside. Definition of the antigenic determinants on oligodendrocytes is of major research interest because it is possible that the oligodendrocyte is the target of immune-mediated injury in MS. In this regard, if MBP is the inciting antigen in MS, then the oligodendrocyte would not be the target of immune-mediated injury. Mature oligodendrocytes do not have MBP on their surface, although prior to myelination, oligodendrocytes express small amounts of MBP on the cytoplasmic side of the membrane surface. Of note is that oligodendrocytes may have a receptor for the Fc portion of immunoglobulin. The Fc portion of immunoglobulin is the "nonspecific" class-determining site of immunoglobulin (i.e., it determines whether an immunoglobulin is IgG or IgM); it is not related to the antigen-combining site of the immunoglobulin molecule. Thus the presence of an Fc-like receptor on oligodendrocytes has complicated attempts to demonstrate specific antioligodendrocyte antibodies in patients with MS since antibody may nonspecifically attach to the oligodendrocyte via the Fc receptor.

Astrocytes The standard marker for astrocytes is glial fibrillary acidic protein (GFAP). GFAP+ cells are found both in fibrous astrocytes (which are primarily in white matter) and in protoplasmic astrocytes (which are primarily in gray matter). Unlike the markers described for neurons and oligodendroglia, which are surface markers, GFAP is an intracellular marker. Two monoclonal antibodies (C1 and M1) have been described which recognize intracellular antigens

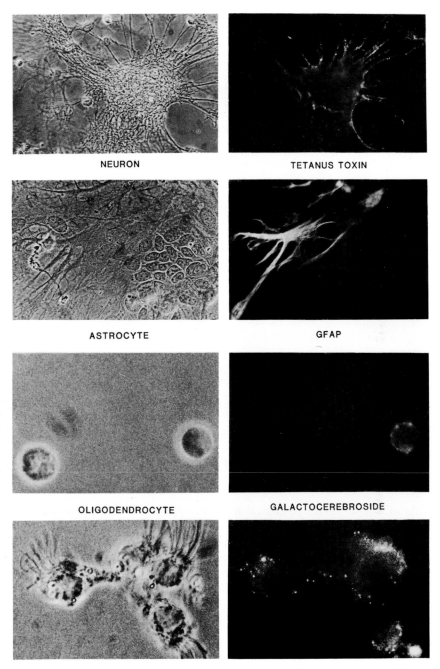

FIGURE 4

Cell types of the nervous system and their antigens. Four major cell types are shown in vitro *under phase and then fluorescent microscopy following staining with appropriate antisera. Tetanus toxin is a surface marker of neurons, glial fibrillary acidic protein (GFAP) an intracellular marker of astrocytes. Note that antigalactocerebroside antibody marks only one of the cells seen under phase microscopy, thus identifying that cell as an oligodendrocyte. The other cell, although morphologically similar to the oligodendrocyte under phase microscopy, is negative for galactocerebroside and thus is not an oligodendrocyte. Ependymal cells are recognized by cilia under phase microscopy and are marked by a specific monoclonal antibody, Epen1.*

NEURON

TETANUS TOXIN

ASTROCYTE

GFAP

OLIGODENDROCYTE

GALACTOCEREBROSIDE

EPENDYMAL CELL

EPEN1 MONOCLONAL ANTIBODY

of astroglial subclasses. Preliminary work with the M1 monoclonal suggests that it may identify a structure that is related to abnormalities in central nervous system development. The M1 monoclonal first appears in white matter astrocytes beginning at postnatal day 7, and by postnatal day 10 it is expressed in Bergmann glial fibers and granular layer astrocytes from which it disappears by the fourth postnatal week. Of note is that the expression of M1 persists abnormally in cerebellar Bergmann glial fibers of adult neurological mutant weaver mice. These results suggest that the structure identified by the M1 monoclonal may in some way be linked to astroglial maturation and illustrates the potential use of monoclonal antibodies for the investiga-

TABLE 5
Cell types of the nervous system and their antigens*

Cell type	Heteroantiserum or marker	Monoclonal antibody
Neuron	Tetanus toxin Cholera toxin Thy 1 (marks a subset of central nervous system neurons and all DRG neurons) Neurotransmitter and peptide markers	A2B5 A4 (central nervous system only) Cholineacetyltransferase Substance P
Oligodendrocyte†	Antigalactocerebroside, anti-myelin basic protein, and anti-oligodendrocyte antisera	01-4 Antigalactocerebroside
Astrocyte‡	Glial fibrillary acidic protein	C1, M1 Ran-2
Ependymal cell	Morphology (cilia)	Epen1 C1 Ran-2
Schwann cell	Ran§	
Fibroblasts	Thy 1 Large external transformation sensitive protein	

* *This list is partial; see references for complete listing.*
† *Oligodendrocytes can also be labeled with antisulfatide, cholera toxin, anti-Gm$_1$, and anti-Gm$_3$, in addition to these standard markers.*
‡ *In addition to these standard markers, a population of astrocytes are labeled with cholera toxin and anti-Gm$_1$. In addition, the S-100 protein is present on astrocytes, oligodendrocytes, Schwann cells, and during early development, on neurons. It has been used as a marker for tumors of glial origin.*
§ *Antigalactocerebroside and antioligodendrocyte heteroantisera cross react with Schwann cells.*

tion of abnormalities of central nervous system differentiation.

Ependymal cells Ependymal cells are easily identified under phase microscopy by their characteristic cilia. Nonetheless, all cells lining the ventricular surface are not ciliated, and there are different subclasses of ependymal cells. A monoclonal antibody prepared by injecting mice with an enriched population of ciliated murine ependymal cells appears to be relatively specific for ependymal cells. Other monoclonals have also been described which recognize ependymal cells. Destruction of ependymal cells may lead to the development of hydrocephalus, and there is evidence that ependymal cells have receptors for a number of viruses. Thus, the definition of antigenic determinants on the ependymal cell surface may lead to a better understanding of the role viruses play in the development of hydrocephalus in the newborn.

Schwann cells, fibroblasts, and microglia
Schwann cells are identified by heteroantisera and by monoclonal antibodies. Fibroblasts are identified by staining with Thy 1 antisera, and microglia in culture are identified by their phagocytic properties (e.g., ingestion of fluoresceinated conjugates). At the present time, microglia are not identified by any conventional markers. Large external transformation sensitive protein (LETS) is found on fibroblasts and leptomeningeal cells but not on neurons or glia.

Antigens which are shared between nervous system and other tissues or between nervous system and infectious agents

One possible mechanism of immune-mediated damage against a nervous system antigen is the sensitization of the immune system against a structure that is antigenically similar to a central nervous system antigen and which is present on another tissue in the body or on an infectious agent.

Early experimental evidence suggested that the central nervous system was an immunologically privileged or isolated site. Thus, if an animal was primed to an antigen by direct inoculation into the central nervous system, when the animal was reexposed (challenged) to the same antigen outside the central nervous system a secondary immune response did not occur. On the other hand, if priming took place outside the central nervous system, the animal would mount an effective secondary immune response when challenged within the central nervous system. More recent data have demonstrated that "isolation" of primary immune responses within the central nervous system is not complete. Nonetheless, it is clear that exposure to a central nervous system antigen in the periphery is an effective way to initiate an anti-central nervous system (autoimmune) response from the peripheral immune system, creating the possibility that an anti-central nervous system immune response could develop following an immune response against an antigen shared between the central nervous system and other tissue or an infectious agent.

Thy 1   Thy 1 was one of the first surface antigens described which is shared between brain and other tissue. Although it has not been implicated in any disease processes, it is one of the best studied examples of an antigen which is shared between nervous system and another tissue. In addition to brain, it is present on T lymphocytes, epidermoid cells, and fibroblastic-cell lines. In fact, the presence of this shared antigen between brain and T cells was initially exploited by immunologists for the preparation of antiserum which identified T cells (i.e., rabbit anti-mouse brain antiserum). In the nervous system, Thy 1 may be a differentiation antigen since it is present in very small amounts in neonatal mouse and rat brain and increases to adult levels by 3 weeks after birth. Similarly, in vitro the appearance of Thy 1 on various neural cell types shows a characteristic developmental sequence. The presence of Thy1 antigen on both lymphocytes and nervous system tissue may reflect a more general phenomenon of shared antigens between the nervous system and the immune system. Thus, lymphocytes have been shown to have receptors for acetylcholine, dopamine, and diazepam. In addition, studies of the molecular structure of the immunoglobulin and Thy 1 molecules have shown prominently shared amino acid sequences between these two molecules.

Acetylcholine receptor   As discussed earlier in this review, acetylcholine receptor (AChR)-like antigens have been demonstrated in the nervous system, in the human thymus, and on the surface of human lymphocytes. Given the known association between thymic abnormalities and myasthenia gravis, these observations raise the possibility that shared antigenic structures between the AChR at the neuromuscular junction and the thymus and/or lymphocyte might have a pathogenic role in the disease.

Sydenham's chorea   Sydenham's chorea, a classic manifestation of rheumatic fever, is associated with group A streptococcus infection. Proteins from group A streptococci cell membranes cross react with cardiac and skeletal muscle, valvular heart tissue, kidney, and skin. Antibodies to heart and muscle sarcolemmal membranes cross react with streptococcal membranes, are present in the sera of acutely ill rheumatic fever patients, and correlate with clinical severity, remissions, and relapses. In an analogous study, Husby et al. demonstrated antibodies against a cytoplasmic structure in caudate and subthalamic neurons in 47 percent of patients with Sydenham's chorea. Titers correlated with disease severity, and antibody was absorbed out with caudate neurons or streptococcal membranes but not by sarcolemmal membranes. These results indicate that there may be a cross reaction between an antigen on the surface of the streptococcal membrane and in the caudate nucleus, and that this antigen does not appear to be shared by sarcolemmal membranes. Although the precise specificity of these autoantibodies in Sydenham's chorea and their actual role in disease pathogenesis remain to be established, they represent one of the best examples of a putative immune response to antigen cross reaction causing a neurologic disease. Of note is that antineuronal antibodies have also been described in lupus erythematosus and in Huntington's chorea. Their role, if any, in these two disorders is unknown.

Paraneoplastic syndromes In a variety of instances, diseases of muscle (dermatomyositis), nerve (sensory neuropathy, dysautonomia), or central nervous system (cerebellar degeneration, encephalomyelitis) are associated with tumors elsewhere in the body. Paraneoplastic syndromes are particularly associated with oat cell carcinomas of the lung and with lymphomas.

In a study of differentiation antigens on human lung tumor (oat cell carcinoma), it was found that the tumor expressed two normal differentiation antigens which were undetectable in normal respiratory epithelium. These antigens were identified by preparing rabbit antiserum against purified plasma membrane fractions of the tumor. One antigen was characteristic of neural crest-derived cells of the peripheral nervous system and was found on Schwann cells but not neurons. This antigen cross reaction between a lung tumor and peripheral nervous system tissue was found on six of six oat cell carcinomas. The other antigen was found on epithelial cells of the digestive system. Although hypothetical, these results offer a potential mechanism to explain the sensory neuropathy that has long been associated with carcinoma of the lung.

Other recent studies have provided evidence that specific autoantibodies in the serum of patients may play a role in two other paraneoplastic diseases: subacute cerebellar degeneration and the myasthenic (Eaton-Lambert) syndrome (see Table 3).

The mechanism of neuropathy in patients with malignant paraproteinemia has been clarified to some degree in recent studies. It had been previously known that a percentage (approximately 5 percent) of patients with monoclonal IgM gammopathy developed peripheral neuropathy. It has been found that, in approximately 50 percent of these patients, the monoclonal IgM antibody reacts specifically with a protein of peripheral nerve myelin identified as myelin-associated glycoprotein (MAG). MAG has recently also been found to be present on the surface of natural killer (null) cells, making MAG yet another example of a shared antigen between the immune and central nervous systems. Why this minor protein (constituting less than 1 percent by weight) of peripheral nerve myelin should be recognized by such a large percentage of paraproteinemias remains unknown.

Shared antigenicity between tumor and normal nervous system tissue is not the only pathophysiologic mechanism to explain the variety of paraneoplastic syndromes known to exist. Examples of other possible etiologies include elaboration of factors from the tumor (which then cause nervous system dysfunction) or direct infection by a virus in an immunocompromised host.

Tumor-associated antigens and immunotherapy Not surprisingly, tumors may express surface antigens which are shared with normal tissue. For example, human gliomas are known to contain both the S-100 and GFAP proteins. Other tumor-associated antigens are present only on immature normal tissue (carcinoembryonic antigen, alpha fetoprotein). Finally, some surface markers on malignant cells are unique to the tumor itself. It is clear that antisera which identify surface markers unique to nervous system tumors might have therapeutic utility. In this regard, a monoclonal antibody specific to neuroblastoma has recently been produced and successfully used as a marker to identify the presence of metastases in patients. Human monoclonal antibodies which react with malignant glioma cells have also been reported (prepared by fusing lymphocytes with a human myeloma line), although their specificity has not yet been determined. Such reagents could theoretically be effective in triggering complement-dependent lysis of tumor cells in vivo or could be used to deliver specific radiotherapy or chemotherapy (by tagging of the antibody with the appropriate drug, toxin, or radioactive element). In the case of human glial tumors in particular, breakdown of the blood-brain barrier in association with tumor growth might facilitate contact of administered antibody with tumor cells. Another possible approach to the immmunotherapy of nervous system tumors might involve sensitization (or priming) of patients against their own tumor cells obtained at surgery. The utility of this approach is speculative, although it is reported that up to 90 percent of human glioma patients lack delayed-type hypersensitivity to subcutaneously administered autologous tumor cells. In vitro assay systems, on the other hand, have suggested that most glioma patients do have humoral and cellular immune reactivity against glioma cell lines.

Cross-reacting antigens and viruses It has long been recognized that viral infection may be associated with autoimmunity. For example, the Guillain-Barré syndrome and acute encephalo-myelitis often follow viral infections. In mice, Theiler's virus infection causes acute neuronal damage, and after clearing of virus from the central nervous system, a late demyelinating disease occurs. Epidemiological evidence suggests that a virus may in some way be an initiating factor in the development of MS.

One mechanism of viral-induced autoimmunity could be the generation of an immune response against antigenic determinants shared between virus and the nervous system. Thus, during the course of an immune response to a virus, antibodies or T cells specific for a viral determinant might also damage central nervous system tissue. Other mechanisms to explain viral-induced autoimmunity include viral-induced changes of cell surface components of the cell that the virus infects, incorporation of normal tissue components when a virus buds from the membrane of a cell, and direct effects of a virus on immunoregulatory cells.

Viral receptors The specificity of viruses for certain areas of the nervous system has long suggested that viral tropism was secondary to the interaction of a specific viral protein with a structure on the surface of a particular cell in the nervous system. The most classic example is that of poliovirus tropism for anterior horn cells in the spinal cord. Similarly, mumps virus has a propensity to infect meningeal cells and cells lining brain cavities, varicella virus can produce focal cerebellitis, herpes virus remains latent in dorsal root ganglia and the fifth cranial nerve nucleus, and herpes simplex encephalitis has a characteristic frontotemporal lobe topography. Although a variety of mechanisms ultimately determine the pattern of viral injury to specific areas of the nervous system, in several instances, viral-receptor interactions are important.

An experimental system being studied in our laboratory has demonstrated both in vivo and in vitro paradigms of focal central nervous system damage secondary to viral-receptor interactions. When reovirus type 3 is injected into newborn mice, it causes a lethal encephalitis in all animals, with destruction of neurons but sparing of ependymal cells. On the other hand, when reovirus type 1 is injected, it does not infect neurons but causes a nonlethal infection of ependymal cells which leads to hydrocephalus in many animals. Reovirus is a segmented double-stranded RNA virus containing 10 genes. When hybrid clones were prepared between the two serotypes to determine which gene was responsible for the differing neurotropism of the two serotypes, it was found that the viral hemagglutinin (HA), encoded for by the S1 gene of the virus, determined viral tropism. Thus, clone 3.HA1 which contains only one gene from type 1 (the S1 gene which encodes the viral HA), and the other nine genes from type 3, behaves identically to reovirus type 1 when injected into animals. Thus, it causes a nonfatal ependymal infection with no damage to neurons. Similarly, the reciprocal clone (clone 1.HA3) causes a fatal encephalitis with neuronal destruction but no ependymal cell damage. These in vivo experiments suggest that the tropism and pattern of neurovirulence of the two reovirus serotypes are secondary to the specific interaction of the viral hemagglutinin with a receptor on the surface of the ependymal or neuronal cell. Furthermore, a receptor for the hemagglutinin of reovirus type 3 exists on a subset of murine and human lymphocytes raising the possibility that the virus may be recognizing a shared receptor between the central nervous system and the immune system.

The structure on the surface of ependymal or neuronal cells to which these viruses bind remains to be identified. Nonetheless, it is assumed that a "viral receptor" on the surface of the cell is not present to provide a route of entry for the virus into the cell but represents a surface structure normally present on the cell which the virus "conveniently" utilizes. Precedents for this have been demonstrated in bacteriophage systems where it is known that certain bacteriophages attach to surface structures which are components of transport systems for low-molecular-weight sugars. A similar situation for a neurotropic virus has recently been suggested. Using an in vitro neuromuscular preparation, investigators have demonstrated that rabies virus appears to utilize AChR for entry into the nervous system. In these experiments, α-bungarotoxin (a compound which binds irreversibly to AChR) blocked entry of rabies virus into the nerves. In other viral systems, investigators have demonstrated that Sendai virus binds to specific gangliosides.

As discussed earlier in this review, the affinity of a virus for a specific structure on the cell surface could lead to the generation of antiidiotypic or antireceptor antibodies which themselves react with the same cell surface structure, as does the virus. Thus, autoantibodies could be generated against viral receptors on nervous system tissue during the course of the normal immune response to the virus. In this regard, antiidiotypic antibodies made against antireovirus type 3 antibodies (reovirus type 3 has affinity for neurons in vivo) have been shown to react with neuronal cells in culture.

In conclusion, advances in understanding immunoregulation and in the mechanisms governing immune response in humans have helped to delineate the pathophysiologic basis of several immune-mediated neurologic diseases. Exploitation of the specificity that is possible with immunologic probes has resulted in major advances in knowledge of nervous system antigens. Continued growth in both of these areas will form the scientific basis for understanding nervous system structure and function in health and disease and for devising effective treatment regimens for patients suffering from a variety of nervous system diseases.

Acknowledgments Supported in part by grants NS17182 and NSAI16998 from the National Institutes of Health. Dr. Hauser is a fellow of the National Multiple Sclerosis Society. We thank Marc Tardieu, Robert Brown, and Marty Raff for helpful criticism and review of the manuscript. We thank Pat Lamy-Gilbreath for her help in the preparation of the manuscript.

References

BARNSTABLE CJ: Monoclonal antibodies which recognize different cell types in the rat retina. Nature 286:231, 1980

BRAUN PE et al: Myelin-associated glycoprotein is the antigen for a monoclonal IgM in polyneuropathy. J Neurochem 39:1261, 1982

BROCKES J (ed): *Neuroimmunology.* New York, Plenum, 1982

DRACHMAN DB: Myasthenia gravis: 1. N Engl J Med 298:136, 1978

———: Myasthenia gravis: 2. N Engl J Med 298:186, 1978

FIELDS KL: Cell type-specific antigens of cells of the central and peripheral nervous system. Curr Top Dev Biol 13:237, 1979

HAUSER SL et al: Intensive immunosuppression in progressive multiple sclerosis: A randomized three-arm study of high dose intravenous cyclophosphamide, plasma exchange, and ACTH. N Engl J Med 308:173, 1983

HUSBY G et al: Antineuronal antibodies in diseases affecting the basal ganglia particularly Sydenham's and Huntington's chorea, in *Clinical Neuroimmunology,* FC Rose (ed). Oxford, Blackwell, 1979, p 90

MCDEVITT HO: Regulation of the immune response by the major histocompatibility system. N Engl J Med 303:1514, 1980

MCKAY R et al (eds): *Monoclonal Antibodies to Neural Antigens.* Cold Spring Harbor Laboratory, 1981, Cold Spring Harbor Reports in the Neurosciences, vol 2

NEWSOM-DAVIS J et al: Thymus cells in myasthenia gravis selectively enhance production of anti-acetylcholine-receptor antibody by autologous blood lymphocytes. N Engl J Med 305:1313, 1981

RAFF MC et al: Cell-type specific markers for distinguishing and studying neurons and the major classes of glial cells in culture. Brain Res 174:283, 1979

REINHERZ EL et al: Loss of suppressor T cells in active multiple sclerosis: Analysis with monoclonal antibodies. N Engl J Med 303:125, 1980

———, SCHLOSSMAN SF: Regulation of the immune response-inducer and suppressor T-lymphocyte subsets in human beings. N Engl J Med 303:370, 1980

TARDIEU et al: Interactions of viruses with cell surface receptors. Int Rev Cytol 80:27, 1982

WEINER HL: Multiple sclerosis, in *Current Neurology,* HR Tyler and DM Dawson (eds). Boston, Houghton-Mifflin, 1978, p 53

ZIPSER B, MCKAY R: Monoclonal antibodies distinguishing identifying neurons in the leech. Nature 289:549, 1981

THE REFRACTORY ANEMIAS

STEPHEN H. ROBINSON

The term *refractory anemia* generally refers to a group of acquired disorders of unknown etiology which share the following features, to a greater or lesser extent: (1) anemia with a normocellular, or more commonly, a hypercellular bone marrow; (2) ineffective erythropoiesis, often with evidence of dyserythropoiesis on inspection of the peripheral blood smear and bone marrow aspirate; (3) frequently, neutropenia and/or thrombocytopenia, so that these patients may be pancytopenic, often with morphologic abnormalities in neutrophil and megakaryocyte as well as in erythroid cell development; (4) variable degrees of iron loading, sometimes associated with the ringed sideroblasts characteristic of refractory sideroblastic anemia; and (5) evolution to acute nonlymphocytic leukemia in some of these patients. These acquired forms of refractory anemia are now considered to be potentially neoplastic disorders of bone marrow cell growth and differentiation and hence part of the myeloproliferative spectrum. In addition, there are rare congenital forms of sideroblastic and dyserythropoietic anemia that are due to metabolic or structural abnormalities of the marrow cells, usually confined to the red cell series.

HISTORY AND CLASSIFICATION

In 1934 Thompson et al. described a group of patients with pancytopenia who differed from the usual patients with aplastic anemia in that there was evidence of active cellular regeneration in the peripheral blood reflected by morphologic changes in the red blood cells, often with some reticulocytosis and the presence of scattered nucleated erythroid cells, together with a normal to hypercellular bone marrow. These authors concluded "that it is quite possible to have serious interference with the normal processes of development, maturation, and delivery of blood cells without evident alteration in the cellular content of the marrow." This is an apt description of the ineffective hematopoiesis that characterizes the disorders we now refer to collectively as refractory anemia.

The term refractory anemia was coined by Rhoads and Barker in 1938 to describe patients with severe anemia and often other cytopenias whose course could not be altered by any known treatment such as iron salts or liver extract. In a classification of refractory anemia published in 1941, Bomford and Rhoads first excluded anemias secondary to underlying disorders such as renal insufficiency, endocrine dysfunction, or cancer. They included the following as subtypes of refractory anemia: aplastic anemia; "pseudoaplastic anemia," referring to patients like those described by Thompson et al. in whom the peripheral blood suggested aplastic anemia but the bone marrow was cellular; some patients with unexplained megaloblastic bone marrow pictures; and an entity they referred to as "leukopenic leukemia." Although the language used to describe these disorders has undergone several transitions, these same entities comprise refractory anemia as the term is generally used today.

In the 1960s Vilter et al. proposed an elaborate classification of refractory anemia which was similar in many respects to that put forth by Bomford and Rhoads but now included refractory sideroblastic anemia. Aplastic anemia was once again included; however, this is now considered to be a separate disorder.

273

More recently, "preleukemia" or "preleukemic syndrome" has been used to refer to patients with refractory anemia because of their propensity to leukemic transformation. Abnormalities in at least two and often all three of the major marrow cell lines (erythroid, granulocytic, and megakaryocytic) have to be present for a disorder to be considered a preleukemic syndrome; thus, the combination of ringed sideroblasts, micromegakaryocytes, and/or impaired granulation of early granulocytic cells would suffice for this diagnosis. What used to be called chronic erythremic myelosis or chronic di Guglielmo's syndrome would fit this definition. The features of chronic erythremic myelosis (including marked erythroid hyperplasia of the bone marrow with megaloblastoid change, nucleated erythroid cells in the peripheral blood, variable cytopenias, a shift to the left in the granulocytic series in the bone marrow, and a predisposition to acute leukemic change) are all possible components of the preleukemic syndrome. The designation "smoldering leukemia" has been used to refer to a subgroup of patients who have a relatively stable, small population of blast cells in the marrow and perhaps the peripheral blood and who often go on to develop overt leukemia.

However, it has become clear that many patients with preleukemia do not undergo leukemic transformation. Therefore, the more descriptive terms *myelodysplastic syndrome* or *hemopoietic dysplasia* have come into use. The French-American-British (FAB) Cooperative Group recently proposed a classification of the myelodysplastic syndromes consisting of five subtypes, in four of which the old designation refractory anemia is retained:

Refractory anemia

Refractory sideroblastic anemia

Refractory anemia with excess of blasts

Chronic myelomonocytic leukemia

Refractory anemia with excess of blasts in transformation

Implicit in this classification is the assumption that these are disorders of bone marrow cell growth which have a neoplastic or potentially neoplastic nature and are often but not invariably associated with abnormalities in multiple marrow cell lines.

This classification does not require that there be abnormalities in more than one cell line for a disorder to be considered one of the myelodysplastic syndromes. Indeed, many patients in the first two categories will present with what appears to be a primary disorder of erythropoiesis. In some of these patients this continues to be the case, whereas in others abnormalities eventually develop in the granulocytic and/or megakaryocytic series. The FAB classification is not without its problems and doubtlessly will be modified with time. However, it serves as a useful framework for the following discussion. We shall first describe features common to all of these entities and then discuss special features that characterize each subgroup.

CLINICAL MANIFESTATIONS

Except for patients with refractory anemia developing after chemotherapy and/or radiotherapy for a previous malignant disease and patients with rare forms of congenital sideroblastic anemia or congenital dyserythropoietic anemia, refractory anemia is usually observed in patients over 50, most often in the elderly. There is no clear predilection with regard to sex. Patients may be asymptomatic and be found to have blood count abnormalities only on routine laboratory examination. They may, however, present with symptoms of anemia such as fatigue and lassitude or cardiac problems such as angina or congestive heart failure. In patients with severe neutropenia there may be recurrent infections affecting particularly the oral cavity, anal area, and respiratory tract. Patients with severe thrombocytopenia may have purpura and excessive bleeding. Unexplained fever may also be a manifestation of acquired refractory anemia.

The physical examination is often normal, although perhaps one-third of patients have moderate splenomegaly and sometimes hepatomegaly. Occasionally there is mild icterus, reflecting the excessive destruction of red cell precursors in the bone marrow. Evidence of hemochromatosis (e.g., bronzing of the skin and/or signs of cardiac, liver, or endocrine abnormalities) is sometimes present, particularly in the sideroblastic subgroup.

LABORATORY FINDINGS

There is moderate to severe anemia in the myelodysplastic syndromes. The red blood cell indices may be normocytic and normochromic but often there is moderate macrocytosis, with mean cell volumes (MCVs) in the high 90s or low 100s. Macrocytosis may be more prominent in the presence of relative folic acid deficiency engendered by the marked erythroid hyperplasia of the bone marrow. Rarely, the red cells are microcytic, in the absence of the usual causes of a microcytic blood picture. The reticulocyte percentage is low, normal, or occasionally slightly elevated, rarely exceeding 3 to 5 percent. The peripheral blood smear may show relatively normal red blood cell morphology, but there is frequently variation in size and shape which can be very striking. Prominent basophilic stippling is often present. Variable numbers of nucleated red blood cells may be found in the blood smear. In the sideroblastic forms of refractory anemia there is typically a hypochromic population of red cells, sometimes relatively small in number, along with round macrocytic cells, giving rise to a dimorphic peripheral blood picture. One may also see erythrocytes containing Pappenheimer bodies, irregular blue inclusions which turn out to be iron deposits when the blood smear is stained with prussian blue; these are most commonly seen in the sideroblastic anemias, especially after splenectomy.

The white blood cell count is usually normal or decreased but is occasionally elevated, especially in chronic myelomonocytic leukemia. The morphology of the circulating white blood cells is usually normal but may be abnormal, especially in disorders with potential leukemic involvement. In these instances there may be Pelger-Huët-like abnormalities in the neutrophils; these cells have hyperchromatic nuclei which are either round and without segmentation or bilobed with a dumbbell or pince-nez appearance. The granulocytes may appear hypogranular and sometimes have bizarre nuclear lobulation. In chronic myelomonocytic leukemia the number of monocytes, some of which may be mature and

some rather immature, is increased. Impaired neutrophil function has been described in some patients with refractory anemia.

The platelet count may be normal, depressed, or elevated. It is commonly decreased in patients with neoplastic forms of refractory anemia. There may be variation in platelet size, and giant platelets may be present on the peripheral blood smear. Qualitative platelet abnormalities have been described in these disorders.

The bone marrow is usually hypercellular, and typically there is erythroid hyperplasia, which is often quite marked. Sometimes, however, the bone marrow is normo- or hypocellular, particularly in patients with refractory anemia following radiotherapy and/or chemotherapy as a prelude to the development of acute nonlymphocytic leukemia; these patients often also have some marrow fibrosis, making the marrow difficult to aspirate.

Despite the ineffectiveness of erythropoiesis, the morphology of the erythroid cells in the bone marrow can be surprisingly normal. On the other hand, it is not uncommon to find evidence of dyserythropoiesis. The red blood cell precursors may have a megaloblastoid appearance (i.e., they appear atypically megaloblastic even though the patient is not deficient in folic acid or vitamin B_{12}). This is presumably a morphologic manifestation of qualitatively abnormal, potentially neoplastic cells. In some instances, however, there is true megaloblastosis due to relative folic acid deficiency as a result of intense erythroid hyperplasia. In addition, the immature red cells may demonstrate multinuclearity, nuclear fragmentation, nuclear lobulation which may be very bizarre, coarse basophilic stippling of the cytoplasm, and irregularities of cytoplasmic staining.

The number of granulocyte precursors in the marrow is variable but is often increased. The morphology of these cells is often normal, but in some instances the cells are hypogranular and in some others the primary azurophilic granules are much larger than normal. The granulocytic series may be shifted to the left, and there may be an increased proportion of blast forms and promyelocytes, especially in patients with refractory anemia with excess of blasts or chronic myelomonocytic leukemia. Even when there are megaloblastoid changes in the erythroid series, it is very unusual to see the giant metamyelocytes and band forms that are characteristic of true megaloblastic anemia, except when there is superimposed folate deficiency.

Similarly, megakaryocytes in the bone marrow may appear normal in number and morphology. In other patients they may be increased or decreased in number. It is not uncommon to find morphological abnormalities of megakaryocytes including small forms, cells containing only a single nonlobulated nucleus, or cells with multiple separate nuclei (referred to as "pawnball" cells by some hematologists), as opposed to the polyploid nuclei of normal megakaryocytes.

Prussian blue stains of the bone marrow reveal an increase in iron stores, often marked in degree. Correspondingly, serum ferritin levels are typically increased. Inspection of individual red blood cell precursors under oil magnification also shows an increased number and size of iron aggregates in the cytoplasm (i.e., there is an increase in sideroblastic iron). In some patients the iron deposits form a partial or complete ring around the nucleus, defining a ringed sideroblast. When 15 percent or more of the nucleated red blood cells in the bone marrow are ringed sideroblasts, we consider the patient to have one of the forms of sideroblastic anemia, a major subcategory of refractory anemia.

The increase in iron stores in the bone marrow in patients with refractory anemia is reflected by an increase in the serum iron concentration, often saturating the total iron binding capacity (TIBC) of serum. The TIBC is usually in the low normal-normal range. The serum iron level may be normal or low in patients in whom the disease has a neoplastic quality (e.g., refractory anemia with excess of blasts) because of the defective reutilization of iron that occurs in a variety of chronic diseases. The serum bilirubin concentration may be mildly or moderately elevated, due predominantly to an increase in the indirect-reacting or unconjugated fraction of bilirubin. Serum LDH levels are typically not increased or are increased only mildly, even when there is marked dyserythropoiesis, in distinction to the often marked elevations observed in the megaloblastic anemias. However, lactic acid dehydrogenase values may be elevated in patients undergoing leukemic change. Serum folic acid levels are normal or occasionally low because of erythroid hyperplasia. Serum vitamin B_{12} levels are normal or sometimes elevated as in various forms of myeloproliferative disease. The leukocyte alkaline phosphatase score is variable and may be normal or either lower or higher than normal. Acquired hemoglobin H disease, increased levels of hemoglobin F, and abnormalities in erythrocytic glycolytic enzymes have all been reported sporadically in patients with refractory anemia, as they have in patients with acute myeloid leukemia and other myeloproliferative disorders.

Measurements of red blood cell survival with ^{51}Cr are normal or show a mild-moderate decrease in the red blood cell life span. Ferrokinetic measurements with ^{59}Fe show a rapid disappearance of iron from the plasma and a high rate of iron turnover but a decreased incorporation of the ^{59}Fe into circulating erythrocytes, a constellation of findings characteristic of ineffective erythropoiesis. Production of carbon monoxide, which is derived from the breakdown of heme, is increased because of the intramedullary destruction of red blood cell precursors. Studies of labeled bile pigment formation from precursors such as glycine-^{14}C demonstrate an increase in the early-labeled peak of bilirubin formation, also compatible with marked ineffective erythropoiesis.

Chromosome preparations of the bone marrow often reveal karyotypic abnormalities. These can be very variable in nature but are often similar to those observed in acute nonlymphocytic leukemia or well-defined preleukemic conditions (e.g., the refractory anemias that occur some time after a patient has received chemotherapy and/or radiotherapy for conditions such as Hodgkin's disease, multiple myeloma, or ovarian carcinoma). Abnormalities in the C group of chromosomes are particularly common. Chromosomal changes often correlate with existing evidence of, or predilection to, leukemic transformation. There is a syndrome, the *5q-syndrome,* in which deletion of much of the long arm of chromosome 5 is associated with macrocytic anemia and thrombocytosis in the peripheral blood and erythroid hypoplasia, dyserythropoiesis, and megakaryocytes with nonlobulated nuclei in the bone marrow. Some of these patients also have an increase in blast forms in the marrow, and of the 15 cases reported as of 1979, 2 have developed acute nonlymphocytic leukemia.

Abnormal growth of bone marrow progenitor cells in vitro has been observed in many patients with refractory anemia. Normal bone marrow cells form colonies of mature cells after several days of culture in semisolid media such as agar or methylcellulose. Colonies formed in the presence of so-called colony-stimulating activity consist of granulocytes and macrophages and are derived from early progenitor cells called *CFU-GM* (colony forming units that are committed to the granulocyte-macrophage pathway of cell development). Marrow cells grown in the presence of erythropoietin form two kinds of colonies of erythroid cells: large irregular burstlike configurations that are derived from a primitive erythroid progenitor cell known as the burst-forming-unit erythroid (BFU-E), and small colonies derived from more mature progenitor cells which are called colony-forming-unit/erythroid (CFU-E). Variable results have been reported for the development of CFU-E-derived colonies in patients with refractory anemia. On the other hand, there is generally a marked decrease in BFU-E colony formation, reflecting either a diminution in the number or, more likely, a defect in the growth of these early erythroid progenitor cells, despite the marked erythroid hyperplasia that is characteristically present in the bone marrow. The formation of granulocyte-macrophage colonies from CFU-GM is also frequently abnormal. The number of these colonies is often reduced, and an increased proportion of CFU-GM is found in the light density fraction after the marrow cells have been subjected to centrifugation in a density gradient. In addition, there is sometimes an increase in small abortive colonies which are referred to as clusters. All of these changes in CFU-GM expression are similar to those observed in patients with acute nonlymphocytic leukemia; indeed, a marked decrease in granulocyte-macrophage colony formation appears to correlate with a leukemic outcome.

DIAGNOSIS

The diagnosis of refractory anemia is reached largely by a process of exclusion. If the marrow appears megaloblastic, one must measure serum folic acid and vitamin B_{12} levels and often give a therapeutic trial of these agents to ensure that one is not dealing with folate or B_{12} deficiency; indeed, some patients with primary refractory anemia may have a partial response to folic acid, as described above.

The findings of mild unconjugated hyperbilirubinemia, morphologic abnormalities of the erythrocytes on the peripheral blood smear, erythroid hyperplasia of the bone marrow, and occasional splenomegaly may suggest that one is dealing with a hemolytic anemia. The reticulocyte count, however, is typically not elevated in refractory anemia and, if it is, the degree of elevation is substantially less than would be expected from the degree of erythroid hyperplasia of the bone marrow. In addition, dyspoietic changes in the marrow will often indicate that one is dealing with refractory anemia. Nevertheless, some patients with primary hemolytic disease (e.g., some patients with immunohemolytic anemia) may have a poor reticulocyte response and a ^{51}Cr-labeled red cell survival study rarely may be necessary to make the distinction from refractory anemia.

Some patients with aplastic anemia may demonstrate marrow "hot pockets," that is, foci of marrow hypercellularity that often contain dyserythropoietic cells. However, the remainder of the marrow should be hypocellular, as would be apparent on the marrow biopsy. This would be further confirmed with the additional one or more biopsies that are required to establish a diagnosis of aplastic anemia. In refractory anemia, on the other hand, the marrow is usually well populated with cells and is often markedly hypercellular.

The constellation of pancytopenia, a hypercellular bone marrow and splenomegaly may suggest a diagnosis of "hypersplenism," leading to a search for primary liver disease with portal hypertension or splenic infiltrative disease such as lymphoma.

The anemia of chronic disease may be mistaken for refractory anemia since the former sometimes occurs in the absence of any discernible evidence of a chronic infectious, inflammatory, or neoplastic problem at the time the anemia is detected. The physician may be tempted to make a diagnosis of refractory anemia because of the apparently idiopathic nature of the hematologic problem. However, characteristic sets of findings with regard to iron metabolism usually suffice to differentiate the two disorders. In the anemia of chronic disease the serum iron concentration is depressed, the TIBC is also low, bone marrow iron stores are normal or increased, and the serum ferritin level is correspondingly elevated, but there is a paucity of intracellular iron in erythroid precursor cells in the bone marrow (i.e., a decrease in bone marrow sideroblasts). In contrast, both the serum iron concentration and sideroblastic iron are generally increased in patients with refractory anemia; in addition, there is often dyspoietic change in one or more of the marrow cell lines. The abnormalities in iron metabolism in the anemia of chronic disease reflect a characteristic defect in iron reutilization; iron released from hemoglobin when senescent erythrocytes are destroyed by cells of the reticuloendothelial-phagocytic system is retained in the storage compartment rather than being liberated into the plasma to be transported to the bone marrow for reincorporation into the hemoglobin of developing erythroid cells. The changes in iron metabolism in refractory anemia, by contrast, reflect increased iron turnover and iron loading due in large part to the ineffective erythropoiesis.

The hereditary dyserythropoietic and sideroblastic anemias must also be differentiated from the various forms of acquired refractory anemia. In contrast to acquired refractory anemia, these hereditary anemias usually occur in the pediatric age group and in a familial setting; however, some patients do not have a positive family history and the problem may sometimes be first detected during adulthood. In these hereditary anemias the white blood cell count and platelet count are typically normal; they may be either normal or abnormal in acquired refractory anemia. Hereditary sideroblastic anemia is discussed further in a later section concerned with the sideroblastic anemias. Hereditary dyserythropoietic anemia has been divided into three subtypes showing the following differential findings:

I–Megaloblastic changes in multinucleated erythroid cells in which the nuclei have internuclear bridges

II–Normoblastic erythroid cells with bi- and multinuclearity, abnormal mitoses, and karyorrhexis

III–Pronounced multinuclearity with up to twelve nuclei per erythroid cell

Patients with type II dyserythropoietic anemia may have a positive acidified serum (Ham) test, a negative sugar-water test, and a high agglutination score with anti-i antibody. A positive Ham test characteristic of paroxysmal nocturnal hemoglobinuria has also been found occasionally in acquired myeloproliferative disorders including forms of refractory anemia. Although it should usually be possible to distinguish congenital dyserythropoietic anemia from acquired refractory anemia on the basis of marrow cytology, family history, and age of onset, the distinction may be difficult in some unusual instances.

Although it may sometimes be difficult to exclude the possibilities mentioned above, the diagnosis of acquired refractory anemia can usually be made on the basis of clinical evidence of ineffective erythropoiesis (anemia and reticulocytopenia with erythroid hyperplasia of the bone marrow); morphologic evidence of abnormalities in differentiation of erythroid, granulocytic, and megakaryocytic cells; and, of course, the pathognomic findings in many of these patients of ringed sideroblasts on iron stain of the bone marrow. The presence of chromosomal abnormalities and abnormal growth of marrow progenitor cells in tissue culture can be very useful. Nevertheless, making the diagnosis of refractory anemia, particularly of the nonsideroblastic variety, can be discomforting to the physician since the diagnosis is made largely by exclusion of other better defined hematologic entities, there is often no specific confirmatory diagnostic test, and the diagnosis carries with it the possibility of eventual leukemic transformation.

ETIOLOGY

In most instances refractory anemia has no definable cause. A few patients with toxic effects of benzene or chloramphenicol will manifest a picture resembling refractory anemia, with erythroid hyperplasia and dyserythropoiesis, usually as a prelude to the development of a hypocellular marrow state. In increasing numbers, patients who have received radiotherapy, chemotherapy usually with alkylating agents, or combined modality therapy for a previous malignant disorder will present with a clinical picture of pancytopenia associated with other manifestations of refractory anemia before they go on to develop acute nonlymphocytic leukemia. In many of these patients the bone marrow is somewhat hypocellular, in contrast to most patients with idiopathic refractory anemia. In addition, there may be some reticulin fibrosis of the marrow, and both ringed sideroblasts and chromosomal abnormalities are common in these patients.

There is evidence for immunologic mechanisms in some patients with refractory anemia. However, this evidence is often inferential or inconclusive, and immunologic factors probably do not play a major role in most patients with these disorders. Admixture of marrow cells from some patients with refractory anemia with normal bone marrow cells suppresses the development of normal CFU-GM-derived granulocyte-macrophage colonies in agar culture. This suggests that the defect in marrow cell growth may sometimes be due to a cell-mediated cytotoxic process. Perhaps related to this phenomenon, it has been possible to increase CFU-GM colony formation in a few patients by the addition of cortisol to their marrow cultures; a positive response predicts that these rare patients have a good chance of responding clinically to steroid therapy. In a case report of a patient with acquired sideroblastic anemia, a good clinical response to azathioprine was attributed to the immunosuppressive properties of this drug, although it might have been due instead to the drug's antineoplastic action. There is also a well-documented report of an unusual case of acquired sideroblastic anemia in a young boy whose serum IgG fraction inhibited erythroid colony formation from CFU-E; both this inhibitory immunoglobulin and the sideroblastic marrow picture disappeared after therapy with cyclophosphamide.

There are several forms of secondary sideroblastic anemia that are associated with exposure to drugs or toxins which impair mitochondrial heme synthesis. Other forms of acquired sideroblastic anemia are associated with a variety of disease states. These are reviewed below under "Refractory Sideroblastic Anemia."

PATHOPHYSIOLOGY

The mechanism of anemia in these disorders is ineffective erythropoiesis (i.e., destruction of abnormal erythroid precursor cells in the bone marrow so that they do not mature into effective, circulating erythrocytes). One can conclude that one is dealing with ineffective erythropoiesis from the disparity between erythroid hyperplasia of the bone marrow and the low or only minimally increased reticulocyte count. Morphologic evidence of dyserythropoiesis, including megaloblastoid change, multinuclearity, and bizarre nuclear configurations, if present, also points to the fact that these erythroid cells are defective and will not mature to the reticulocyte stage. The mild to moderate unconjugated hyperbilirubinemia is largely the result of the intramedullary destruction of young erythroid cells, although there may also be a contribution from some peripheral blood hemolysis.

Disease states characterized by ineffective erythropoiesis are regularly associated with evidence of iron loading including an elevated serum iron concentration, increased intracellular iron deposits in erythroid cells, increased storage iron in the bone marrow, and a high serum ferritin concentration. For reasons that are not entirely clear, ineffective erythropoiesis engenders increased iron absorption from the gut; this is often exacerbated by the need for multiple red blood cell transfusions. Indeed, in some patients with refractory anemia, particularly of the sideroblastic type, hemochromatosis may supervene. This is also true for thalassemia, another disease associated with marked ineffective erythropoiesis and often a large transfusion requirement. Cartwright et al. have demonstrated a high incidence of the HLA-A3 haplotype in patients with primary acquired sideroblastic anemia who develop hemochromatosis. This haplotype is a marker for hereditary hemochromatosis in which two abnormal genes are required to produce clinical disease. Cartwright suggested that hemochromatosis is likely to develop in patients with acquired sideroblastic anemia if they also have a single gene for hemochromatosis, either condition alone being insufficient for the development of parenchymal iron overload. It should be pointed out that hemochromatosis is uncommon in acquired sideroblastic anemia, and the association of HLA haplotypes with the hemochromatosis more frequently encountered in hereditary forms of the disease has not yet been studied.

It is probable that processes similar to ineffective erythropoiesis explain the neutropenia and thrombocytopenia that are seen in many patients with refractory anemia. However, techniques analogous to those for determining the presence of ineffective erythropoiesis (i.e., ferrokinetic measurements and measurements of early-labeled bile pigment formation from isotopic precursors) are not readily available for evaluation of granulocyte and megakaryocyte proliferation.

Ineffective hematopoiesis occurs in a number of hematologic disorders including the megaloblastic anemias, the thalassemia syndromes, and the heterogeneous group of disorders that is subsumed under the category refractory anemia. In the first two categories and in some forms of congenital refractory anemia such as hereditary sideroblastic anemia and hereditary dyserythropoiesis, the ineffective production of erythroid cells is due to a metabolic or structural problem within the cell. The defect in most of the acquired refractory anemias is unknown and the etiology may well be somewhat different from one patient to another. In many of these, however, it would appear that we are dealing with a neoplastic or potentially neoplastic disorder of the bone marrow, one which may be a harbinger of acute leukemic transformation. This concept fits with the fact that all three major cell lines of the bone marrow are sometimes affected and that chromosomal abnormalities and changes in marrow cell growth in vitro similar to those observed in acute nonlymphocytic anemia may be seen in these patients. Moreover, a limited number of studies in black women heterozygous for two different isozymes of glucose-6-phosphate dehydrogenase (G6PD) and who had either sideroblastic or nonsideroblastic refractory anemia have demonstrated only a single G6PD isozyme in the red cells, granulocytes, and platelets. These findings are similar to those in myeloproliferative disorders such as polycythemia vera, indicating that these disorders arise from clonal expansion of a neoplastic pluripotential hemopoietic stem cell which gives rise to all three of these cell lines. It should be kept in mind, however, that many patients with refractory anemia do not develop a leukemic phase. It is also well to remember that pernicious anemia was long considered to be a malignancy until it was found to be a metabolic nutritional disorder.

COURSE AND PROGNOSIS

The course of these patients can be quite variable. Patients with refractory anemia with excess of blasts in transformation are generally in the process of evolution to acute nonlymphocytic anemia, a process which may take a few weeks to several months to complete. Patients with refractory anemia with excess of blasts or chronic myelomonocytic leukemia may have a relatively stable course for a period of several months to even a few years. Indeed, a few such patients recover entirely from their hematologic illness. Many of the others eventually transform to acute nonlymphocytic leukemia, usually over a period of several months to occasionally a few years. Patients with refractory anemia and refractory sideroblastic anemia not having increased blast cells in the marrow have perhaps a 10 to 30 percent chance of developing acute leukemia. Several studies have sought prognostic features which indicate an increased rate of leukemic conversion. These studies were performed in patients with primary acquired sideroblastic anemia and suggested that severe anemia, the presence of leukopenia and thrombocytopenia, or a low serum iron concentration augur poorly; on the other hand, thrombocytosis tends to indicate a nonmalignant course. Chromosomal changes similar to those observed in acute nonlymphocytic leukemia and a marked diminution in granulocyte-macrophage colony formation in marrow culture both tend to predict an eventual leukemic outcome. In fact, they may indicate that leukemia is already present although not yet detectable by morphologic examination of the bone marrow.

In those patients who do not develop acute leukemia, anemia is usually the major problem. In some instances the anemia is mild and the patient's course may be long and relatively benign. In other patients, however, the anemia is quite severe and usually does not respond well to therapy. These patients require repeated transfusions and many develop complications of frequent transfusion therapy such as multiple allo-type antibodies, febrile transfusion reactions, hepatitis, and iron overload.

In a few patients, usually but not invariably those with sideroblastic anemia, hemochromatosis may develop and the patient may suffer from arthropathy, diabetes, cardiac problems, or liver dysfunction. Hemochromatosis is rather unusual except in patients with hereditary forms of sideroblastic anemia. However, it can occur in patients with primary acquired sideroblastic anemia or even nonsideroblastic refractory anemia who have received large amounts of transfused blood or have an HLA haplotype associated with the gene for hereditary hemochromatosis.

Since refractory anemia usually occurs in older patients and may have a benign course, many patients with these disorders eventually die of unrelated disorders or disorders exacerbated by the anemia and its complications (e.g., cardiovascular disease). Other patients with severe neutropenia or thrombocytopenia may succumb to infection or bleeding without developing acute leukemia. Except for those presenting with increased numbers of blast cells in the marrow or blood, only a minority of patients with these "preleukemic" disorders in fact die as the result of acute leukemic transformation.

THERAPY

Treatment for the different forms of refractory anemia is usually not very satisfactory, although various forms of therapy have been more or less successful in occasional patients. In some patients the disorder is so mild as to require no therapy, except perhaps for occasional transfusions. Frequent transfusion therapy is required for many of the others. Some patients do very well even with hematocrits in the mid or low 20s, and it may be possible to manage these patients with few or no transfusions. Since frequent transfusion therapy is associated with numerous complications as outlined in the preceding section, it is best to transfuse patients for symptoms of anemia rather than to maintain an arbitrary hematocrit level.

If the bone marrow shows megaloblastic changes and particularly if the serum folic acid level is low, the patient may profit from the administration of folic acid which may raise the hemoglobin level somewhat but will not restore it to normal. Some patients with refractory sideroblastic anemia will respond to large doses of pyridoxine, 100 to 300 mg per day; the best responses are seen in patients with congenital forms of "pyridoxine-responsive" sideroblastic anemia. A few patients with sideroblastic anemia who fail to respond to pyridoxine may respond to pyridoxal phosphate, 50 mg per day. These agents should be tried for at least 4 to 6 weeks.

Rare patients with refractory anemia will respond to therapy with adrenocortical hormones (e.g., prednisone in the range of 40 to 100 mg per day). Increased granulocyte-macrophage colony formation in vitro when cortisol is added to bone marrow cultures seems to predict a favorable result from steroid therapy. An empirical trial of steroids should be undertaken with caution since many patients seem to do poorly with this form of therapy.

Androgens have been used with generally little success, although an occasional patient may respond well to this form of therapy. Norethandrolone, 200 mg given intramuscularly each week, or oxymetholone, 2 to 3 mg/kg per day by mouth, may be used. These agents may have to be given for 4 to 6 months, although a really good hematologic response usually occurs more rapidly. Liver function tests should be monitored regularly for evidence of cholestatic hepatitis.

Some patients with refractory anemia have been reported to improve after splenectomy. These are anecdotal reports and may well refer to patients with splenomegaly in whom hypersplenism accounted for some of the pancytopenia. It is advisable to document splenic sequestration of ^{51}Cr-labeled red cells before considering removal of the spleen.

Iron overload may become a problem, particularly in patients with sideroblastic anemia. In some of these cases the anemia was so mild that the iron loading could be treated with phlebotomy. In several of these patients a rise in hemoglobin occurred after multiple phlebotomies, suggesting that the iron overload itself had been toxic to the bone marrow. Indeed, in one such patient with the pyridoxine-responsive type of sideroblastic anemia there was decreased activity of two mitochondrial enzymes, δ-aminolevulinic acid (ALA) synthase and ferrochelatase (also called heme synthetase), before iron removal; the activity of the latter enzyme was restored to normal after therapy, indicating that ferrochelatase activity had initially been inhibited by excess iron in the mitochondria. Most patients with refractory sideroblastic anemia are too anemic to withstand phlebotomy. However, newer forms of iron chelation therapy, such as the chronic subcutaneous administration of desferrioxamine, which are proving useful in sickle cell anemia and thalassemia, may also be valuable in patients with sideroblastic anemia who have evidence of hemochromatosis or, on a prospective basis, even those patients who are not yet iron-loaded but require large numbers of transfusions. Based on the earlier experience noted above, it is possible that the anemia as well as the iron overload might be improved in some of these patients.

A small number of patients with refractory anemia with excess of blasts or chronic myelomonocytic leukemia have been treated with aggressive antileukemic regimens. Most of these patients did very poorly, with markedly decreased survival times as compared to untreated patients with the same disorder. However, rare patients experienced complete remissions and had relatively long survivals; these were younger patients who had not had any previous cytotoxic therapy. In general, however, intensive chemotherapy is to be avoided in patients with refractory anemia, many of whom may have a relatively stable course over several years. Indeed, chemotherapy is usually also unsuccessful in patients with refractory anemia who have gone on to develop overt leukemia.

Some patients with refractory anemia have been treated cautiously with agents such as 6-mercaptopurine, with occasional reports of success. More recently, a few patients have been treated with low-dose cytosine arabinoside, 10 to 20 mg/m^2 per day intravenously for a total of 14 to 21 days, sometimes with a good clinical response. This therapy has also had some limited success in the treatment of acute nonlymphocytic leukemia in patients who are not suitable for intensive chemotherapeutic regimens. It has been suggested that treatment with low-dose cytosine arabinoside may work by inducing leukemic cell differentiation. How frequently this mode of therapy will be useful in patients with refractory anemia remains to be determined. It seems unlikely that many will have a durable response, but the treatment has the advantage that it is relatively innocuous.

SUBTYPES OF REFRACTORY ANEMIA

In the following sections we shall describe the features that distinguish the different forms of refractory anemia in the context of the more general discussion presented above.

Refractory anemia

The category of refractory anemia conforms to the foregoing general description and requires little further elaboration. The patient is usually anemic and there may or may not be depression of the white blood cell and/or platelet counts. The bone marrow is usually hypercellular, with erythroid hyperplasia and frequently with evidence of dyserythropoiesis, but the granulocytic and megakaryocytic series often appear normal.

Refractory anemia with excess of blasts

In the condition of refractory anemia with excess of blasts, there are abnormalities of several cell lines both in the peripheral blood and bone marrow. Anemia, neutropenia, and/or thrombocytopenia often coexist in different combinations. The bone marrow is usually hypercellular and shows qualitative abnormalities in multiple cell lines. Ringed sideroblasts are often seen. There is a shift to immature forms in the granulocytic series and the bone marrow may contain 5 to 20 percent blast forms. In addition there may be a small number of blasts (less than 5 percent) in the peripheral blood. This disorder conforms well to the older designations preleukemia or smoldering leukemia. Patients with this disorder often, but not invariably, go on to develop acute nonlymphocytic leukemia over a period of several months to sometimes several years. However, some patients may live for many years with a relatively stable population of blast forms, and full hematologic recovery has been described in a few patients with this disorder.

Chronic myelomonocytic leukemia

Chronic myelomonocytic leukemia is similar to refractory anemia with excess of blasts except for the presence of monocytosis in the peripheral blood and sometimes the bone marrow. The monocytes often appear normal in morphology but may be atypical and young. There may be an increase in mature granulocytes as well. Otherwise, the bone marrow and peripheral blood picture is similar to that in refractory anemia with excess of blasts, and the outcomes of the two disorders are also alike.

Refractory anemia with excess of blasts in transformation

In patients with refractory anemia with excess of blasts in transformation, the peripheral blood contains 5 percent or more blast forms, the bone marrow contains 20 to 30 percent blast forms, and Auer rods may be present in granulocyte precursors. This category presumably represents those patients who are detected during active evolution into a flagrant form of acute nonlymphocytic leukemia.

Refractory sideroblastic anemia

The refractory sideroblastic anemias are defined by the presence of ringed sideroblasts on iron stain of the bone marrow. These are erythroid precursor cells which contain a partial or complete necklace of iron-containing granules around the nucleus. When such ringed sideroblasts make up 15 percent or more of the total erythroid population of the marrow, the patient is considered to have a sideroblastic anemia. The perinuclear distribution of the iron granules indicates that these are mitochondria which are choked with iron, reflecting impairment of heme synthesis in these organelles in which heme synthesis both begins and ends. Some studies have reported a defect in globin synthesis in these disorders, but this is probably a negative-feedback effect of the decreased production of heme.

Although the diagnosis of sideroblastic anemia requires the presence of ringed sideroblasts, the term *sideroblast* actually refers to any nucleated erythroid cell that contains stainable iron granules, and this is true for perhaps 40 percent of the red cell precursors in the normal bone marrow. The siderotic granules in normal cells are aggregates of ferritin in the cytoplasm and reflect the amount of iron available for heme synthesis. The number of sideroblasts and the number and size of the iron granules they contain are increased in many patients with refractory anemia, even of the nonsideroblastic variety (i.e., without ringed sideroblasts), because of increased iron turnover due to ineffective erythropoiesis, probably some decreased utilization of intracellular iron due to impaired red cell maturation, and exogenous iron overload due to increased gastrointestinal absorption and transfusion therapy. In the sideroblastic types of refractory anemia the major abnormality in iron metabolism is in the mitochondria; there is also increased deposition of ferritin in the cytoplasm because of the decrease in mitochondrial heme synthesis as well as the factors mentioned above.

Types of sideroblastic anemia Although primary acquired sideroblastic anemia, also known as idiopathic refractory sideroblastic anemia, is the most common chronic hematologic disorder associated with the presence of ringed sideroblasts in the bone marrow, other causes of this phenomenon exist as outlined in Table 1. There are rare forms of hereditary sideroblastic anemia. These usually conform to a sex-linked pat-

TABLE 1
Types of sideroblastic anemia

I Hereditary sideroblastic anemia
  A Sex-linked type
  B Autosomal recessive type
  C Pyridoxine-responsive type*
II Acquired sideroblastic anemia
  A Primary, or idiopathic, refractory sideroblastic anemia
  B Secondary sideroblastic anemia
    1 Due to drugs or toxins (antituberculosis agents, alcohol, lead, chloramphenicol, nitrogen mustard)
    2 Associated with other conditions (acute nonlymphocytic leukemia, myeloproliferative disorders, hypothyroidism, carcinoma, myeloma, rheumatoid arthritis, polyarteritis nodosa, hemolytic anemia, pernicious anemia, malabsorption, hypothermia)

* A mild response to pyridoxine may be observed in some patients with acquired disease, but the best responses occur in a type of hereditary sideroblastic anemia which is therefore called pyridoxine-responsive anemia.

tern of inheritance, although a few cases have been described in which the pattern of inheritance is that of an autosomal recessive trait. Most forms of sideroblastic anemia are acquired in later life. These may be secondary (related to a drug or toxin or associated with another disease) or primary, also called idiopathic, the latter conforming to the refractory sideroblastic anemia category under primary discussion here.

Several drugs or toxins have been associated with sideroblastic change (i.e., the presence of ringed sideroblasts) which is reversible on withdrawal of the offending agent. This has been observed with antituberculosis drugs, usually some combination of isoniazid, cycloserine, and pyrazinamide. These agents act as antagonists of pyridoxal phosphate which is a cofactor for ALA synthase, the mitochondrial enzyme that is rate-limiting for heme synthesis. Alcoholism, usually in the setting of folic acid depletion, is also frequently associated with reversible sideroblastic change, the precise mechanism of which remains unclear. Chloramphenicol inhibits mitochondrial protein synthesis and thus decreases the activity of ferrochelatase, the mitochondrial enzyme which inserts iron into the protoporphyrin ring to form heme; the mitochondrial cristae become filled with this unused iron, leading to the formation of ringed sideroblasts. Sideroblastic change has also been reported with use of chemotherapeutic agents such as nitrogen mustard; the mechanism is unknown. Finally, chronic lead intoxication is associated with impairment of several enzymes involved in heme synthesis, including ferrochelatase, again leading to potentially reversible impairment of heme synthesis that is sometimes associated with iron loading of the mitochondria.

Sideroblastic changes in the bone marrow also occur sporadically in association with a variety of disease states, as outlined in Table 1. In several of these (e.g., hypothyroidism and rheumatoid arthritis) this is not a simple causal relationship, and treatment of the associated disorder does not necessarily lead to disappearance of the ringed sideroblasts. Ringed sideroblasts, erythroid hypoplasia of the marrow, and thrombocytopenia have been reported to occur with hypothermia; these abnormalities disappeared slowly after the patients regained normal body temperature. Ringed sideroblasts may also be found in

a variety of myeloproliferative disorders, conspicuous among which are the various forms of acute nonlymphocytic leukemia. The relationship between sideroblastic change in the erythroid series and the myeloid leukemias works both ways. The bone marrows of patients presenting with acute nonlymphocytic leukemia may demonstrate sideroblastic change in the residual erythroid cells; this resolves with successful antileukemic therapy. On the other hand, some patients presenting with primary acquired sideroblastic anemia go on to develop acute nonlymphocytic leukemia after a period of several months to many years. In both instances the ringed sideroblasts and the associated defect in heme synthesis appear to reflect an easily discerned defect in biochemical differentiation in neoplastic or quasineoplastic erythroid precursor cells. These, like the leukemic white cell precursors, are descendents of the pluripotential stem cell of the bone marrow, the presumed site of malignant transformation in these patients.

Pyridoxine-responsive anemia Some patients with sideroblastic anemia undergo a partial hematologic response to large doses of pyridoxine, in the range of 100 to 300 mg per day. The best responses are observed in patients with an hereditary form of the disease. Most patients with the primary acquired disorder respond little if at all.

Since pyridoxine responsivity may occur in the various forms of sideroblastic anemia to a greater or lesser extent, it is not yet clear whether pyridoxine-responsive anemia is a single disorder. It is also important to note that this is not pyridoxine deficiency, which is only rarely associated with anemia. In pyridoxine-responsive anemia, unlike a true deficiency state, supraphysiologic doses of pyridoxine are required and do not cause complete reversal of the hematologic changes. Ringed sideroblasts in the marrow and hypochromia of circulating red blood cells usually persist, as does some degree of anemia, and the improvement is usually short-lived if pyridoxine therapy is discontinued.

Nature of the defect in heme synthesis The fundamental defect in primary acquired sideroblastic anemia remains unknown, although it appears to be related to a problem in marrow cell differentiation. In contrast, the inherited forms of sideroblastic anemia, including pyridoxine-responsive anemia, and those that are due directly to drugs or toxins are true metabolic disorders involving defects in the biosynthetic machinery for heme synthesis within the mitochondria of erythroid cells.

Decreased activity of ALA synthase has been described in patients with all forms of sideroblastic anemia. A defect in this key mitochondrial enzyme, which is the initiating and rate-limiting enzyme in heme biosynthesis, would lead to diminished synthesis of heme and consequent retention of iron in these organelles. An accompanying decrease in the activity of another mitochondrial enzyme, ferrochelatase, has been reported in several patients with primary acquired sideroblastic anemia. This would explain the elevation of free erythrocyte protoporphyrin that is found in most subjects with the primary acquired disorder. In contrast, free erythrocyte protoporphyrin is usually lower than normal in the hereditary forms of sideroblastic anemia. Inferential evidence has suggested a defect in the enzyme coproporphyrinogen oxidase in a few such patients described by Heilmeyer et al. many years ago.

Impairment of ALA synthase has also been implicated in the pathogenesis of the pyridoxine-responsive type of hereditary sideroblastic anemia. This is not surprising since the activated form of pyridoxine, pyridoxal phosphate, is a coenzyme for ALA synthase. In addition, a defect in ferrochelatase activity has been described in an instructive patient with pyridoxine-responsive anemia, as mentioned earlier. The activity of ferrochelatase but not ALA synthase increased to normal after excess iron had been removed by phlebotomy and iron chelation therapy. Thus, the ferrochelatase defect appears to have been secondary to iron engorgement of the mitochondria, the latter apparently due to a primary deficit in ALA synthase. It is not clear whether a similar mechanism might account for the decreased ferrochelatase activity that has been observed in some patients with primary acquired sideroblastic anemia. Indeed, the deficiency of ALA synthase that has now been detected in all of the different forms of sideroblastic anemia may not necessarily represent a primary enzyme abnormality but may be a manifestation of a more global mitochondrial defect. One would perhaps expect the latter to be true in primary acquired sideroblastic anemia which often represents a generalized problem in marrow cell growth and differentiation.

Recent work by Aoki et al. has begun to shed some light on this issue. These investigators found diminished activity not only of ALA synthase but also of a series of other mitochondrial enzymes in patients wtih primary acquired sideroblastic anemia; moreover, these defects were present not only in erythroid cells but also in granulocytes. They found somewhat similar abnormalities in patients with hereditary sideroblastic anemia not responsive to pyridoxine and suggested that both of these disorders may be due to some general defect in mitochondrial structure or function. In contrast, patients with the pyridoxine-responsive type of sideroblastic anemia appear to have a primary abnormality in ALA synthase itself, rendering the enzyme molecule susceptible to increased degradation by a protease that is thought to have a regulatory role in mitochondrial enzyme function. Others have described an enzyme with reduced affinity for pyridoxal phosphate. Both of these reported defects are partially overcome both in vitro and in vivo by large doses of pyridoxine.

Clinical and laboratory manifestations The clinical and laboratory manifestations of sideroblastic anemia are similar to those described for refractory anemia in general in the earlier portions of this article. There are, however, a few notable exceptions. There is usually a population of hypochromic red blood cells in the peripheral blood, sometimes rather small in patients with acquired sideroblastic anemia and often quite conspicuous in patients with hereditary forms of this disorder. When these hypochromic cells coexist with normal or macrocytic red blood cells, as typically occurs in the acquired disorder, a characteristic dimorphic blood picture results. The hypochromic cells are presumably the progeny of the ringed sideroblasts in the bone marrow, the latter representing a clone of dysplastic cells, whereas the macrocytes seem to be derived from coexisting clones of normal erythroid progenitor cells which are producing young erythrocytes at an increased rate in response to the anemic stress.

There is frequently dyspoietic change in the red blood cell precursors in the bone marrow and often in the granulocyte and megakaryocyte lines as well; correspondingly, changes in the neutrophil and platelet counts may accompany the anemia. An increase in blast forms may also be present; that is, sideroblastic change is not uncommon in refractory anemia with excess of blasts and chronic myelomonocytic leukemia.

Course, prognosis, and treatment   The clinical course of patients with acquired sideroblastic anemia is quite variable. The disease may be relatively mild and indolent. More commonly, it is severe and difficult to treat, primarily because of the severe anemia which is refractory to most forms of therapy. Treatment is as described for refractory anemia in general. All patients with sideroblastic disease should receive a trial of pyridoxine and perhaps pyridoxal phosphate if pyridoxine is not helpful. Transformation to acute nonlymphocytic leukemia is well described in patients with the acquired form of this disease. This complication may occur in from 7 to perhaps 20 percent of patients, depending on the reported series, and supervenes after several months to many years.

Iron loading is more severe in the sideroblastic anemias than in the other forms of refractory anemia. Hemochromatosis may occur in patients with hereditary forms of this disorder, presumably because of the long survival of these patients, and may occasionally be found in patients with acquired forms of the disease, particularly when there has been a long transfusion history or in association with a gene for hereditary hemochromatosis as marked by the HLA-A3 haplotype.

References

AOKI Y: Multiple enzymatic defects in mitochondria in hematological cells of patients with primary sideroblastic anemia. J Clin Invest 66:43, 1980

BAGBY GC et al: Glucocorticoid therapy in the preleukemic syndrome (hemopoietic dysplasia): Identification or responsive patients using in vitro techniques. Ann Intern Med 92:55, 1980

BENNETT JM et al: Proposals for the classification of the myelodysplastic syndromes. Br J Haematol 51:189, 1982

BERIS P et al: Primary acquired sideroblastic and primary acquired refractory anemia. Semin Hematol 20:101, 1983

BESSIS MC, JENSEN WN: Sideroblastic anemia, mitochondria and erythroblastic iron. Br J Haematol 11:49, 1965

BJORKMAN SE: Chronic refractory anemia with sideroblastic bone marrow: A study of four cases. Blood 11:250, 1956

BOMFORD RR, RHOADS CP: Refractory anaemia. Q J Med 10:175, 1941

BOTTOMLEY SS: Porphyrin and iron metabolism in sideroblastic anemia. Semin Hematol 14:169, 1977

CARTWRIGHT GE et al: Association of HLA-linked hemochromatosis with idiopathic refractory sideroblastic anemia. J Clin Invest 65:980, 1980

CHENG DC et al: Idiopathic refractory sideroblastic anemia: Incidence and risk factors for leukemic transformation. Cancer 44:724, 1979

CHUI DH, CLARKE B: Abnormal erythroid progenitor cells in human preleukemia. Blood 60:362, 1982

CROOKSTON JH et al: Hereditary erythroblastic multinuclearity associated with a positive acidified-serum test: A type of congenital dyserythropoietic anaemia. Br J Haematol 17:11, 1969

DACIE JV et al: Refractory normoblastic anaemia: A clinical and haematological study of seven cases. Br J Haematol 5:56, 1959

DAVIDSON SP et al: Studies in refractory anaemia: III. Refractory anaemias with cellular marrow. Edinburgh Med J 50:431, 1943

GREENBERG PL, MARA B: The preleukemic syndrome: Correlation of in vitro parameters of granulopoiesis with clinical features. Am J Med 66:951, 1979

HEILMEYER L et al: Disturbances in heme synthesis. Springfield, Ill., Charles C. Thomas, 1966, pp 103–178

KAGAN WA et al: Studies on the pathogenesis of refractory anemia. Am J Med 68:381, 1980

KUSHNER JP et al: Idiopathic refractory sideroblastic anemia: Clinical and laboratory investigation of 17 patients and review of the literature. Medicine 50:139, 1971

LINMAN JW, BAGBY GC: The preleukemic syndrome: Clinical and laboratory features, natural course, and management. Blood Cells 2:11, 1976

MACGIBBON BH, MOLLIN DL: Sideroblasts and sideroblastic anaemia. Br J Haematol 11:41, 1965

NOWELL P, FINAN J: Chromosome studies in preleukemic states: 4. Myeloproliferative versus cytopenic disorders. Cancer 42:2554, 1978

O'BRIEN H et al: Recurrent thrombocytopenia, erythroid hypoplasia and sideroblastic anaemia associated with hypothermia. Br J Haematol 51:451, 1982

RHOADS CP, BARKER HW: Refractory anemia. JAMA 110:794, 1938

RITCHEY AK et al: Antibody-mediated acquired sideroblastic anemia: Response to cytotoxic therapy. Blood 54:734, 1979

STREULI RA et al: Dysmyelopoietic syndrome: Sequential clinical and cytogenetic studies. Blood 55:636, 1980

THOMPSON WP et al: An analysis of so-called aplastic anemia. Am J Med Sci 187:77, 1934

VAN DEN BERGH H et al: Distinct hematological disorder with deletion of long arm of no 5 chromosome. Nature 251:437, 1974

VILTER RW et al: Refractory anemia with hyperplastic bone marrow (aregenerative anemia). Semin Hematol 4:175, 1967

SURGICAL APPROACHES TO RHEUMATOID ARTHRITIS

F. RICHARD CONVERY and WAYNE H. AKESON

Any consideration of surgical treatment in the patient with rheumatoid arthritis must be based on an understanding of the differences between these patients compared to most other surgical candidates. The rheumatoid patient is younger, more likely to be female, and frequently without spousal and social support. To place the role of surgery into proper perspective, it is essential to emphasize that rheumatoid arthritis is not solely a joint disease but rather a multisystem connective-tissue disease in which joint destruction may be the most visible but not necessarily the most important expression of the disease. Chronic anemia, osteoporosis, hidden or masked sites of indolent sepsis such as carious teeth and ulcerated nodules, and bones of small size in juvenile rheumatoid arthritis make this a patient population that must be dealt with in a very careful manner. In addition, there is increased susceptibility to postoperative infection which, in joint replacement, is most commonly due to late hematogenous seeding. There is frequently a long history of corticosteroid use or long-term use of nonsteroidal anti-inflammatory drugs, with their well-recognized propensity for inducing peptic ulcer disease.

Surgical intervention in the rheumatoid patient is an adjunctive, although significant, component of the total care of the patient and must be considered in the context of the response, or lack of response, to medical management. In this regard, the rheumatologist is an essential, integral factor in the final decision. With a few exceptions (see below) in which the indications for surgical treatment are absolute, most surgical procedures are undertaken because of failure or expected failure of medical management, as related to the overall expectations of the patient,

and must be based on careful assessment of the cost/benefit ratio. In this context, the principal reference point is not the dollar cost but rather the cost to the patient with respect to the effects on adjacent joints, to the likelihood of further surgery at a later date, and to the risk of possible complications. All of these costs must be balanced against the expectations of benefit from surgery.

The pain of joint disease arises from two separate causes: (1) capsular distention and irritation and (2) erosion of bone. Articular cartilage has no neural tissue, and synovium is poorly innervated by small nerve endings that are thought to be primarily vasomotor in function. However, the capsule of the joint is richly innervated with large pain fibers. The capsule is a mesenchymal tissue and, like the gastrointestinal tract, is extremely sensitive to distention. The capsule of the knee, however, is quite compliant and, unlike the hip or metacarpophalangeal joints, tolerates distention with much less pain. Studies of hand function have shown that grip strength improves when volar subluxation occurs compared to a normally positioned metacarpophalangeal joint in which synovial hypertrophy exists. The subluxation follows capsular destruction resulting from rheumatoid disease which increases the joint volume. Since intraarticular pressure is inversely related to intraarticular volume, it is understandable that pain would decrease and grip strength increase with subluxation. Evaluation of muscle strength in the presence of pain is totally invalid so that grip strength in the rheumatoid hand may be a measurement of pain, not strength. Similarly, the position of maximum volume of the hip is flexion, abduction, and external rotation. A patient with an effusion (e.g., septic arthritis) will automatically place the limb in this position.

The second pain mechanism in joint disease is due to osseous destruction with exposure of subchondral bone, which is thought to cause the dull, aching pain of advanced disease. In addition, the incongruities of osseous destruction cause intermittent capsular stretching that produces a sharp transitory pain. The patient will say that the hip or knee catches and buckles. Frequent falls or the fear of falling is often a motivating factor in the desire to undergo surgical treatment. The buckling or giving way of the knee is more than simple mechanical locking. The incongruities of the articular surface cause a sudden stretch of the capsule, usually just before heel strike. Stretching the capsule causes a reflex inhibition of the quadriceps and increased muscle activity in the hamstrings. Accordingly, just before placing the foot on the ground in preparation for weight bearing, the patient suddenly experiences sharp pain, relaxation of the quadriceps, and increased hamstring activity, all of which contribute to instability and potential falls.

INDICATIONS FOR OPERATIVE INTERVENTION

In the majority of rheumatoid patients, the primary indication for surgical treatment is pain unresponsive to medical management. This dictates that the patient has had an "adequate" trial of nonoperative treatment. The criteria of an adequate trial of conservative treatment are relatively proportional to the magnitude of the operative procedure. For example, treatment with anti-inflammatory medication and intraarticular steroids is advisable before recommending synovectomy of the knee for a large or ruptured popliteal cyst. Conversely, surgical release of a carpal tunnel syndrome is recommended after a relatively short trial of medication and/or splinting.

Improvement in function is an important but usually a secondary goal in the indications for arthroplasty. The functional improvement gained is more directly related to pain relief than to improvement in alignment, position, or range of motion. However, since it is not possible to quantitate the degree of pain objectively or

to separate pain from suffering, it is necessary to evaluate pain on a functional basis. Specifically, alterations in life-style caused by limitations in walking, inability to carry out occupational or household duties, failure to sleep comfortably at night, and inability to engage in recreational activities are important determinants in the decision to recommend operative intervention.

In polyarticular disease it is not uncommon for the global disability to be a summation of several joints. Although rheumatoid arthritis is a symmetric polyarthritis, the severity of joint destruction in patients in whom surgical treatment is a consideration is usually asymmetric. In the upper extremity this asymmetry has been related to dominance, and "unilateral rheumatoid arthritis" (seen when the disease occurs following hemiplegia) suggests that the asymmetry is of functional origin. Regardless of the cause, the lesser degree of destruction in the opposite side will allow the patient to compensate initially by shifting load to the side of lesser involvement and thereby to decrease symptoms from the more involved side. With time and further bilateral joint destruction, the need to compensate increases, and the ability to compensate decreases to a point where the global disability becomes intolerable. Likewise, the use of external support (i.e., cane or crutches) may initially allow satisfactory function, but with increasing upper extremity joint destruction, this compensation may no longer be effective. It is frequently at this point that the patient is referred to the surgeon. Under these circumstances, it is current practice to recommend simultaneous or closely spaced multiple arthroplasties. Several studies support the conclusion that bilateral or multiple procedures during a single hospitalization are both functionally and economically desirable. Furthermore, there are patients in whom symmetrical deformities of major-degree, bilateral, severe restriction-of-motion or symmetrical-disabling symptomatology dictate the need for simultaneous procedures in order to achieve maximum benefit. For example, a patient with bilateral fixed flexion deformities of the knee in whom the deformity is completely corrected by total knee replacement in only one knee will continue to stand with both knees flexed at the original angle. If this posture is allowed to persist, the operated knee will develop a flexion deformity that matches the unoperated knee. In a similar manner, a very stiff hip on the opposite side will limit the range of motion gained following hip replacement. Conversely, it is not uncommon to see a patient with bilateral involvement and symmetrical symptoms but very asymmetrical radiographic destruction. In addition, the less involved joint from a radiographic standpoint may be the more symptomatic. In this situation, in either the hips or the knees, joint replacement of the more severely destroyed joint will provide a means by which the patient can again compensate and the need for replacement of the less involved joint may be deferred for some time.

It should be clear from the foregoing that in the majority of patients the indications for surgical intervention are elective, and the final decision is based primarily on the ratio of the expected benefit balanced against the estimated risk. There are, however, certain situations in which the indications are not elective but absolute.

ABSOLUTE INDICATIONS FOR SURGICAL INTERVENTION

Cervical instability

Instability (motion increased beyond normal limits between vertebral segments) is common in the cervical spine but is most unusual in the thoracic or lumbar spine of the rheumatoid patient. Forty percent of patients with chronic rheumatoid arthritis will have increased motion between the first and second cervical vertebrae (Fig. 1). Although the forward displacement of the anterior arch of C1 (which normally measures up to 4 mm between the posterior rim of the anterior arch and the anterior edge of the odontoid) tends to increase with time, the incidence of neurological deficits is quite low (1 to 2 percent) and does not seem to correlate with increasing displacement. Even though the incidence of spinal cord compression is relatively low, evidence that it is present is an absolute indication for reduction and posterior cervical arthrodesis. A history of recurrent urinary tract infections should arouse suspicion of spinal cord involvement. The presence of ankle clonus, hyperreflexia, and pathological reflexes demands ex-

peditious evaluation because complete quadriplegia can occur if stabilization is not achieved. The extent of the arthrodesis is determined by the presence or absence of adjacent instability. Subaxial displacement, most commonly at C3, C4, and C5, is almost as common as atlantoaxial instability and, if present, must be included in the arthrodesis. Likewise, the less common superior migration of the odontoid into the foramen magnum (platybasia) requires extension of the arthrodesis to the occiput. There is no indication for decompressive laminectomy in cervical instability due to rheumatoid arthritis because it will lead to further instability or, if performed in conjunction with arthrodesis, will unnecessarily compound the already recognized difficulty of achieving a solid fusion.

Tendon rupture

Rupture of the extensor tendons of the wrist, infrapatellar tendon, and Achilles tendon is relatively common in rheumatoid arthritis. Although spontaneous ruptures of the Achilles tendon and infrapatellar tendon are more often associated with systemic lupus erythematosus, the injudicious use of local injections of corticosteroid preparations can precipitate a traumatic rupture of these large tendons. Rupture of the extensor tendons at the dorsum of the wrist is caused by direct synovial invasion, attrition due to abrading action across a subluxated wrist or distal radial ulnar joint, or deterioration of blood supply. The ruptures occur just distal to, or beneath, the extensor retinaculum, which is a tight nonyielding compartment. Proliferation of the tenosynovium within this compartment compresses the blood supply which enters the tendons via the vincula. Because of these factors, necrosis of tendons may be quite extensive and usually precludes direct end-to-end repair. Therefore, a side-to-side repair utilizing an intact tendon or a tendon transfer is required. A synovectomy of the dorsal compartment is routinely performed, and an arthroplasty of the distal radial ulnar joint is frequently included with the repair. The patient is characteristically surprised by the tendon rupture, because it occurs with minimal trauma, is not painful, and occurs abruptly without any appreciable prerupture symptoms except for persistent synovial prolif-

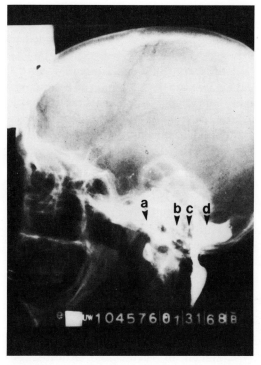 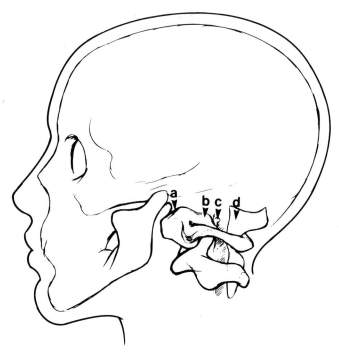

FIGURE 1

Atlantoaxial subluxation. The myelogram demonstrates the narrowing of the spinal canal. The patient had a Brown-Séquard syndrome: (a) the anterior arch *of the atlas, (b) the displaced odontoid, (c) the spinal cord, (d) the myelographic dye column which is indented by the posterior arch of the atlas.*

eration. The high probability that rupture will occur in the opposite hand in a patient with known rupture is a strong indication for prophylactic synovectomy of the opposite wrist.

Compression of the posterior interosseous nerve, the deep motor branch of the radial nerve, results from synovial proliferation at the elbow. Compression of this nerve results in inability to extend the metacarpophalangeal joints and the thumb. In contrast to extensor tendon rupture, which is acute and painless, posterior interosseous nerve palsy is painful, evolves slowly, and is associated with paresthesias.

Peripheral nerve compression

Paresthetic pain and hypesthesia in the distribution of a peripheral nerve in a patient with rheumatoid arthritis indicate the likelihood of nerve compression secondary to proliferative synovitis. If peripheral nerve compression is confirmed by clinical and electrical diagnostic techniques, aggressive treatment is indicated. If

motor function is intact, symptoms may be reversed by the use of local and systemic anti-inflammatory agents and splinting and by decreased activity. If these conservative measures are unsuccessful, or if motor loss is present, surgical decompression is clearly indicated.

Peripheral nerve compression occurs most commonly in the upper extremity and is associated with unrestrained proliferative synovitis in tight restraining canals. Median nerve compression (i.e., the carpal tunnel syndrome) is the most common, but compression of the ulnar nerve at the elbow is also observed frequently. This is caused by distention of the capsule beneath the ulnar collateral ligament which forms the floor of the cubital canal. Another potential site of entrapment of the ulnar nerve is at the wrist, the so-called ulnar carpal tunnel syndrome. This is an uncommon diagnosis in rheumatoid arthritis, possibly because the lesion is uncommon or, equally, because it is easily missed. The deep motor branch of the ulnar nerve has no sensory component and does not supply the muscles of the hypothenar eminence. Accordingly, the patient presents with weakness and atrophy of the intrinsic muscles of the hand, no sensory loss, and little or no pain; in rheumatoid arthritis this situation does not stimulate thoughts of ulnar nerve compression. Although much less common, compression of the posterior interosseous nerve (the motor branch of the radial nerve) just distal to the elbow is important in the differential diagnosis of extensor tendon rupture (see above).

With the exception of the tarsal tunnel syndrome (compression of the tibial nerve medial to the ankle joint), peripheral neuropathy due to synovial proliferation is relatively uncommon in the lower extremities. A neuropathy in the lower extremities is more commonly associated with vasculitis or is caused by external compression. Findings of upper motor neuron dysfunction are usually related to cervical spine instability.

SYNOVECTOMY

For the better part of 20 years, between 1950 and 1970, synovectomy was the mainstay of surgical treatment for rheumatoid arthritis. The knee was by far the most common joint treated in this way, although synovectomy of the dorsum of the wrist, the metacarpophalangeal joints, and the elbow was also performed commonly. In addition, there were sporadic reports of a small number of synovectomies done in the shoulder, hip, and ankle. The rationale for synovectomy is twofold: (1) palliative, to relieve pain, and (2) prophylactic, to prevent or delay progressive joint destruction. Short-term studies consistently reported satisfactory results in approximately three-quarters or more of patients when relief of pain was the primary objective. The prophylactic concept, although enthusiastically endorsed, has never been adequately demonstrated. A consistent finding in all of the reported series was that the quality of the result was directly proportional to the degree of joint destruction present.

In the past 10 years, two developments have occurred which have severely curtailed the application of this procedure. First, total knee replacement, when successful, is far more effective and is feasible in joints destroyed beyond the point at which synovectomy could be expected to succeed. At the time of its greatest popularity,

there were only two alternatives to synovectomy of the knee: arthrodesis or primitive interpositional arthroplasties. The limitations of arthrodesis are significant, and the early arthroplasties were rarely successful more than 50 percent of the time. In this setting, synovectomy was a viable option. The second factor that has decreased the indications for synovectomy has been the growth and development of the specialty of rheumatology. The use of progressively more effective anti-inflammatory medications by a greater number of well-trained rheumatologists has added greatly to the control of inflammation. The better control of inflammation, however, has not been reflected in a decrease in the rate of joint destruction. Nevertheless, the net result has been the control of symptoms until the joint destruction has progressed beyond the point where synovectomy could be successful and where prosthetic arthroplasty is more appropriate.

In sum, synovectomy is a procedure that reduces inflammation but not joint destruction, and the rheumatologist is much more effective in the control of inflammation than was the case heretofore. In the future, however, the pendulum may again swing back to synovectomy, which historically has waxed and waned in popularity, because of the technical feasibility of arthroscopic synovectomy. This technique has only recently been developed, and already there are enthusiasts for its application. The short hospitalization, low morbidity, and easy postoperative rehabilitation makes this an attractive option. The many patients who are responding poorly to medical management and are not candidates for joint replacement may benefit from arthroscopic synovectomy. It does seem likely that this procedure will find a place in the comprehensive management of rheumatoid arthritis, but all the evidence to date indicates that it will be a temporizing palliative supplement to medical treatment rather than a definitive surgical procedure.

REGIONAL CONSIDERATIONS

Shoulder

The shoulder joint is highly mobile and, because of its inherent lack of osseous stability, requires effective muscle and ligamentous support for normal function. The muscles about the shoulder are particularly susceptible to disuse atrophy, and the ligamentous support is especially vulnerable to the inflammatory process of rheumatoid arthritis. These two factors, plus the need for great mobility, are the major reasons why progress in shoulder arthroplasty has been so slow compared to other joints.

The primary function of the shoulder is to position the hand. For most activities of daily living, the extreme range of motion is not necessary but maintenance of strength and motion are essential components of conservative treatment to relieve or prevent pain. Because the muscles of the shoulder are so susceptible to disuse atrophy, and because of the propensity of the joint to develop contracture as the result of disuse, maintenance of motion is essential. In rheumatoid arthritis as well as in the "frozen shoulder" from other causes, the contracture causes pain in addition to that caused by inflammation and joint destruction. The resting position, with the arm at the side, is the most comfortable for the patient. This positioning for comfort, however, reinforces the cycle of atrophy and stiffness which progressively increases limitation of motion that further impairs function.

Brisement and manipulation   Most patients with a shoulder contracture will regain motion and obtain relief of pain from a progressive exercise program. Occasionally, however, a shoulder will not respond to exercise alone, and manipulation under anesthesia should be considered. After induction of general anesthesia, a brisement (breaking up of the ankylosis) is done. The procedure is not without hazard, as torsional stress on the humerus can easily cause a spiral fracture. The expected benefit must be carefully balanced against the degree of osteoporosis and, hence, the risk of fracture. If the shoulder is particularly tight or osteoporosis unduly severe, an open release of the subscapularis tendon followed by gentle manipulation under direct vision is preferable.

Arthrodesis   Prior to present-day joint replacement, arthrodesis (fusion) of the glenohumeral joint was thought to be a helpful procedure for the patient with advanced rheumatoid destruc-

tion. This was in part due to the lack of a suitable alternative. If a solid fusion was obtained, complete relief of pain from the glenohumeral joint was achieved and motion of the scapulothoracic articulation allowed intermediate-range shoulder function. The patients, however, were usually less enthusiastic about the result than the surgeon. Personal hygiene was a particular problem, symmetrical disease precluded bilateral arthrodesis, and frequently the pull of the arm on the suprascapular muscles after arthrodesis produced an aching, unpleasant discomfort. In addition, the recommended position of the arthrodesis (30 to 40° of abduction) made turning over in bed difficult. For these reasons, arthrodesis of the shoulder was not done frequently and now is performed only rarely.

Resection arthroplasty   Resection of the humeral head (Jones procedure) creates a pseudoarthrosis which is a relatively successful operation for chronic dislocation but has been done only occasionally as a primary procedure in rheumatoid arthritis, most commonly for late-stage septic arthritis. In the future, as shoulder replacement becomes more common, resection arthroplasty may be the preferred salvage procedure for complications of postoperative infection. Few primary procedures of this type have been done in rheumatoid arthritis because the functional results are poor.

Prosthetic arthroplasty   In no other joint in the body are the results of joint replacement so dependent upon the presence of, or lack of damage to, the stabilizing muscles. The absence or lack of function of the rotator cuff preoperatively is of such significance that it is currently the practice to classify results of shoulder replacement according to the preoperative expectations. The patient with rheumatoid arthritis in whom the rotator cuff is particularly susceptible to the inflammatory destruction of the disease is in a category of limited expectations preoperatively.

The very early destruction of the rotator cuff as is seen in patients with rheumatoid arthritis has led to the development of inherently stable or fixed-fulcrum prostheses designed to substitute for the absent musculotendonous cuff. These prostheses have not been particularly successful and are associated with a high risk of complication such as loosening, dislocation, and fracture. Accordingly, an unconstrained or semiconstrained implant with limited expectations seems more appropriate. Significant relief of pain is usually achieved and increased function as a consequence of pain relief occurs, but only a very modest increase in range of motion can be expected.

Elbow

Ulnar nerve transposition The ulnar nerve runs in a sulcus between the medial epicondyle and the olecranon where it is vulnerable to the effects of exposure to proliferating synovium from the joint below. The nerve is firmly fixed in this groove, and if compressed in this region by synovium or scar, the typical findings of an ulnar palsy will result. Although less common than the carpal tunnel syndrome, ulnar nerve palsy is an extremely serious complication. Persistent ulnar paresthesias, numbness, and motor weakness in the face of good medical management require decompression. The differential diagnosis of ulnar nerve entrapment at the elbow includes instability of the low cervical spine (which is uncommon in rheumatoid arthritis) and compression distal to the groove, such as in the canal of Guyon at the wrist. The badly disabled patient uses the forearm and elbow to assist in transfers and ambulation. These activities, especially with the forearm in pronation, may apply pressure on the nerve just distal to the groove where it passes between the two heads of the flexor carpi ulnaris. Decompression, therefore, requires more than simple release of the nerve from its constriction in the groove, but also transfer of the nerve to a position anterior to the medial epicondyle. Most surgeons recommend rerouting the nerve beneath the origin of flexor muscles arising from the medial epicondyle.

Synovectomy and radial head excision Synovectomy of the elbow, combined with excision of the radial head, can be symptomatically and functionally helpful even in the face of significant erosion of the radiohumeral articulation. In reality, this is an excisional arthroplasty in addition to a synovectomy. The outcome, however, is compromised by the presence of erosions at the humeroulnar articulation (i.e., at the olecranon

notch). In an effort to avoid elbow replacement, many surgeons will expose this articulation through a second medial incision, prophylactically transfer the ulnar nerve, and debride the humeroulnar articulation. The results are surprisingly good, even in the face of fairly significant osseous erosion. The decision to recommend a synovectomy and radial head excision rather than elbow replacement is difficult, and the final recommendation is flavored heavily by the individual surgeon's experience with elbow replacement.

Total elbow replacement The overall results of elbow replacement have not been as uniformly successful as in the case of the total joint replacement of the hip. Prosthetic replacement of the elbow is, in many respects, similar to the present state of the art in shoulder replacement. The indication for elbow replacement is primarily pain, but with present-day implants a significant increase in range of motion (but not a return to normal range of motion) can be expected.

Wrist

Carpal tunnel syndrome Compression of the median nerve by proliferating synovium beneath the transverse carpal ligament is a frequent, and in many patients the initial, manifestation of rheumatoid arthritis. Unlike the carpal tunnel syndrome in a nonrheumatoid population in which conservative measures are at least temporarily effective, patients with rheumatoid arthritis usually require surgical release and synovectomy. The simplicity of the procedure compared to the devastating effects on hand function due to progression of median nerve damage, including loss of sensation in the median nerve distribution and loss of strength in the thenar muscles, make carpal tunnel release one of the more commonly performed operations. This is especially true in the early stages of the disease when synovial proliferation is at its maximum. Later, when advanced destruction of bone and cartilage has occurred, the inflammatory process decreases and carpal tunnel compression decreases as well.

Dorsal synovectomy and radioulnar arthroplasty Surgical removal of the extraarticular synovium from around the extensor tendons of the wrist seems to be an effective procedure with a low rate of recurrence in contrast to intraarticular synovectomy elsewhere. The procedure is widely believed to reduce the incidence of extensor tendon rupture, although conclusive evidence for this is lacking. Excision of the distal ulna is usually also performed to relieve a bony prominence causing attritional changes in the ulnar extensors.

Radioulnar arthroplasty, in which a sufficient segment of distal ulnar diaphysis is excised to allow easy reduction of the distal ulna into proper alignment with the shortened radial side of the joint, is a procedure of significant benefit which is sometimes overlooked. This relatively uncomplicated procedure can be quite helpful and will postpone or eliminate the need for more extensive reconstruction of the radiocarpal joint.

Arthrodesis The primary purpose of the wrist is to provide a base from which the hand functions. Good hand function requires a pain-free wrist in the appropriate position. Arthrodesis can achieve both of these requirements and, in properly selected patients, can be a very satisfactory procedure. Wrist arthrodesis is permanent, will not require revision, and will not become infected by hematogenous bacterial seeding, a significant concern in total joint replacement. Despite these very significant considerations, arthrodesis is not commonly done in rheumatoid patients. The need for slight wrist flexion to maintain personal hygiene, the usual bilateral involvement, and the availability of alternative procedures limit this procedure to a relatively small number of patients. The ideal patient for wrist arthrodesis has pauciarticular disease, has a wrist with good motion on the opposite side, is relatively young, and has high functional requirements in which strong power grip is necessary. Advanced osseous destruction of the carpus, absent or paralyzed wrist extensors, or sepsis, each of which eliminates a consideration of total wrist replacement, are situations in which arthrodesis of the wrist is a feasible consideration.

Total wrist replacement Total replacement of the wrist, utilizing nonlinked metal and polyethylene components secured with polymethyl methacrylate (bone cement), is a relatively new procedure that has not yet been done in large numbers of patients (Fig. 2). Although there have been problems, the early results are encouraging.

Hand

The most significant changes seen in the past 20 years have been a distinct shift away from soft-tissue realignment procedures, a greater acceptance of implant arthroplasty, and a narrowing of operative indications toward relief of pain as the paramount indication for operative intervention. The soft-tissue procedures, so popular in the 1960s and early 1970s, are now rarely done as independent procedures because of high recurrence rates but are frequently done as adjunctive components of more elaborate hand reconstruction.

Soft-tissue procedures Synovectomy of the metacarpophalangeal and proximal interphalangeal joints of the hand, once very popular procedures, are now only rarely indicated. The rate of recurrent synovitis, short-term relief of pain, and frequent loss of motion following synovectomy of these joints far outweigh the short-term benefits achieved.

Resection arthroplasty of the metacarpal heads provides an immediate restoration of normal appearance. Despite the satisfactory cosmetic result, however, functional improvement is modest; the benefits of the procedure are more clearly related to relief of pain than to the improvement in position.

In the late 1960s, a flexible silicone rubber implant was introduced by Swanson and modified by Neibauer and has remained the standard to date. The silastic implants are inherently stable, but the correction of severe deformities requires a meticulous balance of the soft tissues, sophisticated postoperative splinting, and a carefully supervised exercise program. If these prerequisites are fulfilled, properly performed silastic arthroplasty will correct advanced deformities and provide excellent relief of pain originating from the metacarpophalangeal joint, and the patient can expect 30 to 75° of active range of motion. Postoperative complications are relatively uncommon and include recurrent deformity, fatigue fracture of the implant, infection,

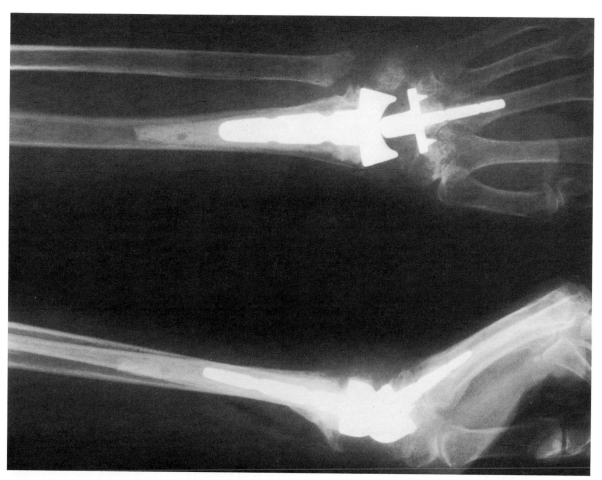

FIGURE 2
Total wrist replacement. This particular design is from the University of Arizona.

and occasional incisional skin necrosis, especially in the patient with atrophic skin. In contrast to joint replacement elsewhere, the occurrence of implant fracture is not usually a major problem because soft-tissue stability achieved by the time of fracture is frequently adequate.

In no other anatomical region, however, is there a more direct relationship between the functional result obtained and the status of the adjacent joints. In the care of the wrist, the important requirements are functional position and stability; position and modest motion are most important for the metacarpophalangeal joints, whereas at the proximal interphalangeal joints a large range of motion is crucial to function and becomes progressively more important from the index to the little finger.

The motion obtained following metacarpophalangeal arthroplasty is directly related to the motion present in the proximal interphalangeal joints. That is, the less motion present in the proximal interphalangeal joints the more motion can be expected postoperatively in the metacarpophalangeal joints. At least 45° of flexion in the proximal interphalangeal joints is necessary for a satisfactory functional result following metacarpophalangeal arthroplasty. On the other hand, significant flexion deformities at the interphalangeal joints are not detrimental to the functional outcome if there is sufficient flexion range beyond the contracture.

In view of the very real need for motion in the proximal interphalangeal joints, it is not surprising that silastic implants have been designed and placed in these joints. Unfortunately, silastic implant arthroplasty of the proximal interphalangeal joints has not been nearly as successful as in the metacarpophalangeal joints. Usually, the range of motion obtained is disappointing, frequently it is not increased, and occasionally postoperative motion is actually decreased. If arthroplasty is considered, it is essential that the flexor and extensor mechanisms are functional, otherwise arthrodesis is more appropriate.

Arthrodesis If advanced destruction occurs in the distal interphalangeal joint, arthrodesis is the procedure of choice. Arthrodesis might be required, for example, in a patient with painful destruction of the distal interphalangeal joint of the index finger. Strong pinch would not be possible on either the side or the tip of the index finger. Arthrodesis would restore this function along with reconstruction of adjacent joints in the fingers and thumb as necessary. Not infrequently, the amount of destruction in the proximal interphalangeal joint is such that adequate motor control is lost. In this situation, arthrodesis rather than arthroplasty is indicated.

The metacarpophalangeal joint of the thumb requires special comment. It is frequently destroyed by the rheumatoid process, and there is volar subluxation of the proximal phalanx. The volar subluxation creates a relative shortening of the thumb. Because of the shortening, the flexor pollicis longus becomes relatively lengthened and weakened, compromising thumb-to-index pinch which requires appreciable force. The "lengthened" flexor pollicis longus cannot generate the appropriate force because of the volar instability, and attempted pinch produces hyperextension of the thumb interphalangeal joint. Combined volar subluxation at the metacarpophalangeal joint and hyperextension of the interphalangeal joint produces the "swan neck" deformity of the thumb. Treatment of this deformity is directed not at the hyperextension of the interphalangeal joint but at the subluxated metacarpophalangeal joint. Arthrodesis of this joint in the reduced position restores the relative length of the thumb and provides a firm base across which the flexor pollicis longus can function to prevent interphalangeal hyperextension. It is possible to demonstrate this effect by reducing and stabilizing the metacarpophalangeal joint during strong thumb-to-index pinch.

Hip

The evaluation of hip disease as well as disease in other joints in the lower extremity begins with an assessment of gait. Prerequisites to gait evaluation are an understanding of the normal gait cycle and the mechanics of the hip.

The gait cycle (Fig. 3) Normal and pathologic gait is divided into two phases: stance phase and swing phase. Stance phase begins when the heel

FIGURE 3
The gait cycle. Note the two periods of double-limb support at the beginning and end of the stance phase.

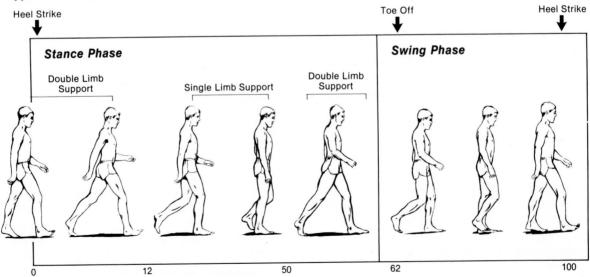

strikes the floor (heel strike) and ends when the toe leaves the floor (toe-off). Swing phase begins with toe-off and ends at heel strike. Stance phase is subdivided into a period of double-limb support and single-limb support. Single-limb support occurs in the midportion of stance phase, and double-limb support occurs at the beginning and end of the stance phase. The description is facilitated by referring to Fig. 3 and considering the right limb. At the time of heel strike, stance phase has begun, but the left foot is still on the ground prior to toe-off; the patient is in the double-limb support phase. At the time of toe-off on the left (opposite) side, all weight is borne on the right limb and the patient is in single-limb support. Single-limb support ends with heel strike of the left limb, at which time the patient is again in the double-limb support phase.

An antalgic gait (a pain-relieving gait) is commonly observed in arthritic patients. The stance phase, which normally accounts for approximately 60 percent of the gait cycle, is increased in an antalgic gait in an effort to relieve pain. The period of double-limb support is increased by a shortened swing phase on the opposite side and is also associated with a decrease in the period of single-limb support on the involved side. The total percent of the stance phase increases with the severity of the limp.

Hip mechanics (Fig. 4) The abductors, the gluteus medius and minimus, are the crucial muscles of the hip. They are crucial not because they abduct the limb, a relatively unimportant function, but because they stabilize the hip (i.e., they maintain the pelvis level when the opposite limb is off the floor). This is accomplished by a simple lever system. The fulcrum of the lever system is the femoral head. In single-limb stance the abductors, which arise from the ilium and insert on the greater trochanter, keep the pelvis from dropping on the opposite side by generating force on a short lever from the fulcrum of the femoral head to the greater trochanter. Resisting this force is the body weight (minus the weight of the stance limb) which works through a lever extending from the fulcrum of the femoral head to the center of gravity. The ratio of the body-weight lever arm to the abductor lever arm is approximately 3:1. Therefore, the joint reaction force is the summation of the body weight (minus

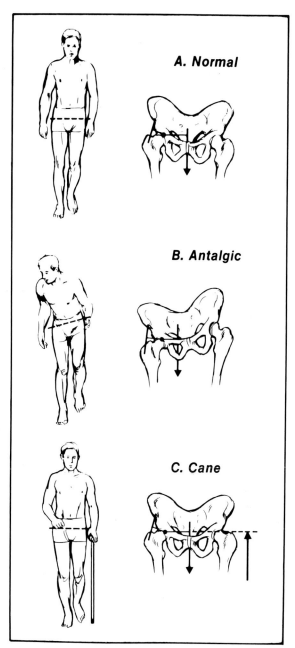

FIGURE 4

Mechanics of the hip. The antalgic gait (B) shifts the center of gravity toward the involved hip to shorten the body-weight lever arm.

the weight of the stance limb) times three, plus the abductor force required to balance the level system. When the weight of the supporting limb is subtracted, the force on the hip in single-limb stance is approximately three times the body weight.

With this lever system in mind, it is easy to understand the seemingly inappropriate shift of the body weight toward the side of a symptomatic hip. In doing this, the patient shifts the center of gravity toward the symptomatic hip, decreases the length of the body-weight lever arm, decreases the amount of abductor force needed to balance the shortened body-weight lever arm, and in this way decreases the summation of forces upon the hip. A patient with a painful hip has a coxalgic gait which is the combination of decreased single-limb support phase and a shift of the center of gravity toward the involved side. A Trendelenburg gait (or, as it is sometimes called, an abductor lurch) is the shift of the body weight only. A positive Trendelenburg sign is a tilting downward of the opposite side of the pelvis with a shift of the center of gravity toward the fulcrum (hip joint). The patient does this to compensate for weakness of the abductors or to decrease the joint reaction force. The well-recognized difficulty of quantitating the degree of hip pain is made much easier by an objective assessment of the patient's gait.

The lever system also explains the rationale for the use of a cane on the side opposite the symptomatic hip. When a patient pushes down on a cane, an equal and reactive force is applied in the opposite direction. A moment is created with a long lever arm extending horizontally from the cane to the fulcrum at the head of the opposite femur which markedly reduces the abductor force, and hence, reduces the joint reaction force.

Total hip replacement In approximately 15 years, total hip replacement has become the standard against which other joint replacements are compared and has made obsolete all of the previously done reconstructive procedures for arthritic destruction of the hip. When introduced to this country in 1968 and 1969, the procedure was restricted to the elderly patient (older than 65) with incapacitating hip pain in whom functional demands were relatively low and would predictably decline with advancing age. This restriction, however, applied primarily to the nonrheumatoid patient; even then, age restrictions were lower for patients with rheumatoid arthritis because of the polyarticular involvement which limited functional potential, "the restraints of the disease." Very rapidly, however, due to the excellence of outcome following hip replacement and also because of relative dissatisfaction with alternative reconstructive procedures, age as well as most other restrictions was rapidly ignored.

For at least the next 5 to 7 years it was only rarely that alternative procedures were considered, much less performed. In part, because of this unbridled enthusiasm, large clinical series evolved which demonstrated quite clearly the capabilities and limitations of joint replacement. Initial concerns relative to high infection rates and rapid wear of the high-density-polyethylene bearing surface have not materialized, but loosening of the polymethylmethacrylate and bone interface is approaching epidemic proportions. Failure of the bone-cement interface is a multifactorial problem that results in the return of pain and may eventually lead to fracture of the metal prosthesis and, if severe enough, requires revision of the joint replacement with lowered expectations for success compared to primary replacement. Some of the risk factors which relate to the incidence of loosening include age below 50, weight above 80 k (200 lb), vigorous activity following replacement, and revision of previous prosthetic joint surgery. It is widely believed that recent improvements in cement technique, prosthetic design, and patient selection will reduce the likelihood of loosening, but this has yet to be demonstrated unequivocally because of the lengthy observation periods required for determination of loosening rates.

The patient with rheumatoid arthritis undergoing total hip replacement is less likely to develop loosening than a nonrheumatoid counterpart, but by the very nature of the disease there are additional risks. To begin with, the patient is likely to be younger (the average age of rheumatoid patients undergoing hip replacement is usually about 55 compared to a nonrheumatoid population of about 65), so implant longevity is a concern. The age problem is amplified further in patients with juvenile rheumatoid arthritis and youthful patients treated with corticosteroids who frequently develop avascular necrosis requiring hip replacement, even though the rheumatoid disease elsewhere in the body is relatively mild. Despite the adverse age factor, the rheumatoid patient is relatively privileged with respect to loosening. Conversely, the rheumatoid patient is at higher risk of infection than the general population. This risk is not as significant in the immediate postoperative period, but tends to be a late complication due to hematogenous seeding. Comparative studies between patients with osteoarthritis and rheumatoid arthritis have shown that the incidence of postoperative infection is about 1 to 2 percent in both types of arthritis when there has been no previous surgery. In studies of late-developing infection, the rheumatoid patients have infection rates of 6 to 8 percent. This factor is of special concern to the internist or rheumatologist following the patient long after joint replacement surgery, because occult or obvious infections elsewhere (teeth, urinary tract, foot ulcers, and ingrown toenails) must be treated aggressively and antibiotics must be used early to protect the implant. The data relative to late hematogenous seeding come from clinical studies of hip replacement, but it is logical to extrapolate the findings to all joint replacements.

The development of fatigue fractures following hip replacement in the rheumatoid patient may produce diagnostic difficulty. The clinical presentation, however, is quite typical. Characteristically, following joint replacement the patient will become more ambulatory. Osteoporotic bone resulting from preoperative disuse and corticosteroids may be unable to carry the load, and a fatigue fracture may result. This is particularly common in the pubic or ischial rami but is also seen in the distal tibia and os calcis. The spontaneous atraumatic onset of pain in the groin, ankle, or foot is frequently attributed to a flare-up of underlying joint disease. The diagnosis is supported by radiographs which are not diagnostic initially. Fatigue fractures do not become apparent radiographically for 2 to 3 weeks after the onset of pain, but a bone scan is diagnostic and can discriminate between a periarticular fatigue fracture and increased joint inflammation.

Alternative procedures

Surface replacement   Cemented double-cup arthroplasty or surface replacement of the hip was developed initially in Europe and modifications were introduced in the United States in the mid-1970s. The intent of this concept was to pro-

vide an operation that would serve better the needs of the functionally active younger patients and that would preserve bone stock for later revision, which was assumed to be inevitable in this patient population. Unfortunately, neither of these objectives has been achieved. By cementing a cup on the head of the femur rather than amputating the head and neck of the femur as is done in conventional hip replacement, the procedure does, indeed, preserve more of the proximal femur. The large cup on the femoral head, however, dictates the need for a large acetabular component which requires removal of more pelvic bone than in conventional hip replacement. It was recognized quite early that surface replacement was not an improvement compared to conventional hip replacement for the patient with rheumatoid arthritis. More recently, convincing data have been presented that clearly demonstrate the inferior quality of outcome in patients with nonrheumatoid joint disease. The procedure is technically demanding, intraoperative and early postoperative complications are greater, and the incidence of loosening is equal to or perhaps greater than in conventional replacement. In summary, it now seems quite clear that surface replacement of the hip offers no significant advantage and subjects the patient to a set of adverse circumstances greater than with conventional replacement.

Arthrodesis and cup arthroplasty   The failure of total hip replacement to provide long-term relief of pain and satisfactory function in the young patient with advanced destruction of the hip has stimulated the orthopedic community to reassess two procedures which for the past decade have been of interest only to the historian. Arthrodesis of the hip is a definitive procedure providing pain relief that does not require revision. However, arthrodesis transmits stresses normally absorbed by the hip to the adjacent joints, and long-term studies have demonstrated that these mechanical changes have an adverse effect on the knees and, to a lesser extent, the lumbar spine. Because it is known that excessive stresses applied to a joint with existing inflammation lead to accelerated destruction over and above that arising from the basic disease process, arthrodesis of the hip is contraindicated in patients with rheumatoid arthritis. The best evidence that supports the above concept is the well-recognized unilateral rheumatoid arthritis seen in patients with preexisting hemiplegia and the adverse effects on the knee of leg-length inequality.

Another procedure which is being reassessed in youthful patients is cup arthroplasty. This arthroplasty, in which a metal cup is interposed between the head of the femur and the acetabulum after removing all cartilage and subchondral bone, was the standard procedure for reconstruction of the hip in the United States from the mid-1930s to the late 1960s. Even at the zenith of its popularity, however, the indications for the procedure were quite limited. It was relatively satisfactory in elderly females with unilateral osteoarthritis and limited functional expectations. The outcome was quite unsatisfactory in patients with bilateral disease, in younger patients, and in active males. Even in ideally selected patients, prolonged hospitalization (5 to 6 weeks), prolonged rehabilitative exercises, and lifelong stress protection were necessary to achieve a satisfactory result. Total hip replacement almost completely eliminated the use of cup arthroplasty.

Resection arthroplasty (girdlestone pseudarthrosis)

Resection arthroplasty consists of resection of the head and neck of the femur at the intertrochanteric line, excision of the lateral aspect of the acetabulum to create an osteotomy line parallel to the intertrochanteric line, and transfer of the iliopsoas tendon from the lesser to the greater trochanter. It is the classic salvage procedure for failure of hip arthroplasties. The procedure provides relief of pain and is often successful in controlling deep sepsis, but involves significant functional limitations for the patient. Skeletal traction for 4 to 6 weeks postoperatively is required and is particularly detrimental to the patient with atrophic muscles, which atrophy further during the imposed bed rest. One to three inches of shortening is expected, and the fulcrum for the hip lever system is lost. Occasionally, especially after sepsis and with a pain-free functional contralateral hip, a patient may be able to ambulate well with only one cane. More often, especially in the patient with rheumatoid arthritis, one or two crutches are required. Despite these inherent limitations, a girdlestone pseudar-

throsis may be the only solution when uncontrolled sepsis or inadequate bone stock for a revision procedure exists.

Synovectomy and intertrochanteric osteotomy of the femur

As discussed previously the present indications for synovectomy are extremely narrow. Even when the enthusiasm for synovectomy was at its peak, it was rarely done for hip disease. The resultant postoperative loss of motion, the inability to completely remove the synovium without dislocating the femoral head, and the inherent risk of avascular necrosis were, and remain, valid reasons to avoid this procedure in rheumatoid arthritis.

Intertrochanteric osteotomy of the femur with or without displacement was a popular and effective procedure for the patient with early degenerative arthritis of the hip prior to the development of total hip replacement. This procedure is done only in degenerative arthritis, and there is no reason to expect that it would be beneficial for the patient with rheumatoid arthritis.

Knee

Synovectomy and popliteal cysts

Today, for the reasons outlined earlier, synovectomy of the knee is rarely done. There may, however, be an occasional patient in whom synovectomy is indicated. For example, if symptomatic popliteal cysts do not respond to medical treatment and the articular surface is still intact, it is the treatment of choice.

Popliteal cysts are common manifestations of all arthritic diseases of the knee but are particularly common in rheumatoid arthritis. The cysts develop in response to intraarticular pressure and serve to decompress the joint. They are, in effect, a herniation of the joint capsule. Differential pressure measurements have shown that there is a one-way flow of synovial fluid from the joint into the cysts. The so-called ball-valve effect explains the not uncommon finding of a large popliteal cyst in the absence of an appreciable joint effusion. Not infrequently, the cyst will rupture with extravasation of synovial fluid into the posterior compartment of the leg (Fig. 5). At the time of rupture, the patient perceives a sharp lancinating pain down the back of the leg which is followed by severe swelling and inflammation

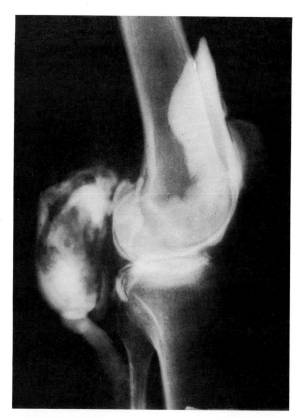

FIGURE 5

A ruptured popliteal cyst showing extension of the arthrographic dye into the posterior compartment of the leg. Note the absence of a large intraarticular effusion.

of the calf. To the uninitiated, the clinical presentation is that of acute thrombophlebitis, and these patients are too frequently treated with anticoagulants. Since patients with rheumatoid arthritis are relatively free from thrombophlebitis, there is validity to the axiom that a patient with rheumatoid arthritis does not have thrombophlebitis until an arthrogram has been obtained.

The treatment of popliteal cysts, whether ruptured or simply large and symptomatic, is the treatment of the intraarticular inflammation. They usually can be controlled by systemic anti-inflammatory medication but occasionally may require intraarticular corticosteroid injections. If these measures are unsuccessful, and the joint is well preserved, anterior synovectomy is appropriate. Conversely, if there is significant destruction of articular cartilage and bone, knee replacement is a more suitable alternative.

Total knee replacement Since first introduced 10 years ago, the evolution of total knee replacement has been quite rapid. The number of modifications and variations has seemed almost infinite, but the net result has been the development of a prosthetic arthroplasty that is reliable and reproducible. At the present time, it is clear that the results of knee replacement are equivalent to those achieved by hip replacement and some centers report short-term success rates of as high as 95 percent. The patient with rheumatoid arthritis undergoing knee replacement is, however, different than the general population. Following knee replacement, as well as hip replacement, the patient with rheumatoid arthritis is relatively less likely to develop component loosening or thrombophlebitis than is a nonrheumatoid counterpart. Conversely, the rheumatoid patient is at greater risk for infectious complications and periprosthetic fracture of the femur or tibia.

Over the past 10 years, with all of the changes and modifications that have occurred, some basic principles of knee replacement have evolved that are the basis of contemporary usage. These are:

1 The rate of the bone-cement interface failure (prosthetic loosening) is directly proportional to the degree of implant restraint.

2 Soft-tissue balance by appropriate release and reenforcement is critical.

3 The central axis of the implant must be in line with the mechanical axis of the leg, and the articulating surfaces must be perpendicular to the central axis of the body. The mechanical axis is a line from the center of the femoral head to the center of the ankle joint.

4 Metal-on-metal articulations are contraindicated.

5 Infection rates are relatively proportional to the size of the implant.

6 Resurfacing of the patella in most patients is an essential feature.

7 Intensive postoperative rehabilitation is essential to a satisfactory outcome, which can be facilitated by continuous passive motion.

Preoperative preparation and postoperative rehabilitation are far more important in knee compared to hip replacement; therefore, patient selection and motivation are critical. Postoperative pain following hip replacement is surprisingly modest, and because the hip is inherently stable, relatively little physical therapy is required. Motion of the postoperative knee replacement is usually instituted within 2 to 3 days following surgery, and is quite painful. It is essential that the patient be able to tolerate the pain and that a talented physical therapist be available to assist the patient in obtaining motion. In addition, quadriceps strength is necessary for stability and many times a prolonged rebuilding program is required to regain muscle strength.

Arthrodesis and pseudarthrosis Arthrodesis of the knee is the procedure of choice in neuropathic arthropathy, but in rheumatoid arthritis it is strictly a salvage procedure. The awkwardness of gait, the increased transmission of forces to adjacent joints, and the difficulty arising from a chair (which may be impossible because of severe destruction of the opposite knee) are compelling reasons why arthrodesis is not recommended as a primary procedure in polyarticular disease. In some situations, most commonly uncontrolled sepsis, it may be the only alternative.

High tibial osteotomy and patellectomy High tibial osteotomy and patellectomy are recommended only in degenerative arthritis and are not appropriate for patients with rheumatoid arthritis.

Foot and ankle

The foot is basically a tripod in which three-point load bearing occurs at the os calcis and on either side of the forefoot. Two arches connect the feet of the tripod. The transverse arch runs through the metacarpal heads to form the base and the longitudinal plantar arch connects the base to the apex. The ankle joint is almost a pure hinge joint with an axis of rotation set at 25 to 30° external to the coronal plane, around which flexion and extension occur. Rotation about the longitudinal axis occurs primarily at the subtalar joint (the talocalcaneal joint) and is termed inversion and eversion. Abduction and adduction occur at the midtarsal joints. Rotation of the forefoot, pronation and supination, is a combined motion of eversion and abduction or inversion and adduc-

tion respectively. Reversal of the transverse metacarpal arch from its normal plantar concavity to plantar convexity is the beginning of the typical forefoot deformity of rheumatoid arthritis. The base of the tripod now has only one point instead of the normal two points of weight bearing, and force is concentrated on the middle three metatarsal heads, producing the well-recognized syndrome of metatarsalgia.

Metatarsal head resection The advanced forefoot deformity in which the transverse arch has been reversed, the metatarsophalangeal joints have been dislocated with the proximal phalanges pushing down on the dorsal surface of the metatarsal heads, and painful calluses have developed over the subcutaneous metatarsal heads, is exquisitely painful. The patient describes a sensation of walking on stones. Simple excision of the metatarsal heads is one of the oldest, most common, and still most successful procedures for the patient with rheumatoid arthritis. It is not appropriate when conservative measures such as metatarsal bars or pads and shoe modifications are effective, but in advanced deformities it is reliable. After metatarsal head resection, the patient lacks push-off, an important component of normal gait, and walks flat-footed. Since a flat-footed gait has been preoperatively imposed on the patient by the metatarsal pain, it is rarely noticed postoperatively. Such a gait is a helpful indicator of the proper timing for surgical intervention.

Advanced forefoot deformities tend to be symmetrical, but if not, it is probably best to defer surgical treatment until bilateral intervention is justified. This solves the shoe problem, can be done under a single anesthetic, and only minimally increases hospitalization time and duration of recovery.

Triple arthrodesis Destruction of the subtalar joint usually results in an everted hind foot (calcaneovalgus) and pronation of the forefoot. The midtarsal joints are also usually involved and abnormal weight bearing along the medial border of the foot causes the buildup of painful calluses. Occasionally, the hind foot will invert (calcaneovarus) with a supination deformity leading to increased weight bearing along the lateral border of the foot. In either of these situations, triple arthrodesis or one of its modifications is the procedure of choice to correct the deformity. Corrective wedge resections of the subtalar joint and appropriate alignment of the mid foot by resection of the talonavicular and calcaneocuboid joints is done to place the os calcis in neutral or slight valgus balance and the forefoot in neutral balance. Plaster immobilization for approximately 3 months is required to obtain arthrodesis.

Total ankle replacement and arthrodesis

(Fig. 6) Rheumatoid arthritis involves the ankle joint, but the ankle is relatively less frequently

FIGURE 6

Total ankle replacement. This design is from the University of California, Irvine.

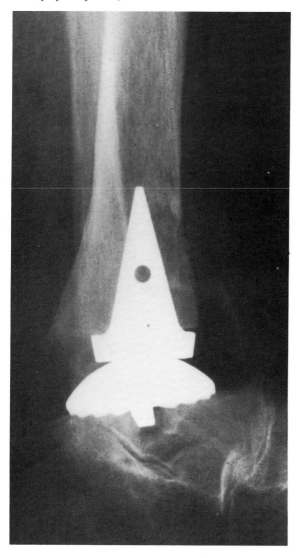

and less severely affected than other joints. The great majority of ankles requiring reconstruction are the result of trauma and are seen in younger people with isolated joint disease.

In the early 1970s during the expansionist period of total joint replacement, numerous total ankle joint replacements were introduced for all types of arthritis. It quickly became apparent that, although suitable for the elderly and sedentary patient, ankle replacement was not a viable alternative to arthrodesis in the young, active patient. Arthrodesis of the ankle results in a pain-free joint, does not alter gait except on inclines, and is durable. In the young patient with traumatic arthritis, arthrodesis is the procedure of choice. The patient with rheumatoid arthritis and severe ankle destruction presents an entirely different problem. Functional demands are less and the hind foot below the ankle usually is severely involved and potentially may require triple arthrodesis. For these reasons, total ankle replacement is usually preferable to arthrodesis in the rheumatoid patient with advanced joint destruction.

References

BLOUNT WP: Don't throw away the cane. J Bone Joint Surg (USA) 38A:695, 1956

CONATY JP, MONGAN ES: Cervical fusion in rheumatoid arthritis. J Bone Joint Surg 63A:1218, 1981

CONVERY FR, CONVERY MM: Examination of the joints, in *Textbook of Rheumatology,* WN Kelley et al (eds). Philadelphia, Saunders, 1981

DEMOTTAZ JD et al: Clinical study of total ankle replacement with gait analysis. J Bone Joint Surg 61A:976, 1979

FLATT AE: *Care of the Arthritic Hand,* 4th ed. St. Louis, Mosby, 1983

FRANKEL VH, NORDIN M: *Basic Biomechanics of the Skeletal System.* Philadelphia, Lea & Febiger, 1980

FREEMAN, MAR (ed): *Arthritis of the Knee: Clinical Features and Surgical Management.* New York, Springer-Verlag, 1980

GSCHWEND N: *Surgical Treatment of Rheumatoid Arthritis.* Philadelphia, Saunders, 1980

INGLIS AE (ed): *Symposium on Total Joint Replacement of the Upper Extremity.* St. Louis, Mosby, 1982

LASKIN RS: Total condylar knee replacement in rheumatoid arthritis: A review of one hundred and seventeen knees. J Bone Joint Surg 63A:29, 1981

Multicenter evaluation of synovectomy in the treatment of rheumatoid arthritis: Report of results at the end of three years. Arthritis Rheum 20:765, 1977

Neer CS et al: Recent experience in total shoulder replacement. J Bone Joint Surg (USA) 64A:319, 1982

Poss R et al: Complication of total hip replacement arthroplasty in patients with rheumatoid arthritis. J Bone Joint Surg (USA) 58A:1130, 1976

Ranawat CS Symposium: Total knee replacement. Clin Orthop 6:101. 1983

Sheon RP et al: *Soft Tissue Rheumatic Pain: Recognition, Management, Prevention.* Philadelphia, Lea § Febiger, 1982

Sledge CB: Introduction to the surgical management of arthritis, in *Textbook of Rheumatology.* WN Kelley et al (eds). Philadelphia, Saunders, 1981